American Holistic Nurses' Association

Guide to Common Chronic Conditions

DI005402

American Holistic Nurses' Association

Guide to Common Chronic Conditions

Self-Care Options to Complement Your Doctor's Advice

Carolyn Chambers Clark, A.R.N.P., Ed.D., H.N.C.

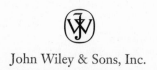

John Wiley & Sons, Inc.

Copyright © 2003 by Carolyn Chambers Clark. All rights reserved

Published by John Wiley & Sons, Inc., Hoboken, New Jersey
Published simultaneously in Canada

Design and production by Navta Associates, Inc.

No part of this publication may be reproduced, stored in a retrieval system, or transmitted in any form or by any means, electronic, mechanical, photocopying, recording, scanning, or otherwise, except as permitted under Section 107 or 108 of the 1976 United States Copyright Act, without either the prior written permission of the Publisher, or authorization through payment of the appropriate per-copy fee to the Copyright Clearance Center, 222 Rosewood Drive, Danvers, MA 01923., (978) 750-8400, fax (978) 750-4470. Requests to the Publisher for permission should be addressed to the Permissions Department, John Wiley & Sons, Inc., 111 River Street, Hoboken, NJ 07030, (201) 748-6011, fax (201) 748-6008, email: permcoordinator@wiley.com.

Limit of Liability/Disclaimer of Warranty: While the publisher and author have used their best efforts in preparing this book, they make no representations or warranties with respect to the accuracy or completeness of the contents of this book and specifically disclaim any implied warranties of merchantability or fitness for a particular purpose. No warranty may be created or extended by sales representatives or written sales materials. The advice and strategies contained herein may not be suitable for your situation. You should consult with a professional where appropriate. Neither the publisher nor author shall be liable for any loss of profit or any other commercial damages, including but not limited to special, incidental, consequential, or other damages.

For general information about our other products and services, please contact our Customer Care Department within the United States at (800) 762-2974, outside the United States at (317) 572-3993 or fax (317) 572-4002.

Wiley also publishes its books in a variety of electronic formats. Some content that appears in print may not be available in electronic books.

Library of Congress Cataloging-in-Publication Data:

Clark, Carolyn Chambers.
    American Holistic Nurses' Association complete guide to mind, body, and spirit care for common chronic conditions / Carolyn Chambers Clark.
        p. ; cm.
Includes bibliographical references and index.
    ISBN 0-471-21296-2 (pbk.)
    1. Holistic nursing. 2. Chronically ill—Care. [DNLM: 1. Chronic Disease—Popular Works. 2. Health Promotion—Popular Works.
3. Psychophysiology—Popular Works. 4. Risk Factors—Popular Works.
WT 500 C592a 2002] I. Title: Complete guide to mind, body, and spirit care for common chronic conditions. II. Title.
    RT42 .C575 2002
    616—dc21

                                                            2002014034

Printed in the United States of America

10 9 8 7 6 5 4 3 2 1

This book is dedicated to my grandson, Niall,
who is just beginning his journey toward self-care.

Contents

Foreword

Do you worry that your medical care is becoming depersonalized? While medicine can produce astounding results—we're now able to transplant a heart, or compose a shiny, new hip out of an alloy that would take us fifteen minutes to learn how to pronounce—it can make you, the patient, feel like no one person is overseeing and responsible for your care.

Think of it this way: the doctor in the ER, who perhaps first recognizes the broken hip, then will send you to an orthopedist. He or she will be responsible for putting in the new hip—but then you must seek the advice of an entirely new doctor, a physiatrist who will help you to take charge of your rehab.

I work in the emergency room, so I can't paint an accurate picture of what your surgery would entail, although I may be responsible for your diagnosis. The same kind of thing holds true for the other doctors in the picture. And your general practitioner, who sees you back in the office after you've gone through the procedure, may have only a faint appreciation of what you've just been through.

There is one person who can help you keep on top of it all. Not only you but also we, the doctors, can turn to our trusty counterparts and coequal professionals, the nurses, who are so adept and concerned about making you aware of the big picture and how to make sense of it all. Thank God for nurses.

The real difference between a doctor and a nurse is perspective. Doctors don't feel their job is done until a diagnosis is made and a plan of action is reached. But nurses haven't done their job until you know how to manage the illness you've got. That means learning the prescribed medications and the nonmedication treatments, it means learning the role you may have played in achieving the state you're in, and it means finding out what you can do to stop the progress of your disease and/or improve your condition in all possible ways.

As a stalwart member of the American Holistic Nurses' Association (AHNA), Carolyn Chambers Clark, a nurse practitioner with a doctorate in education, has prepared an important work for you that focuses on your body, mind, and spirit. This holistic book takes you beyond what I may say or do to inform you of the diagnoses for twenty serious, chronic conditions, and teaches you to see the condition as a process. And once you understand where you are as a point along a spectrum from health to illness, you can learn self-care measures to work in concert with your doctor's prescriptions and muster the energy to get back to health again.

Julian B. Orenstein, M.D.
Potomac, Maryland

Acknowledgments

A big "thank you" to all the people who contributed to this project:

to Julian Orenstein, who served as medical consultant

to Elizabeth Zack, my editor at Wiley, for her valuable help in preparing the manuscript; and to Jenny Bent, my literary agent.

I am grateful to my many teachers and colleagues who informed my work: Hildegard Peplau, Janice Manaser Geller, Sheila Rouslin Welt, Phyllis Class, Shirley Smoyak, Elizabeth Maloney, Halbert Dunn, Dee Krieger, Jean Penny, Susan DiFabio, and Judith Ackerhalt.

Finally, I thank the many clients who have asked important questions and reported significant results.

American Holistic Nurses' Association

Guide to Common Chronic Conditions

Why You May Need This Book

You may need this book for three very important reasons:

1. Your healthcare practitioner may not have the time to explain everything to you.
2. A medical approach is not always, and often is not, a holistic self-care approach that takes into account all the things you can do to get well and stay well.
3. You find yourself wanting more medical information, so you look on the Internet and listen to TV or radio and even scan the newspapers, only to discover conflicting and incorrect information.

Here Are the Answers to Your Questions

You're not feeling well and you go to the doctor. As usual, there are many patients in the waiting room and you barely catch a glimpse of your harried doctor. After you've waited for quite a while, the doctor examines you quickly, gives you a diagnosis, scribbles a prescription, and rushes off to the next patient. You're there, prescription in hand, not 100 percent sure what's really wrong with you, how you got that way, or what to do about it other than to have your prescription filled. Down the hall, you stop a nurse, who explains it all to you, plus tells you what to watch out for when you take the medication. The nurse also suggests some other

1

things you can do to feel more comfortable. You leave feeling calmer and with some understanding of what to do and why.

Maybe another familiar situation occurs when you're in the hospital for surgery. You wait all morning to see the doctor because you have a thousand questions to ask. The doctor hurries in, asks you how you are, and then rushes out. You watch the doctor leave, realizing you didn't ask any of the questions you wanted to ask.

A little while later, a nurse comes by and asks if you need anything. Before you know it, you're asking all the questions you forgot to ask your doctor. By the time the nurse leaves, you feel a whole lot better. Someone cares. The nurse has time to listen and give you answers to your questions in words you can understand.

We all know that doctors are busy people. They are in the business of curing, and that takes a lot of time. Nurses are busy, too, but they are in the business of *caring*. That's their job. They soothe your feverish brow, give you the lowdown on your condition, translate your doctor's orders, tell you the side effects of the medications your doctor prescribes, listen to your woes, and suggest treatments that fit right in with what your doctor has ordered. In this sense, nurses are the perfect complement to doctors, and their advice can add a lot to what your doctor says.

You Have a Right to Know about Measures You Can Take to Be Well

That's what this book is meant to do: give you some answers; talk to you in language you can understand; explain side effects or unwanted reactions to your medicines, treatments, or surgery; and add a few simple, safe things you can add to your daily regime to help you feel better—kind of like wrapping a warm, cozy blanket around you. It's okay, the nurse is in and is listening to you, maybe even anticipating your questions.

This book takes the stance that health is not a drive-through window. You have a very important role to play in getting well and staying well. The top three killers—heart disease, cancer, and stroke—have one thing in common: they're all strongly influenced by lifestyle or what you do. You can take charge and get well by eating right, exercising, and reducing your stress, among other actions. The specifics of how to do these appear for each condition.

Some strategies, such as losing weight and keeping it off, may mean a change in the way you think about food, from "I need to have French fries and burgers every day" to "Food is a medicine, a healing source."

The book provides safe procedures to use instead of always reaching for a pill. Just because a drug is legal doesn't mean it's *safe*. As pharmaceutical companies push more and more aggressively to sell their drugs on television and in other ways, they play down the side effects and dangers of their drugs. Remember: advertisements help make money; they don't protect you from harm.

Today, physicians and even many nurse practitioners are feeling the pressure from their bosses and insurance companies. The time they can take with you during your visits with them shrinks. They may barely have the time to tell you what medication to take or what surgery is suggested and have little time to listen to your concerns.

This book maintains that self-help information is as important in many cases as pills and procedures. It contends that you are an important individual deserving of a holistic approach. What does that mean? It means taking into account that your body parts are connected into a unique whole person, that healing and not just curing is valuable, and that there is always something you can do despite your diagnosis.

Why a Nurse?

A nurse is the perfect person to explain your doctor's orders because the education a nurse receives for giving you care is similar to the model used to educate doctors. Nurses are taught medical care, but they are also taught to focus on *your reactions* to your illness or condition. They see you as a total person, in the context of your family, occupation, and culture, not only a collection of symptoms. This holistic approach helps nurses tune into your reactions to what's happening to you and help you learn how to deal with them.

The American Holistic Nurses' Association

The American Holistic Nurses' Association (AHNA) is the voice of holistic nursing practice in the United States and in other parts of the world. Its members embrace caring and healing in their work with clients and also integrate these concepts in their lives. The AHNA believes that health and disease are part of the human experience and that disease and distress can provide opportunities for you to increase your awareness of the interconnectedness of your body, mind, and spirit. Two of the AHNA's objectives are to:

1. encourage nurses to be wellness role models for their patients and clients

2. improve the quality of healthcare by promoting education, participation, and self-responsibility for wellness in their patients and clients (Dossey 2001)

The AHNA has developed a certification program leading to the title holistic nurse certified (HNC), which means that those who pass the certification exam are board-certified to provide care for you that enhances your body, mind, and spirit. Holistic nurses not only care *for* you, they also care *about* you, and are dedicated to teaching you how to provide high-level self-care that complements your doctor's medical care.

What Do Nurses Know?

In medical school, medical students learn about how to diagnose what's wrong with you and what medications and treatments may help. In nursing school, nurses learn about medical conditions and their treatments, but they also learn a lot more. They are interested in helping you attain a balance, whether it's to find what's lacking in your diet or whether you need an exercise program or how to obtain support from family or others. One of the things nurses are absolute experts on is nutrition. Physicians receive very little, if any, education on nutrition in medical school. Some other areas nurses are experts in are how to:

- protect you from infection
- communicate with you and your family in a way that helps you grow
- teach you about the effects of what you eat on how well you heal
- promote health and well-being and prevent illness in the home, hospital, school, and community
- teach you to control your symptoms, especially pain
- include you in decisions about your care
- prepare you for medical procedures in a way that reduces your anxiety

- work effectively with your sexuality issues and concerns
- teach you about labor, birth, and caring for a child
- identify domestic violence
- teach you about complementary and alternative therapies
- support your right to be treated with kindness and respect

Why I'm the Right Nurse to Write This Book

Now that you know what nurses do, you can see that a nurse is the perfect person to write this book. You may still wonder why I'm the person writing it. Here are some of my reasons:

I've been a registered nurse since 1964, when I graduated from the University of Wisconsin. Since then, I've added a couple of graduate degrees (M.S. from Rutgers University and Ed.D. from Columbia University); worked in numerous hospitals, clinics, and private practice situations; taught and supervised nursing students; and even started my own wellness institute. I'm a Fellow of the American Academy of Nursing, a Certified Holistic Nurse, a Diplomate of the American Board of Forensic Nursing, and a Fellow and Advisory Board Member of the American Association of Integrative Medicine (AAIM).

I've also been writing nursing and health-related texts for twenty years, and three of the texts (*The Encyclopedia of Complementary Health Practice, Integrating Complementary Procedures into Practice*, and *Wellness Practitioner*) won Book of the Year awards from the *American Journal of Nursing.* And I've taken and taught many research courses, so I can tell you about the studies that provide significant evidence, and which indicate steps you should take to enhance your wellness.

During all of these experiences, I've met clients, sometimes even those in my own family, who asked me questions about medications, treatments, or surgery. They feel comfortable asking me, and to tell the truth, it makes me feel good to help them. Because I know you're out there with valid questions about the treatment your doctor orders for you, I've written this book.

For the medical diagnosis and treatment, I worked with a medical consultant to make sure I didn't make any assumptions about medical diagnosis or treatment. For a special seal of approval, I went to the American Holistic Nurses' Association, the largest organization for nurses worldwide that takes a truly holistic, mind/body/spirit orientation to your care.

The Conditions You'll Find in This Book

The twenty chronic conditions in this book are listed alphabetically for easy reference. First, the doctor's likely comments and prescription for that condition are presented. Below that, the nurse's thorough explanation of the condition and symptoms; what might have led to them; possible side effects of medications or treatments; how the condition can be prevented; and finally, complementary therapies or self-care procedures you can take to enhance comfort and healing are presented.

I've chosen to cover these conditions because they're chronic and because there's a lot you can do *beyond* the standard medical treatment to help yourself. Self-care advice in this book is backed by research. Studies that support the validity of each self-care approach can be found in the References at the back of the book.

Throughout the book, you will find references to milligrams (mg or mgm) and micrograms (mcg), primarily referring to vitamins and minerals. Read labels carefully so you do not confuse the two dosages.

Remember, a holistic approach means you are actively involved in self-care that complements your doctor's treatment. Take advantage of the information in this book, apply it to your daily activities, and be well!

CONDITIONS

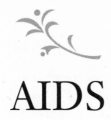

AIDS

AIDS stands for acquired immune deficiency syndrome. It is believed that a virus called HIV causes AIDS. It is probable that HIV is necessary, but not sufficient in and of itself, to cause the onset of AIDS. The virus probably needs help bringing about AIDS. It is also probable that people with weak immune systems are more susceptible to AIDS and viruses.

Some people with signs of full-blown generalized immune deficiency test negative for HIV antibodies, leading researchers to think there is another factor operating. Compelling evidence has demonstrated that nutritional deficiencies can affect immunity before and after acquiring AIDS. Nutritional deficiency could be the factor that dictates whether someone is susceptible to AIDS.

The HIV virus can be passed during the sharing of needles by intravenous drug users, by blood transfusion, or by the use of blood products that are infected. Although blood is carefully screened, it is possible for infected blood to occasionally pass through the screening process.

It is also possible for dentists and healthcare workers who come into close contact with the bodily fluids of contagious persons to become infected under certain circumstances. That is why healthcare workers and dentists, and even police officers, now routinely use rubber or other protective gloves to prevent them from coming in contact with blood products, saliva, or other bodily fluids. For your own safety, ask your healthcare worker and dentist to change their gloves prior to working on you.

Babies of mothers with the HIV virus can become infected during pregnancy or birth or through breast-feeding. (Sexual contact has now surpassed intravenous drug use as the leading means of transmission among women.)

Your Risks for Developing AIDS

The highest-risk practice is receptive anal or vaginal intercourse without a condom. The use of alcohol or mood-altering drugs may lead to engaging in high-risk sexual encounter because the use of these substances limits impulse control and impairs decision-making.

If you fall in either of the categories that follow, your risk for developing AIDS also is great:

1. You inject recreational drugs into your veins.
2. You are a man and have sex with men. This group represents the largest proportion (60 percent) of men diagnosed with AIDS.

If you have recurrent vaginal candidiasis (yeast infections), pelvic inflammatory disease, precancerous changes in your cervix (cervical dysplasia), yeast infections of the mouth or throat, or any sexually transmitted disease (genital ulcers and warts, and herpes virus infection), your risk for AIDS also is increased.

How the Doctor Diagnoses AIDS

The medical criteria for a diagnosis of full-blown AIDS require the presence of one or more opportunistic infections or cancers known to be associated with HIV infection. Testing HIV-positive does not mean you have AIDS. It only means that you have been *exposed* to HIV and have built up antibodies to the virus. Only 50 to 60 percent of people exposed to HIV have actually developed AIDS. If you do test positive for HIV, arrange for repeat testing as soon as you can. No laboratory or blood test is 100 percent reliable, so have two tests done.

What the Doctor Will Probably Prescribe

According to the *Merck Manual*, AZT is a potent inhibitor of the human immunodeficiency virus (HIV), but it is not a cure for the infection. The drug is toxic and can suppress bone marrow. This effect is seen mostly in established AIDS and often requires dosage modifications or a temporary end to therapy. Side effects of the drug can include anemia (and other blood disorders), nausea, vomiting, muscle pain, headaches, liver abnormalities, anxiety, tremors, and confusion. The long-term toxicity of this drug is unknown, but the risk for children born to HIV-infected women who take AZT is nearly three times greater than in the general population, according to a study reported in the *Journal of Acquired Immune Deficiency Syndrome*. Other widely used drugs for HIV are 3TC and Combivir. There are many other drugs that are used, so be sure to check a *Physicians' Desk Reference* (available at the reference desk of your local library) for actions and side effects.

Self-Care Measures You Can Take

Treatment is very expensive, and the new drugs aren't working as well as once thought. *Prevention* remains the best hope against AIDS. The problem is, many people do not support the most common prevention measures, which include using condoms, providing safe and clean needle exchange programs for drug addicts, and educating people about how unprotected sexual intercourse and intravenous drug injections can lead to AIDS. If these steps are not for you, consider actions to strengthen your immune system so that even if you do come in contact with the virus, your body's natural processes will fight it successfully. Below you will find ways to enhance your immune system.

Eat Foods and Take Supplements Containing Important Vitamins

Vitamins C (1,000 mg/day) and E (800 mg/day) were found to reduce stress and infectious organisms, according to a study published in *AIDS*. Foods high in vitamin C include green peppers, honeydew melons, cooked broccoli or Brussels sprouts, cooked kale, cantaloupes, strawberries, papayas, cooked cauliflower, oranges, watercress, raspberries, parsley, raw cabbage, grapefruit, blackberries, lemons, onions, sprouts, spinach, and tomatoes. Foods high in vitamin E include wheat germ, peanuts, outer leaves of cabbage, leafy portions of broccoli and cauliflower, raw spinach, asparagus, whole grains (rice, wheat, or oats), cold pressed wheat germ or safflower oil, cornmeal, eggs, and sweet potatoes.

Selenium is an essential trace element important to the optimum function of the immune system. It's best to get your vitamins and minerals from foods, but selenium is one nutrient you might have to get in a mineral pill, since many of our soils have been depleted of the nutrient. According to a study reported in *AIDS Research in the Human Retroviruses,* selenium supplementation can suppress the human immunodeficiency virus type 1, while a study reported in *Alternative Medicine Review* found that selenium levels are highly significant in reducing death due to AIDS. A review of studies in *Nutrition Review* suggested that taking additional selenium can increase the immune defense of HIV-infected patients.

Vitamin B_{12} also can protect against HIV, according to a report in *Alternative Medical Review.* A study reported in the *European Journal of Clinical Investigation* concluded that even people with advanced AIDS can also benefit from high doses of NAC (N-acetylcysteine) and vitamin C.

Other nutrients that may be helpful are vitamin A, zinc, and magnesium, according to a study reported in *Alternative Medicine Review.* Foods high in vitamin A include carrots, broccoli, kale, turnip greens, watercress, beets, dandelion greens, spinach, eggs, papaya, parsley, red peppers, pumpkin, yellow squash, apricots, and cantaloupes. Some foods rich in zinc are pumpkin seeds, whole grains, oysters, herring, liver, eggs, nuts, and wheat germ. Magnesium can be found in whole grain breads and cereals, fresh peas, brown rice, soy flour, wheat germ, nuts, Swiss chard, figs, green leafy vegetables, and citrus fruits.

It's important to keep your liver and immune system as healthy as possible when you are stressing them by taking drugs or fighting off infection. To assist with liver and lymphatic cleansing, drink a combination of olive oil and lemon juice. Blend the following: 1 washed whole lemon (pulp, rind, seeds, and all) with 1 tablespoon of extra virgin olive oil and 1½ cups of distilled water. Strain the blend through a wire strainer to remove the pulp, which is discarded. Divide the juice into four equal portions and consume one with each of the three daily meals and the last one before bedtime. This will stimulate lymphatic flow, increase the flow of bile from your liver and gallbladder, and help digest essential fatty acids in your intestine.

Use Distilled Water

Recent tests have shown that cryptosporidium, a waterborne parasite, is commonly found in lakes, rivers, and some reservoirs across the country, according to the Centers for Disease Control and Prevention.

Because of this danger, Robert Morris, a cryptosporidium expert at the University of Wisconsin Medical School, suggests that anyone with AIDS should definitely not drink tap water. Two federal agencies also have warned that drinking tap water could be fatal to Americans with weakened immune systems and that they should take precautions such as boiling water before consuming it, or better yet, drink distilled water.

Drink Your Vitamins and Minerals

If you have difficulty digesting your food or if you want your vitamins and minerals to get right into your bloodstream, "drink" your vitamins and minerals. Make a "green drink" daily: put a cup or two of a green lettuce (except iceberg) in a blender. Add a handful of parsley and another of fresh spinach or kale. Fill the blender with pineapple juice and blend until frothy. Ingest it slowly, chewing each mouthful (to get the digestive juices in your mouth flowing).

Also, make carrot juice 1 to 3 times a day. You can buy a juicer at your local health food store. Wash carrots and cut their ends off. Put a glass measuring cup (enough to hold 2 cups) under the spout. Put 5 to 6 or enough carrots in the top of the juicer to make at least 8 ounces. Add a handful of fresh spinach or parsley to the juicer and then another carrot or two. Juice. Drink slowly, chewing.

Try Herbs

Echinacea and ginseng have been shown to stimulate the immune system, according to a report published in *Immunopharmacology*. Extracts of *Echinacea purpurea* and *Panax ginseng* were shown to enhance cellular immunity in both healthy individuals and patients with AIDS. (Do not use Siberian ginseng if you have low blood sugar, high blood pressure, or a heart condition.) Some other natural products that can protect against AIDS, according to *Medical Research Review*, are blue-green algae, glycyrrhizin (extracted from the licorice root *Glycyrrhiza radix*), and the spice curcumin. You can find all of them at your health food store, but don't take licorice root more than seven days in a row, and avoid it if you have high blood pressure.

Chinese herbs also have shown promise. A research study reported in *Life Sciences* found that each of twenty Chinese herbs showed varying ability to inhibit various aspects of the AIDS virus type 1. Another report, in *Virology*, concluded that astragalus and other Chinese herbs dramatically decreased the infectiousness of HIV-1. (Do not use astragalus if you have a fever.)

Saint-John's-wort has also shown promise for AIDS, according to studies reported in *Life Science*, the *Journal of Pharmaceutical Pharmacology*, and *Phytomedicine*. All those studies conclude that Saint-John's-wort is safe and effective.

Aloe vera juice also contains ingredients that can boost your immune system, according to a report in the *Journal of Agriculture and Food Chemistry*. Never try make your own aloe vera juice. You might get the laxative portion, which is located right next to the leaf. Use only the commercially prepared aloe juice, available in half-gallon and gallon jugs in your health food store. It contains the healing portion of aloe.

Note: If you choose to investigate herbs, be sure you don't mix them with prescribed medications without consulting with a healthcare practitioner who is an expert in herbs and who knows about herb-drug interactions.

Use Castor Oil Packs to Assist in Healing

People with AIDS may need to prevent liver overload. Large amounts of toxic AIDS medications can tax the liver. Conditions that tax or compromise the immune system may benefit from castor oil packs. Your skin is a living organ that absorbs external substances, so make sure that any oil used on your body is cold-pressed and of the highest quality. It is not exactly known how castor oil packs work, but they may affect the lymphatic system, which filters toxins out of your body.

Check with your local health food store for cold-pressed castor oil. Warm the oil and dip a clean piece of natural cotton or flannel in it. Place the castor oil packs on sores and leave them there for an hour; then dispose of the packs.

Learn Stress Management Procedures

One study that took place at the University of Florida's College of Medicine and the university's Brain Institute provides evidence that stress is very important to the development and severity of HIV-AIDS. For every severe stress a patient with AIDS reported in a six-month period, the risk of early disease progression doubled.

A study reported in the *Journal of Consulting and Clinical Psychology* concluded that a ten-week group cognitive-behavioral stress management program for HIV-positive gay men decreased their anxiety and depression about their symptoms and enhanced some immunological measures.

So reducing your stress level could be an important action to take if you have AIDS or are at risk for developing it. See pages 88–89 for a sample relaxation script. You also can purchase relaxation/guided imagery self-help tapes at many bookstores, or make an appointment with a psychologist or nurse practitioner skilled in stress management procedures.

Exercise to Increase Healthy Muscle

Wasting, or loss of muscle mass, and abnormal distribution of body fat occur with AIDS. A report in *Tufts Nutrition* described an eight-week intensive progressive resistance training program for people with AIDS. The twenty-four people who completed the study had significant increases in strength, increased their lean body mass, and reduced fat. Those participants suffering from wasting were also able to gain weight, mostly in lean body mass. If body wasting is a problem for you, consider finding a similar program or hire a personal trainer to help you develop an intensive resistance training program.

Take Special Actions If You're Pregnant

There are plenty of reasons to make sure your unborn infant is properly nourished. Now there's another one. A long-term study reported in the *Journal of Acquired Immune Deficiency Syndrome Human Retrovirology* found that infants born to women with vitamin A deficiency consistently have lower weight and height for their ages. Taking large doses of vitamin A is not a good idea because it is oil-soluble, and the vitamin will stay in the body and could do harm. The best approach is to eat foods rich in vitamin A, including carrots, broccoli, kale, turnip greens, watercress, beets, dandelion greens, spinach, eggs, papaya, parsley, red peppers, fish, sweet potatoes, pumpkin, yellow squash, apricots, cantaloupes, and organ meats (such as liver and sweetbreads).

A study published in the *Journal of Pediatric Gastroenterology and Nutrition* found that when HIV-infected pregnant women took vitamin A and beta-carotene, their newborn infants had an improved digestive system. Another study, published in the *American Journal of Public Health,* concluded that vitamin A supplements for children of HIV-infected women kept the babies alive and reduced their diarrhea.

Enjoy Massage and Enhance Your Immune System

A National Institute of Health study by Dr. Tiffany Field showed that massage helped HIV-exposed infants to gain weight and stay calm. Another study, published in the *International Journal of Neuroscience*, found that massage therapy helped HIV adolescents improve their immune function.

Use Distance Healing

A study reported in the *Western Journal of Medicine* found that AIDS patients paired with distance healers acquired significantly fewer new AIDS-related illnesses, had lower illness severity, and required significantly fewer doctor visits, fewer hospitalizations, and fewer days of hospitalization. They also had a significantly improved mood compared to a group of controls who did not receive distance healing.

Try Self-Hypnosis

Self-hypnosis was shown to significantly influence immunity in a study reported in the *International Journal of Psychophysiology*. If you have AIDS, you might want to find a psychologist or psychiatric/mental health nurse practitioner with hypnosis skills.

Use Affirmations

Optimism and positive thinking have been shown to affect disease progression. Being chronically hostile, depressed, and apathetic can lead to disease. In *The Self-Healing Personality*, Friedman found that hardy people have self-healing personalities that make them resilient and healthy.

Affirmations use positive thinking and optimism, so consider using one or more of the following affirmations. Be sure to write or speak them at least twenty times a day to replace the negative thoughts that may be holding back your self-healing personality:

- I am powerful and capable.
- I am loved.
- I love and appreciate myself.

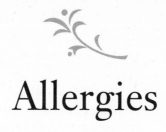

Allergies

When the doctor tells you that you have an allergy, it means your body is overreacting to something (called an *allergen*) with a response usually saved for dangerous substances such as viruses. Usually your immune system can tell the difference between a threat, such as a virus, and some harmless substance, such as food or pollen. When your immune system can't discriminate, it attacks the harmless food, pollen, animal dander, or whatever, as if they were threats to health. Allergies can range from mildly bothersome to life-threatening. Once you are exposed to an allergen, your immune system releases a chemical called histamine, which is why your doctor prescribes an antihistamine.

An *allergy* is an unusual reaction or sensitivity to a substance. What conditions are caused by allergies? You can include hay fever, asthma, hives, itching, difficulty breathing, sneezing or a runny nose, and headaches, and sometimes stomach aches, migraine headaches, leg and joint pains, excessive fatigue and irritability, pallor, and dark circles under your eyes. Bed-wetting also has been associated with allergy. If you suffer from allergies, you may also have sinusitis and more frequent colds because allergens can block and swell your nasal passages and sinus cavities.

If you have an allergy to house dust mites, feathers, animal dander, or fungi, you will probably have symptoms such as sinus infections or nasal polyps, and a nose that may run unpredictably throughout the year.

If you can't control the source of your allergy, your doctor may suggest surgery.

If you are allergic to windborne pollens from trees, grass, weeds, or fungi, you may notice itching in your nose, the roof of your mouth, your throat, and/or your eyes. You may sneeze, tear, have red eyes, and also have a watery discharge coming from your nose. Headaches, feeling irritable, losing your appetite, feeling depressed, and having difficulty sleeping also are common.

If you have a food allergy, you may have had symptoms since childhood, including eczema, diarrhea, cramps, constipation, and so on. At first you may have had a skin rash, but by the end of your first year of life, your symptoms probably switched to breathing problems. By then you probably developed reactions to specific foods. It is now believed that food intolerance may be responsible for some cases of irritable bowel syndrome, pain, cramps, and diarrhea. You may be very sensitive to allergens in nuts, legumes, seeds, or shellfish. Milk is another common allergen that can produce breathing difficulty in some people. *Food additives* also start allergic reactions in some people. The most common additives that people are allergic to are monosodium glutamate (MSG), metabisulfite, and the yellow dye called tartrazin. It's possible to suffer from a food-induced migraine, too.

Your Risk for Developing Allergies

A number of factors have to mesh for an allergy to develop. If you have the genetic makeup for a sensitivity to animal dander and are around animals, you could develop an allergy. The same holds true for food allergies. In fact, eating the same foods day after day can result in a sensitivity to those foods. This is one reason why it's important to eat a variety of foods. Not only can you ward off food sensitivities, but also you will be more apt to take in a wider variety of vitamins and minerals.

A whole new field of medicine called clinical ecology unravels environmental causes of mental and physical ills. The theory is that allergies are similar to addictions and people can become addicted to common foods such as corn, wheat, beef, coffee, tea, and tobacco. For those susceptible, every chemical (gas from your kitchen stove, the glue that holds your carpeting to the floor, commercial household cleaners, pesticides, supermarket food additives, dyes used in foods and medicines, and just about any substance you are sensitive to) can result in allergic symptoms. To lower your risks, avoid gas stoves, carpeting, commercial household cleaners, pesticides, supermarket food additives, and foods and medicines that contain dyes.

Stress is another factor in allergies. If you stay calm, your reaction to an allergen may be lessened. Tension, fatigue, worry, and poor general health can trigger allergic symptoms and make them worse.

How the Doctor Diagnoses an Allergy

Your doctor may use specific tests to make sure that you have an allergy. By asking questions, called taking a history, the doctor can make the best diagnosis, one that is more valuable than tests in determining whether you have an allergy. The doctor may ask you how old you were when the allergic symptoms started (childhood asthma is more likely to be due to an allergy than if the symptoms first appeared at age thirty), if your symptoms start at about the beginning of a pollen season, if they started after you were exposed to an animal or dust, or if your symptoms appear when you're in specific environments (e.g., at home, school, or work). All of this information can provide helpful clues. You also may be asked if you notice your symptoms occur when you're around cigarette smoke, other pollutants, cold air, or when you're exercising, drinking alcoholic beverages, taking certain drugs, or feeling stressed.

If what you tell your doctor points to an allergy, skin tests may be ordered. The solutions the doctor uses for a skin test are made from extracts of substances you inhale, eat, or inject (windborne tree, grass, and weed pollens; house dust mites; animal dander and fluids; insect venom; foods; and some drugs).

If you have a skin inflammation or can't bear being pricked, you may be given a radioallergosorbent *(RAST)* test, which detects the presence of allergen-specific substances in your blood. A known allergen is mixed with your blood serum and tested. If your serum sticks to the allergen, it is a sign you are allergic to the substance.

For a food allergy, you may be placed on an elimination diet to see if your symptoms improve. Foods are systematically eliminated so you can eat only certain foods. If your symptoms improve after a specific food is eliminated, the doctor may ask you to eat the food again to see if it re-creates the symptom. Common food allergens include milk, eggs, shellfish, nuts, wheat, peanuts, soybeans, chocolate, and all foods containing these ingredients, but other foods also may be culprits.

What the Doctor Will Probably Prescribe

The best way to treat an allergy is to eliminate the allergen. You may be asked to change your diet or occupation, stop taking a drug, or remove a household pet. Heating certain foods may help if you're allergic to them (e.g., warming milk may reduce its allergic qualities). If complete avoidance of the allergen is impossible, reducing your exposure to that substance may help. For example, if you are allergic to dust, you can remove dust-collecting furniture, carpets, and draperies and use plastic covers over your mattress and pillows. Frequent wet-mopping and dusting will reduce the high humidity favorable to dust mites. Installing a high-efficiency air filter also can help.

When you can't control the allergen sufficiently to relieve your symptoms, the doctor may decide to use an injection of an extract of the allergen in increasing doses. The injections are never given into a vein or muscle, but into the skin, and may be required year-round to provide relief. If the dose of the injections is not increased gradually, you may experience symptoms ranging from a mild cough or sneezing to itching, severe asthma, or even shock. In certain cases, antihistamines may be prescribed.

What If Your Doctor Prescribes an Antihistamine?

If your doctor prescribes an antihistamine, your reaction to it may differ depending on the kind you take. Always be sure to take the prescribed amount at the prescribed times. You will find common negative reactions to antihistamines listed below, as well as other drugs and conditions that should be avoided. Be aware that these are only the *known* precautions and interactions. If you're taking a number of other medications, there may be no way to know what kind of interaction could take place between or among the various drugs. To protect yourself, always be sure to tell your doctor about any drugs, supplements, or herbs you are taking in case any negative reactions might occur.

COMMON ANTIHISTAMINES

Advil cold and sinus, Allegra-d, Aquatab, Benadryl Allergy/ Congestion, Bromfed, Claritin-d 24 hour, Deconamine Sr, Deconsall, Dimetapp, Drixoral cold 7 allergy, Duratuss, Duravent, Exgest la, Extex la, Nasalcrom a allergy prevention pack, Neo-Synephrine, Pediacare infants' decongestant, Phenergan vc, Poly-histine-d, Rondec, Ryna-12s, Rynatan, Semprex-d, Sudafed, Tavist-d, Triaminic syrup, Trinalin, and Tylenol sinus.

Many of these antihistamine drugs cannot be taken if you have high blood pressure; diabetes; glaucoma; an enlarged prostate; arteriosclerosis (hardening of the arteries); a history of bronchospasm; or if you have heart, thyroid, kidney, or liver conditions, or stomach intestinal or urinary obstruction. You also may need to avoid some antihistamines if you are taking (or have taken in the past two weeks) the antidepressants Nardil or Parnate; tricyclic antidepressants (e.g., Anafranil, Elavil, Ludiomil, Norpramin, Pamelor, Remeron, Sinequan, Surmontil, or Tofranil); beta-blockers for your heart (Acebutolol, Atenolol, Betaxolol, Bisoprolol, Carteolol, Carvedilol, Labetalol, Metroprolol, Nadolol, Penbutolol, Pindolol, Propranolol, or Timolol); other central nervous system depressants (e.g., amphetamines, pemoline, provigil, or Ritalin, chlordiazepoxide, diazepam, clorazepate, flurazepam, halazepam, prazepam, clonazepam, quazepam, alprazolam, lorazepam, oxazepam, temazepam, or triazolam); drugs to thin your blood (e.g., aspirin, Aggrenox, Bufferin, Coumadin, Ecotrin, Fragmin, or Heparin Sodium); or drugs to lower your blood pressure. Immediately stop taking any histamine if you notice any problems with your eyes or liver. Don't take antihistamines if you're pregnant, nursing, or elderly. Also, avoid them if you're taking pain relievers or if you drink alcohol in any form.

Some of the bad reactions you could have, depending on the antihistamine you take, are convulsions, depression of your central nervous system, itching, rash, upper respiratory infection, breathing difficulties, headache, drowsiness, weakness, thickening of throat secretions, lowered blood pressure, heart palpitations, nasal discomfort, nasal congestion, jaundice, blood dysfunction, lack of appetite, throat irritation, stomach irritation or ulcers, stomach and/or intestinal upset or bleeding, nervousness, dizziness, dry mouth, blurry vision, unusual skin sensations (prickling, creeping, or tingling), abdominal or back pain, trouble sleeping or urinating, tremor, and/or weakness.

What If Your Doctor Prescribes Prednisone or Another Steroid?

If you are diagnosed with hay fever, and if nasal symptoms do not subside, a steroid (systemic corticosteroid) called prednisone may be used, with a gradual reduction in dosage over one week to zero. This medication cannot be taken over a long period of time or if you have tuberculosis, hypothyroidism, liver conditions (cirrhosis), herpes simplex in the eyes, kidney problems, ulcerative colitis, diverticulitis, peptic ulcer, high blood pressure, osteoporosis, diabetes, or are a nursing mother. Also, it cannot be given if you are taking barbiturates (e.g., Butalbital, alurate elixir, belap elixir, buff-a-comp, butabarbital sodium elixir or tablets, buticaps, butisol sodium elixir, carbrital, donnatal, donphen, kinesed, levsin/phenobarbital, mebaral, nembutal, oxoids, plexonal, or repan) or hydantoins (dilantin). Adverse reactions include a masking of infection, glaucoma, cataracts, secondary infections, high blood pressure, muscle changes, osteoporosis, stomach ulcer, skin atrophy, depletion of needed minerals (potassium, sodium, and calcium), increased pressure in your cranium, and carbohydrate intolerance.

There are other steroids that may be prescribed. These potent drugs are often in the form of nasal sprays. Some of their names are Beconase AQ, Flonase, Nasacort, Nasalide, Nasarel, Nasonex, Rhinocort Aqua, and Vancenase AQ. These drugs are usually given only for a few weeks because some of them can result in impaired wound healing, fungal overgrowth, nosebleeds, infections, or glaucoma.

Taking steroids by inhaler can increase your chances of developing cataracts on your eyes, according to a study reported in the journal *Epidemiology*. Heavy users of inhaled steroids aged forty or older had an 80 percent higher risk of developing cataracts than those who had not used steroids.

Be Wary of Nebulizers

University of Florida studies provide evidence than an antibacterial agent added to some asthma medications can cause airway constriction, making an asthma attack worse. The chemical *benzalkonium chloride*, or BAC, is added to some albuterol solutions given by a nebulizer. Albuterol is considered the most effective medicine for quickly opening the airways, but when BAC is added, the reverse may occur. To be safe, if you use a nebulizer, make sure it comes in a bottle with a lid that breaks off (BAC is found only in screw-cap container products).

If you use an inhaler often, be aware that this is dangerous. They are meant to be used *occasionally* to relieve an acute asthma attack. Not only do inhalers become less effective over time, but you also may suffer from serious side effects, including increased heart rate and blood pressure, anxiety, restlessness and insomnia. Using inhalers frequently can even worsen asthma, so please follow directions and do not misuse them.

Other Drugs and Foods That Can Aggravate Asthma or Allergies

According to the book *Prescription Alternatives*, some of the medicines that can cause or aggravate asthma are beta-blockers (propranolol, timolol) and moricizine, Dramamine, Dimetabs, anti-Parkinson's drugs, psychiatric drugs (phenothiazines and lithium), antiviral drugs used to treat AIDS (cidofovir and protease inhibitors), barbiturates, anti-anxiety drugs (Valium, Dalmane), cephalosporin and sulfonamide antibiotics, cholinesterase inhibitors used to treat Alzheimer's, narcotics, Prozac, Luvox, Paxil, tricyclic antidepressants, weight-loss drugs (e.g., dexfenfluramine), Nytol, Sleep-Eze, Sominex, Tylenol PM, ibuprofen-related anti-inflammatory drugs, Ismelin, and other drugs to lower blood pressure. Yellow dye no. 5 and red colorings in many pills, liquid drugs, and food products can also set off allergic reactions.

If you're taking albuterol (Proventil, Ventolin, Repetabs, Volmax, Airet), Isoetharine (Arm-a-Med Isoetharine, Beta-2, Bronkosol), Isoproterenol (Isuprel Glossets, Isuprel, Medihaler-Iso, Dispos-a-Med), Metaproterenol Sulfate (Alupent, Metaprel), or Terbutaline Sulfate (Brethine, Bircanyl), mood swings, fatigue, nightmares, aggressive behavior, increased appetite, the "jitters," nasal congestion, increased saliva, muscle cramps, discoloration of your teeth, inflammation of your eyes or eyelids, or nosebleeds can occur. Talk to your healthcare practitioner about these drugs if you have glaucoma, diabetes, high blood pressure, heart disease, history of stroke, hyperthyroidism, are elderly, or have a history of seizures or psychoneurotic illness, as dosages may need to be reevaluated. You may not want to take any of these drugs if you have a dangerous heart arrhythmia or heart blockage or narrow-angle glaucoma. If you are going to have surgery, tell your doctor. He will make sure you don't have any of them in your system while you are under general anesthesia.

Avoid foods that may interfere with any of the mentioned drugs, including any meat, fish, or dairy product that has been sitting around more than a few days (check freshness dates when you buy them), aged cheese, wine and pickles, avocados, sour cream, pickled fish, flavor enhancers such as hydrolyzed vegetable protein (check ingredients in all canned, jarred, and bottled food), raisins, chocolate, sausages, pepperoni, salami, bologna, tofu, soy sauce, teriyaki sauce, miso, tomatoes, wine, beer, liqueurs, champagne, and yeast (check all breads, cakes, and canned food ingredients). If you take these drugs and eat any of these foods, it could cause a serious reaction.

Only a sampling of the drugs that may be prescribed for you if you have asthma or an allergy have been listed, so become an informed consumer. Your local library has a recent copy of the *Physicians' Desk Reference (PDR)* at the reference desk. Look up the drugs you are taking or plan to take and see what the precautions and side effects are. With so many medications on the market, it may be nearly impossible for your physician to keep up with all precautions, interactions, and dangers.

If you're concerned about taking medicines that have strong negative effects, get a second opinion. Consider seeing a healthcare practitioner who is knowledgeable about alternative treatments.

If you do decide to take medications, be aware that research carried out by Professor Philipe Camus of the University Medical Center of Dijon, France, shows that there are more than three hundred "problem" drugs that can cause irreversible damage to the lungs. Even more drugs could be implicated. What can you do? Consult with your healthcare practitioner at the slightest abnormal breathing or lung symptom and immediately stop taking the suspect product until you see your doctor.

Self-Care Measures You Can Take

An antihistamine or some other medication may work just fine for you, but remember, they only treat your *symptoms*. The underlying cause of the problem is still there and can recur. Also keep in mind that allergies are often hard to diagnose and difficult to treat, so complementary approaches have become very popular. Remember, though, for severe allergies see your doctor if:

- *You have violent stomach cramps, bloating, diarrhea, or vomiting.* This might mean you have food poisoning or a serious allergic reaction.
- *You suddenly develop skin welts, intense flushing and itching, and your heart beats rapidly.* This could be a sign of anaphylactic shock.
- *Your breathing is extremely difficult or painful.* This could be an asthma or heart attack.

If you don't have any of these serious reactions, you might want to consider the complementary approach. This approach to allergies is based on the theory that there is an underlying process that leads to your symptoms. The theory also says that there is a communication pathway between your brain and your symptoms. This pathway explains the links among what you eat and/or what environmental toxins you are exposed to, stress, and your immune system.

Environmental Actions You Might Want to Take

If you have allergies to pollen and mold spores, you might want to buy a high-efficiency particulate air cleaner *(HEPA filter)*. It can remove the pollen and mold spores that may be setting off your allergic responses. Using a vacuum cleaner with a HEPA filter can eliminate many airborne allergens, too. Turning on the air conditioner in your car and at home and then cleaning damp areas with bleach or a citrus cleaner also may help. Avoiding household pets and/or giving them frequent baths can reduce noxious dander that creates allergic responses in you. Also, keep pets outside as much as possible.

You also may be allergic to the glues and content of carpets. If you are, consider removing rugs in your house and installing tile or wood floors. Wall-to-wall carpeting also invites roaches and their waste products. Carpeting plus increased insulation and sealed windows can lead to symptoms of "sick building syndrome," including eye, nose, throat, and skin irritation, headache, fatigue, and breathing problems. Chronic colds and dull headaches have also have been associated with sick building syndrome.

Consider covering pillows, mattresses, box springs, and furniture with plastic casings. Be sure to wash all linens in hot water to kill dust mites. Keep the windows in your house shut to keep outdoor allergens outside. Use a dehumidifier for damp spaces. Avoid heaters, including wood-burning stoves and fireplaces that release irritating particles.

Carbonless paper, toners (from laser printers and copy machines), adhesive floor coverings, and smoking can increase symptoms. Permanent-press clothes (containing formaldehyde) have been associated with allergies, too. Look at the concentration of a rash to see if it matches areas where your permanent-press clothes fit tightly. To avoid allergic responses, wear natural fiber clothing such as cotton, silk, or wool.

While you may be allergic to dogs or cats, a bird also can be a source of allergens. Bird antigens linger in a house for as long as eighteen months. The best action you can take if you have lung irritations (hypersensitivity pneumonitis) is to avoid the room in which a bird was kept. Other actions you can take, to make your bedroom allergyproof: encase your mattress in allergenproof plastic; wash your sheets, blankets, pillowcases, and mattress pads every week in water that is at least at 140°F; and use hypoallergenic bedding materials.

Start a Food Diary to Eliminate Offending Foods

If you suspect a food allergy, start a *food diary* to record all the foods, beverages, medications/drugs, and supplements you take. Also record the time of day you took them and your mood and symptoms for six hours after you took them. Any of the following symptoms could suggest a food allergy: warmth, itchiness, head stuffiness, headache, fatigue, stomach upset, canker sores, chronic diarrhea or gas, ulcers, bladder infections, bed-wetting, kidney disease, chronic infections, frequent ear infections, anxiety, depression, insomnia, irritability, mental confusion, joint pain, low back pain, asthma, chronic bronchitis, wheezing, acne, hives, rashes, itching, sinusitis, watery swelling from edema, fainting, fatigue, headache, hypoglycemia, itchy nose or throat, or migraines.

In young children, bed-wetting, sleep disorders, excessive coughing, bad breath, "growing pains," abdominal pains, constant runny nose, nausea, recurring middle ear infections, ringing in the ears, or hyperactivity could mean a food allergy. Food additives such as yellow dye no. 5 (tetrazine) and benzoates can increase the production of mast cells, elevating the possibility of an allergy. The following food additives also have been associated with allergies and/or asthma: azo dyes and food colorings, salicylates, aspartame, benzoates, nitrites, sorbic acid, hydoxytoluene, sulfites, gallates, polysorbates, and vegetable gums.

Avoid Processed and Dairy Foods

Stay away from processed foods, as they often contain allergy-producing preservatives such as BHA and BHT. Dairy foods generate additional mucus, which can aggravate sinus infection and add to digestive problems. They are to be avoided (Clark 2001).

Eat a Low-Salt Diet

Salt has been implicated as an asthma aggravator for some men. In a study conducted by Carey, Locke, and Cookson, men on a low-sodium regime used their bronchodilators less often; were able to exhale more air; and had fewer symptoms, such as wheezing.

Drink Enough Water

Many people who suffer from acute asthma attacks do so because they are dehydrated, according to a report in *The Clinical Advisor*. So drink at least ten glasses of water a day without fail to stay well.

Take Selenium

Selenium supplementation improves cellular oxidative defense, counteracting the inflammation and disordered respiration associated with asthma, according to a study in *Allergy*. Due to the poor quality of soil in the Northeast, Florida, parts of Washington and Oregon, and parts of the Midwest, selenium may have to be taken as a supplement (50–70 micrograms a day), although seafoods, whole-grain breads and cereals, asparagus, garlic, and mushrooms may contain some selenium.

Increase Fatty Acid Foods and Decrease Saturated Fats

Fatty acids are important protectors against the inflammation of allergies because of their ability to form prostaglandins, substances that control many body actions such as blood pressure, muscle contraction, kidney function, stomach secretion, intestinal absorption, and contractions of the uterus. While fatty acids protect you from allergies, animal foods (meat and dairy products) can irritate them because they contain saturated fats and arachidonic acid, both of which can increase your allergic response. If you eat less meat, eggs, and cheese and more cold-water fish (mackerel, herring, sardines, and salmon) and use flaxseed oil, you can reduce inflammatory/allergic responses. A study published in the *Medical Journal of Australia* concluded that consumption of oily fish may protect against asthma in childhood.

Rotate Offending Foods

By rotating offending foods so you only eat them once every five days or more, your allergic reactions can be reduced. Keep a food diary and examine it and see when you have bothersome symptoms. Do your symptoms occur after eating certain foods? The most common food allergens include milk, cheese, yeast, wheat, rye, corn, soybeans, eggs, oranges, white potatoes, peanuts, chocolate, various spices, beef, coffee, tomatoes, malt, and pork. You may have to examine can and container labels for ingredients when you eat processed foods. For example, you may find that corn or malt syrup is included as one of the ingredients in your favorite food, or that a canned tomato sauce is flavored with cheese or beef. It's not always possible to identify what substances in processed foods may be causing the allergic reaction, so if you can, try to eat unprocessed foods. Reach for the fresh form of whatever food you plan to eat whenever possible. Caffeinated and decaffeinated beverages and sugar can overstimulate the immune system and may aggravate your allergies. You may be sensitive to one or more of these foods or food substances or to something else.

It also may be important to buy organically produced foods. They will not contain toxic pesticide residues or be genetically engineered, both of which could increase allergic responses.

Eat More Fruits, Vegetables, Grains, and Seeds

In a study conducted by Carey and colleagues, children who ate an Indian diet (more vegetables, less meat, and fewer additives and packaged and processed foods) had fewer symptoms of allergy and asthma than Indian youngsters eating a mostly Western diet. The children with fewer symptoms did not eat meat, fish, eggs, green peas, soybeans, salt, sugar, coffee, ordinary tea, chocolate, potatoes, grains, apples, citrus fruits, or dairy products. They maintained a vegetarian diet and drank only nonchlorinated tap water.

Ellwood and colleagues came to the same conclusions in their study of children and teenagers in fifty-six countries. They confirmed Carey's findings and reported their results in the *European Respiratory Journal*.

Berries and onions have been shown to produce antiasthmatic effects. You may want to try them to see if they help control your allergic symptoms.

A study by Soutar and colleagues found an increased risk for allergic symptoms in individuals who had low food intakes of zinc, magnesium, manganese, and vitamin C. A study published in the *Archives of Pediatrics & Adolescent Medicine* reported that vitamin C may block the effect of exercise-induced asthma. Try eating a lot of foods high in these minerals and vitamin C to see if your symptoms subside. Some foods high in zinc include oysters, herring, nuts, wheat germ, and liver. Whole-grain bread and cereals, brown rice, wheat germ, nuts, Swiss chard, figs, and green leafy vegetables are high in magnesium. Nuts, seeds, whole grains, fruits and vegetables, dry beans, and peas and oatmeal are high in manganese. Green peppers, honeydew melons, cooked broccoli or Brussels sprouts, kale, cantaloupes, strawberries, papayas, cooked cauliflower, oranges, watercress, raspberries, parsley, raw cabbage, blackberries, onions, spinach, tomatoes, and rose hip tea or powder contain vitamin C.

Citrus fruits or vitamin C and bioflavonoid supplements contain natural antihistamines. If you usually sip on coffee, tea, or soda, try squeezing a lemon, grapefruit, or orange (or all three) in a quart or two of filtered water and drinking that throughout your day (unless your food diary shows that you react to citrus fruits). Onions also can build your immune system and help heal lung tissue.

A study that appeared in *Lancet* found that eating foods high in vitamin E (olive oil, wheat germ, whole-grain cereals, fruits, green vegetables, and fish) may protect you from asthma, since the condition is related to increased levels of oxidants. Vitamin E is an antioxidant that reduces levels of these harmful compounds.

Drink Fresh Juices

If you don't have a juicer, buy one. Most health food stores sell them. Wash seven or eight carrots, cut off the tops and stems, and put the cleaned carrots through the juicer. This will remove the indigestible fiber and many of the toxins from pesticides while providing you with an easy-to-digest, pleasing drink. Add 1 or 2 radishes to the juicer and mix them into the carrot juice. Drink several glasses a day. This juice will reduce mucus, especially if you eat fewer mucus-forming foods such as dairy foods, white bread, cheese, cookies, pies, cakes, and sugary cereals.

Heat Things Up

Capsicum (from cayenne or hot chilies) may be helpful because it can boost your immune system and circulation, clean your blood, and thin bronchial secretions. Also, try eating ¼ to ½ teaspoon of fresh, ground horseradish pulp (without the juice) mixed with lemon juice between meals to clear your sinuses.

Try a Saltwater Solution

The Women's Health Advocate (April 1998) suggests that a saltwater solution may help. Combine 1 quart of boiled water, 1½ to 3 heaping teaspoons of table salt, and 1 rounded teaspoon of baking soda. If your nose is dry, add 1 tablespoon of white Karo syrup or glycerine. Mix the ingredients in a 1-quart glass jar with a lid. Warm the solution in a microwave or on the stove in a pot. Make sure it isn't too hot, then place a small amount in a baby bulb syringe. Bend over the sink and squirt the solution into one nostril and then into the other one. Repeat two or three times. Discard the unused solution and clean the syringe in warm, soapy water.

Take Pantothenic Acid

Pantothenic acid is one of the B vitamins. It acts as a heart protector, may improve circulation, helps the body store sugar, eliminates waste by-products (ketones), and plays an important role in various body processes, especially the production and breakdown of fatty acids. It also may be helpful in clearing the head of congestion. Since it is water-soluble, unneeded amounts of the ingested vitamin are eliminated in the urine and do not accumulate in the body. There are no known side effects.

If You're Pregnant, Consider Breast-Feeding

Breast-feeding also can reduce allergic symptoms in your children. A study by Marini and colleagues showed that breast-feeding, followed by hypoallergenic weaning and avoidance of parental smoking for the first two years of life, resulted in infants with fewer allergic symptoms. A study published in the *British Medical Journal* verified the importance of breast-feeding, at least for the first four months of life.

Get Your Kids to Lose Weight

Children who are overweight or obese are significantly more likely to be diagnosed with asthma, according to analysis of a ten-year investigation called the Children's Health Study. If you have children or grandchildren who are overweight, feed them fewer processed sweet and fatty foods, and give them more fruit and vegetables.

Think Carefully about Taking Replacement Hormones

If you're a woman nearing menopause, think carefully about taking replacement hormones. A study published in the *American Journal of Respiratory & Critical Care Medicine* found that women who never used replacement hormones had a significantly lower risk of asthma than women who take HRT.

Investigate Herbs

Some herbs also have anti-inflammatory, immune-system-building, respiratory-soothing, and antimucus effects. Consult a herbalist about using fenugreek, rose hips, saw palmetto, boswellia, chamomile, eyebright, garlic, gingko, licorice, sage, fennel, thyme, or pau d'arco teas or capsules. Eucalyptus oil used in a mister or nebulizer also can help, as can drinking 2 to 4 ounces of aloe juice a day.

Ginger tea also has been used successfully to reduce sinus inflammation. The steam from grated ginger is simmered in water and then breathed in for five to seven minutes, two to three times a day until symptoms subside. Unlike drugs that treat symptoms, herbs may strengthen the immune system. Once it has been strengthened, it may be possible to gradually reintroduce an allergen and get no allergic response. Astragalus, licorice, pau d'arco, ginseng, ginger, and garlic may tone your immune system so it doesn't react to safe substances with an allergic response. *Note:* Always talk with your doctor or healthcare professional if you are taking or plan to take a herb, to make sure it will not interact poorly with the medications you are taking.

Consider Homeopathic Remedies

Homeopathic remedies also may help. Reilly and colleagues used homeopathically prepared dilutions of grass pollens or dust mites in the treatment of nasal allergies. The group who received the highly diluted preparations improved considerably more than those given a placebo that did not contain the allergens.

Runny noses, itchy throats, and sneezes may be helped by the homeopathic remedies *Arsenicum album* or sabadilla. Homeopathic remedies for temporary relief of allergies include monkshood, windflower, eyebright, red onion, trioxide of arsenic, phosphate of iron, iodide of potassium, quicksilver, and poison nut. Since most allergies are long-term problems, they require consultation with a trained homeopathic practitioner. Since most homeopathic remedies are so highly diluted that little if any of the original substance remains in the treatment, it is unlikely that there will be a reaction with prescribed or over-the-counter drugs. To be sure, let your healthcare practitioner or physician know that you are planning to use or are using a homeopathic remedy.

Exercise Daily

According to a 2001 study in the *American Journal of Public Health*, physical activity, especially walking and more vigorous activity, can enhance your quality of life and help you to live longer, especially if you have difficulty breathing. Start slowly and be sure to begin an exercise program under the supervision of your physician, but move, even if it's only a walk or two around your house at the start.

Try Yoga

A study of the effect of a yoga therapy program on chronic bronchial asthma found that yoga could reduce symptoms and drug requirements. Look into local yoga programs in your area.

Keep Calm

Strong emotion can trigger an asthma attack. A study reported in *Psychosomatic Medicine* found that people with asthma have more problems breathing when they are feeling anxiety, anger, depression, and even happiness or elation. Finding a way to reduce stress, be it positive or negative, will help.

The first step is to identify what triggers asthma attacks. Once that is achieved, you can take steps to reduce the effects of these triggers. A strategy that may work for you may include practicing yoga or guided imagery, or taking B vitamins. (See later in this chapter.)

Try Writing about Stressful Experiences to Reduce Symptoms

A study in the *Journal of the American Medical Association* showed that writing about the most stressful events in your life could reduce asthma symptoms. Spend at least twenty minutes a day on three consecutive days writing about the most stressful event you've ever encountered. It could reduce your asthma symptoms for four months or longer.

Apply Gentle Pressure to Key Acupuncture Points

Stress and allergies can play havoc with your energy flow. Two acupuncture points named K-27 (Kidney 27) are on the front of the body, where the first rib, collarbone, and breastbone come together. To find the location:

1. Place your fingers on either of your collarbones and slowly follow it toward the center of your chest. When you feel a small depression or hole, this is where the three bones come together and K-27 is located.

2. Now put your index and middle finger of one hand on either side of your belly button. Place the index finger of your other hand on K-27 on the right side of your body.

3. At the same time, apply gentle pressure to both areas and rub in a rotary fashion for fifteen to twenty seconds.

4. Move your top index finger over to the left K-27 point and rub both places again for fifteen to twenty seconds.

Get Aromatherapy Massage

An aromatherapy massage can be calming for adults or children, thereby helping to open up constricted breathing passages. Dilute 5 drops of essential lavender oil in 2 tablespoons of vegetable oil; then massage the back in long, sweeping movements. Start at the base of the spine, with your hands on either side of the vertebrae. Move up the back slowly in upward strokes, coming over the shoulder and down the sides of the body.

Try Guided Imagery

James Halpern, M.D., has shown that guided imagery can help participants discontinue their allergy medicine. Another physician, William Mundy, M.D., has used guided imagery to treat allergies as well as depression and unhappiness. It used to be thought that body chemistry dictates behavior and symptoms and that feelings and thoughts were separate entities, but due to Candace Pert and her work with psychoneuroimmunology, it is now agreed that body chemistry interacts back and forth with your symptoms and feelings. Mind and body chatter back and forth, using the language of biochemicals.

Pert's work at the National Institute of Mental Health showed that a certain kind of white blood cells are equipped with the molecular equivalent of antennae that are tuned in to receive messages from the brain. A mosaic of evidence suggests that our body systems communicate with one another through messengers carried back and forth on tiny molecules. These biochemical messengers, now called neurotransmitters, neuropeptides, lymphokines, and by other tongue-twisting terms, are informational substances that have a powerful effect on your moods and emotions. Based on these ideas, it is possible that by changing your thoughts and feelings, you can change your body's responses as what you think and feel are relayed to your immune system.

Results of a small study published in *Brain and Behavioral Immunity* showed that a combination of relaxation, guided imagery, and self-esteem workshops reduced the number of asthmatic episodes and the use of bronchodilator medication in asthmatic children, compared to what had happened six months prior to the intervention.

You might want to use the following script to teach your immune system not to react to allergens. Record the directions into a recorder, pausing often, especially at the ". . ." marks, and speak in a slow monotone. When you've made the tape that sounds right for you, play it back to yourself when you're in a quiet, safe place. Remember to play it several times a day so it will be firmly planted in your mind and body, and follow its directions.

1. Loosen your clothes, close your eyes, and let yourself relax in a comfortable chair.

2. Allow a relaxing warmth to spread from the tips of your toes throughout your body. . . . Take your time . . . breathing in relaxation . . . and comfort.

3. Think of yourself as a cartoonist, and picture the little particles of allergens that have plagued you in the past. Make them colored or polka-dotted or however you wish to see them. . . . Take your time . . . making sure you have them pictured exactly as you wish to see them. . . .

4. Now imagine a six-inch-thick Plexiglas wall that separates you completely from those allergen particles. . . .

5. While you're sitting safely behind that six-inch-thick Plexiglas . . . imagine yourself on the other side of that wall, having an allergy attack. You are separated from that person, but can clearly see what's happening. There are allergic molecules circulating around you on the other side of that Plexiglas shield, while you remain safe and protected, behind your Plexiglas shield. . . .

6. When you have the picture of you on the other side of the Plexiglas having an attack, shift your attention to some peaceful, quiet, and soothing place. . . . Smell the smells you associate with that spot. . . . Hear the sounds you associate with that spot. . . . Feel the sensations you associate with that place. . . . See the sights you associate with that spot. . . .

7. Notice that there are certain particles in that air . . . particles that come in through your lungs and into your mouth. . . . They smell and taste good and healthy. . . .

8. Picture those particles becoming part of you, filling every cell of your body with peace and relaxation . . . calm and serene . . . totally relaxed and healthy . . . totally surrounded by the healthy molecules, keeping you safe from harm.

9. Now look through that Plexiglas protective shield and see yourself over there, behind it, having that allergic attack. . . . You remain behind your shield, safe and healthy.

10. In your mind's eye, reach through that Plexiglas shield and get a handful of those allergic particles . . . See how calm and safe you remain, even though you're holding those allergic molecules in

your hand. If at any time you lose that feeling of calm safety, just dissolve those allergic molecules and take yourself in your mind's eye to that safe and comfortable spot you pictured before. . . . Stay there until you feel safe and comfortable again, then come back and reach through that Plexiglas shield and get another handful of allergic particles.

11. See how those allergic molecules just disappear . . . swallowed up by the healthy molecules surrounding every part of you . . . keeping you healthy, calm, safe. . . .

12. Reach through that Plexiglas shield and grab another handful of allergic particles. . . . Notice how they can't touch you . . . you are totally protected by your healthy molecules . . . staying safe, healthy, and comfortable. . . .

13. When you're ready, grab a small bucket of those allergic molecules, watching them disappear as they are surrounded by the healthy, comforting molecules surrounding you . . . take your time . . . let the allergic molecules blend with yours while you stay healthy, calm, and comfortable.

14. Bask in your success of having blended the allergic molecules with your healthy, safe, and calming molecules . . . picture the blended healthy and happy you, no longer concerned at all about the allergy particles, completely safe and healthy. . . . You're in a bubble of healthy, happy, and safe particles. . . .

15. When you're ready, slowly lift up the Plexiglas shield . . . keeping relaxed and comfortable, totally safe and healthy in your bubble. . . .

16. Notice how the allergic molecules are slowly moving toward your safe and healthy bubble, but you don't mind because you feel safe and healthy, protected behind your bubble . . . and there you are, breathing easily and enjoying that you no longer have any problems with the allergic particles . . . in fact, the two bubbles have met and blended and you continue to feel safe, comfortable, and healthy. . . . Realize that the allergic particles are now harmless and simply part of the things your body can handle easily and every day in a healthy and routine way. . . . Take your time to experience how good it feels to be free of things that used to bother you . . . to be totally in control of how good you feel . . . to be healthy, comfortable, and secure. . . .

Use Hypnosis or Storytelling, Too

A study published in the *American Journal of Clinical Hypnosis* reported that by applying hypnosis in a preschool family education program, physician visits for asthma were reduced and parents reported increased confidence in self-management skills. Symptom severity was also reduced.

In the study, symptom severity also was reduced through storytelling, imagery, and relaxation. Many activities such as reading, driving, and watching TV can bring on a hypnotic state of relaxation and focused attention.

Hypnosis is an exaggerated form of body relaxation and focused attention that uses suggestion. It is easily learned and practiced once you learn the method. Ask your doctor for a referral to a trained hypnosis practitioner or nurse practitioner with hypnosis skills and make an appointment to learn the procedure. Once learned, you can practice it on your own.

If you have a child diagnosed with asthma, try reading or telling calming stories, perhaps finding ideas in the preceding guided imagery script. For example, depending on the age of the child, you could tell a story about a fairy princess who can't breathe and she finds a wizard who provides her with a Plexiglas shield from the dog (trees, flowers, or whatever) and she lives happily ever after. The idea is to tell the story in a monotone voice, using plenty of pauses and calming phrases. You also can talk to your local librarian, who can help you find stories that are relaxing and calming. Read them to your child prior to bedtime or at times of stress to ward off asthma attacks. The same idea can be used with adults, only use stories appropriate for an older audience.

Alzheimer's Disease

Alzheimer's disease is one of the most common causes of the loss of mental function known as dementia. This type of dementia proceeds in stages, gradually destroying memory, judgment, reason, language, and eventually the ability to carry out simple tasks daily tasks. Personality may change, people may have difficulty feeding themselves or their pets, and they may buy outrageous products that they later wonder why they bought or if they bought them. People with Alzheimer's may wander, be agitated, and become quite aggressive.

In the mid-1970s, scientists discovered that levels of a neurotransmitter called acetylcholine fell sharply in people with this condition. Acetylcholine is a critical in the process of forming memories, and it also is used by neurons in the hippocampus and cerebral cortex.

Research also has shown that there may be a problem in glucose metabolism, or in having too much calcium in the neurons. Other possible causes include aluminum, zinc, foodborne poisons, and/or viruses.

A metaphysical explanation for Alzheimer's is that the person who develops the condition refuses to deal with the world as it is, with hopelessness, helplessness, and anger abounding. Affirmations may help. (See "Affirmations Could Help" for specific affirmations.)

Your Risk for Developing Alzheimer's Disease

Risk factors for Alzheimer's include age. The risk of suffering from the condition rises exponentially with age, doubling in each decade after age sixty-five. If you have relatives who developed Alzheimer's, you are more likely to develop the condition, as three genes have been discovered that help explain why family history is a risk factor.

Head injury also may be a risk factor. Some studies have found that people who suffered traumatic head injuries early in life were more likely to develop Alzheimer's. Also, the more years of formal education you have, the less likely you are to develop Alzheimer's. Lower educational levels may increase the risk. Gender also is important. Women have a higher risk of developing this condition, but that may because they have longer life spans on the average than men. Eating a high-fat diet during early and mid-adulthood also may increase the risk of developing the condition according to Grace Petot, an assistant professor emeritus of nutrition at Case Western Reserve University School of Medicine in Cleveland. Participants in her study who consumed the highest-fat diets (more than 40 percent of calories from fat) had an up to twenty-nine times greater risk of developing Alzheimer's disease than those who ate a lower-fat diet.

Living alone may be a risk factor for dementia and Alzheimer's disease. Individuals without spouses or cohabitants have a twofold increased risk of dementia and almost a threefold increased risk of Alzheimer's according to a study in *Neurology*. Cohabiting with another person usually means more social contacts and leisure activities, more brain stimulation, and a greater likelihood of better nutrition. All of these factors are important for preventing Alzheimer's.

How the Doctor Diagnoses Alzheimer's Disease

Your doctor can make a diagnosis of the condition in four ways. The first and most important way is through a detailed history. You will be asked questions about how and when symptoms developed, your medical history and your family's medical history, your emotional state, and your living environment.

A physical exam and laboratory tests will provide more information to help identify possible causes. A computed tomograph (CT) scan or magnetic resonance imaging (MRI) can detect strokes or tumors that could be causing symptoms of dementia. It also can show evidence of shrinkage in the cortex and the hippocampus, key memory centers in the brain. Neuropsychological testing will be conducted, which consists of being asked to answer questions or complete tasks that measure memory, language skills, ability to do arithmetic, and other abilities related to brain functioning. The results can help your doctor decide if you have Alzheimer's.

Not everyone with impaired memory has Alzheimer's. At the World Alzheimer Congress 2000 in Washington, D.C., Gunhild Waldemar, M.D., examined 785 patients with memory problems. Only 43 percent had Alzheimer's disease or some other form of dementia. Six percent had amnesia, 11 percent had some other kind of cognitive deficit, 28 percent had no serious thinking deficit, and 12 percent could not be diagnosed. Six percent of the patients diagnosed with Alzheimer's also had another condition—depression, high blood pressure, thyroid disease, alcohol dependence—that was treatable and that contributed to memory loss. Thirty-five percent of the individuals she evaluated had a potentially treatable condition that could impair memory.

Additionally, other factors can mimic Alzheimer's, including a low level of vitamin B_{12} in the nerve tissue. This vitamin affects nerve tissue and the creation of neurotransmitters, the messengers that bring information to and from the brain. For this reason, it is important not to accept a diagnosis of Alzheimer's until a course of vitamin B_{12} treatment has been instigated and all other possibilities have been eliminated.

What the Doctor Will Probably Prescribe

To date, no effective drug has been found to treat Alzheimer's, but there are many theories. The discovery that the neurotransmitter acetylcholine declines in Alzheimer's led naturally to the hypothesis that replacing acetylcholine could stop the condition from advancing. Many of the experimental drugs developed to date are cholinesterase inhibitors, including donepezil, rivastigmine, and metrifonate. They are designed to suppress cholinesterase so that acetylcholine will not be broken down as quickly.

The theory that there is a rise in calcium levels in neurons led to the belief that calcium channel blockers might fill this role, so they may be prescribed, but there is no research to show that they will help. Still another theory is that there is a possible link between estrogen and Alzheimer's, because in a study of thousands of women, those who had taken estrogen after menopause had lower rates of Alzheimer's than those who had not taken hormones. Some doctors may prescribe estrogen, but keep in mind that the study showed only an *association* between estrogen and lower rates of Alzheimer's and did not prove causation. Also be aware that estrogens are linked with cancer.

A study reported in *International Clinical Psychoparmacology* found that although a drug called Cerebrolysin was associated with some improvement in thinking, adverse events, due to side effects, were recorded in 43 percent of the individuals receiving the drug.

Alzheimer's rates may be lower among people who take anti-inflammatory drugs than those who do not. Still another theory about calcium imbalance points to out-of-control molecules called free radicals. The agents that disarm them, antioxidants, are abundant in fruits and vegetables.

Self-Care Measures You Can Take

There are a number of things you can do to prevent and/or treat Alzheimer's. *The more active you are in self-care measures, the more likely you are to control your symptoms.*

Change What You Eat

Eat low-fat foods. Stop eating fried foods and those with saturated fats (meats, cheese, pastries, cakes, and pies). Start eating more low-fat foods, including fruits, vegetables, and whole grains. Read labels of processed foods for the amount of saturated fat, and choose low-fat options.

A deficiency in vitamin B_{12} and an overabundance of homocysteine (a type of amino acid, a building block of protein that can injure blood vessel linings) can cause dementia and severe nerve damage. According to a report in the *American Journal of Clinical Nutrition*, with age, your digestive tract becomes less efficient in absorbing vitamin B_{12}. It may be important to eat more foods containing vitamin B_{12} to overcome the lack of efficiency of your digestive tract. Foods high in this vitamin include sardines, mackerel, trout, herring, eggs, some cheese, nutritional yeast, crab, crayfish, clams, oysters, sea vegetables (kombu, dulse, kelp, wakame), and fermented soyfoods (tempeh, natto, and miso). Limit your coffee intake. Five or more cups of coffee a day raises homocysteine significantly, producing negative effects for your heart.

Oxidative stress probably plays a key role in the dementia that occurs in Alzheimer's disease. Plant foods contain flavonoids, powerful antioxidant substances. To protect yourself against harmful oxidative stress, eat at least five servings of fruits and vegetables every day.

A lack of folate also may be involved in the development of Alzheimer's according to a study reported in *Neurology*, so it makes sense to eat foods rich in this substance. Foods to concentrate on include asparagus, desiccated or fresh liver, fresh dark green uncooked vegetables, wheat bran, turnips, potatoes, orange juice, black-eyed peas, lima beans, watermelons, oysters, and cantaloupes.

Drink more green tea. It exerts a protective effect against brain injury, according to a study reported in *Brain Research Bulletin*.

Drink filtered or distilled water. Aluminum in drinking water is correlated with Alzheimer's disease, according to a recent study reported in the *American Journal of Epidemiology*. Also, reduce consumption of foods or drugs that contain aluminum, including antacids, buffered aspirin, and aluminum cookware. Fluoridated drinking water may be especially bad for you. Studies in *Brain Research* and the *Archives of Physiology and Biochemistry* provided evidence that aluminum fluoride, which is used to fluoridate drinking water, alters nerves and blood vessels in the brain.

Minerals compete with each other in your body, so by increasing your consumption of magnesium and/or magnesium-rich foods, there will be less chance of aluminum absorption. Magnesium-rich foods include whole grain breads and cereals, fresh peas, brown rice, soy flour, wheat germ, nuts, Swiss chard, figs, green leafy vegetables, and citrus fruits.

Be Careful of Inhaling Aluminum

The amount of aluminum you get in your daily food may pass harmlessly out of the body, but still it's best not to cook with aluminum pots. Switch to iron, stainless steel, glass, or porcelain-coated cookware.

Aluminum that you inhale may be completely absorbed because the olfactory nerves in the nasal cavity lead directly to your brain. For this reason you may want to discontinue the use of spray-on antiperspirants, hair sprays, cleaning solutions, hobby sprays, and paints and glues.

Consider Taking Beneficial Supplements

Pycnogenol is a supplement that may help. Research reported in the *Biological Pharmacy Bulletin* reports that the supplement may be useful to prevent and/or treat neurodegenerative conditions such as Alzheimer's disease.

Acetyl-L-carnitine is another supplement to consider. A report in *Molecular Psychiatry* summarized the importance of this supplement: it contains both acetyl and carnitine, both of which have neurobiological properties that have been shown to have beneficial effects in combating Alzheimer's disease.

Antioxidants can function as powerful protectants. A study in the *New England Journal of Medicine* concluded that the progression of Alzheimer's in patients with moderately severe impairment is slowed equally well with vitamin E or selegiline, a monoamine oxidase inhibitor. According to a report in the *Journal of Neural Transmission*, vitamin E (alpha-tocopherol) in both its natural and synthetic form has been shown to protect neurons against the oxidative cell death caused by Alzheimer's disease.

Vitamin C is another antioxidant that can help. A report in *Free Radicals in Biological Medicine* reported that supplementation with vitamin C and E together significantly decreases oxidation, a factor in Alzheimer's disease.

A study of older men (aged seventy-one to ninety-three) reported in *Neurology* found that participants who took both vitamin C and E supplements at least once a week were 88 percent less likely to have vascular dementia (speech, language, and visual disturbances, paralysis and mental impairment) and a 20 percent greater chance of having better cognitive (thinking) function than those who didn't, even four years later! You might be best off taking the supplements in an ongoing fashion, because participants in the study who took the supplements over a six-year period showed a 75 percent greater chance of better mental performance.

Alzheimer's is associated with deficiency of a brain chemical, acetylcholine. Lecithin (made from soy) and choline (a supplement) are precursors to this chemical, so taking them daily could help.

Investigate Herbs

According to the journal *Alternative Therapies in Health and Medicine* one herb that has been show to be useful and safe in the treatment of Alzheimer's is ginkgo biloba. Used for thousands of years in traditional Chinese medicine, the herb now has been shown to treat failing memory, age-related dementias, and poor blood flow to the head and brain. A study in the *International Journal of Neuropsychopharmacology* found that healthy participants who took gingko biloba showed significant improvements in speed of working memory and processing information.

A study reported in the *Psychopharmacology Bulletin* concluded that the herb has a significant effect on the central nervous system and may treat insufficient blood flow to the brain. Another study, in *Phytomedicine*, showed that gingko is equally effective as a cholinesterase inhibitor (donepezil, rivastigmine, and metrifonate).

Ginkgo also benefits Alzheimer's patients, according to a study in the *Journal of the American Medical Association*. The ginkgo extract improved thinking and social function.

Note: Use of any herbs needs to be carefully coordinated with other medications you are taking. Be sure to consult with a healthcare practitioner who is an expert in herbs, since ginkgo can interact with aspirin and antiplatelet drugs and can increase clotting time. Follow the dosage directions on the bottle.

Lower Your Blood Pressure

Although most age-related dementia is due to Alzheimer's, the second most frequent cause is high blood pressure. If you're overweight, lose weight by eating low-fat foods and increasing exercise. Make sure you eat breakfast so you'll eat less in the evening, when you won't be as active and it can turn to fat. Also, take a stress reduction class to learn how to control stress and anger, and consider getting massage, which can lower the body's level of cortisol, an indicator of stress.

Keep Your Mind Stimulated

Adults with hobbies that exercise their minds, such as reading, jigsaw puzzles or chess, are protected more than twice as much from Alzheimer's disease as those whose leisure is limited to TV watching. A study published in the *Proceedings of the National Academy of Sciences* found that unused brainpower is lost brainpower. Every day be sure to read, do a puzzle, play a musical instrument or a board game, knit, or do wood-work. Physical activities such as baseball, football, bike riding, swimming, walking, or skating also stimulate your brain and may help ward off Alzheimer's. One study, reported in the *American Journal of Alzheimer's Disease and Other Dementias*, found that even the Bingo did the trick!

Stop Smoking

Smoking raises homocysteine and depletes antioxidant vitamins that may protect the brain, so find a way to stop smoking if you don't want to develop Alzheimer's.

Listen to Music

Listening to music you prefer can work better than medication for agi-tated movement, according to reports in the *Journal of the American Psychiatric Nurses Association, International Psychogeriatrics*, and the *Journal of Gerontological Nursing*. Play music you prefer at the first sign of agitation.

Exercise Helps

Exercise can help improve energy, circulation, stamina, and mood, according to a report in *Gerontology*. If you or a family member have Alzheimer's, you may have the desire, but not the wherewithal, to plan it. Someone else may need to lead the exercise. Many nursing homes have seated range-of-motion programs. Even frail people can participate in these, and memory loss, mobility, balance, flexibility, and knee and hip strength have been shown to improve in a three-times-a-week program according to reports in the *Journal of Gerontology* and the *American Journal of Alzheimer's Disease*. At home, dancing, walking and mild stretching can be employed. It is best to complete the activity regularly, at the same time of day and in the same vicinity, to minimize confusion.

Consider Touch to Reduce Agitation

Nurses have long used touch and massage to help patients relax. It is important to approach an agitated person in a gentle, unhurried manner. Sometimes just holding hands and talking softly will reduce agitation. Gently stroking the patient from earlobe to chin in an unhurried manner can bring calm and may stimulate memory, according to a report in the *Journal of Gerontological Nursing*.

Massage also can enhance relaxation as well as reduce blood pressure. A study in the *International Journal of Nursing Practice* showed that massage also could lessen anxiety and lower the body's level of cortisol, an indicator of stress.

Gentle hand massage using lotion with a scent familiar to the patient can reduce anxiety and agitation, according to a study reported in the *International Journal of Nursing Practice*. If the patient is at home, use a lotion familiar to the person with Alzheimer's. Hold some in your hands to warm it, and then gently massage the back. If a family member is already in a nursing home, bring in lotion that is familiar for the nurse to use. Massage with lotion can increase alertness and contentment, reduce stress levels and agitation, and improve sleep. Family caregivers providing massage reported that their sleeping patterns improved, too, and that they felt more calm and less stressed.

Foot massage with acupressure reduced patient wandering and increased periods of calm according to a study in *Image: Journal of Nursing Scholarship*. If a family member is a resident in a nursing home, ask that he or she receive foot massage. If there are no nurses or massage therapists available to give a foot massage, investigate having one come into the nursing home on a consultant basis. You may have to coordinate this with your doctor. If the family member is at home, you can have a massage therapist come in, or try using lotion yourself to gently rub the family member's feet.

Slow stroking massage also has been used to reduce Alzheimer's symptoms. A report in the *Journal of Gerontological Nursing* found that slow-stroke massage reduced pacing, wandering, and resisting in individuals with Alzheimer's.

Affirmations Could Help

While still healthy or during early stages of the condition, practice affirmations. Say or write the following statements at least twenty times a day, and place the sayings on 3 × 5 cards in prominent places:

- I forgive and release the past.
- I accept a life of complete joy.
- I move forward into a new and better way of experiencing life.

FOR CAREGIVERS

Connecting with People Who Have Alzheimer's Disease

It's easy to get upset when talking to someone who's agitated, but it's essential not to take that behavior personally. Let your loved one express frustrations. Even if the words don't make total sense, the speech and inflection may hold clues to what is meant.

Give your loved ones as much control over their daily lives as possible. Ask "What do you want to wear today?" and hold up two outfits. Ask "What do you want to eat for breakfast?" and hold up an egg and a box of cereal (or whatever choices there are). Do the same for lunch and dinner. It is important to assume that some of what you say and do is getting through to your loved one. This gives the message that you care for and respect the person.

Provide signs, pictures, and familiar objects that can guide a family member who wanders. Offer toileting every two hours. Consider getting an ID bracelet, or an alarm device designed to sound when your loved one rises from a bed or chair unassisted, to ensure safer walking. Regular vision and hearing assessments to confirm that eyeglasses are clean and operational and hearing aids are working can decrease misinterpretation of the environment.

Introduce yourself and your relationship regularly during the day, and keep a clock nearby so you can say the time aloud, especially when you notice that the memory of your loved one is failing. Photo albums with familiar pictures, favorite foods, personal memorabilia, and preferred music can provide comfort.

An unpublished 1998 study by a geriatric nursing researcher at the University of Rochester found that rocking chairs calm dementia sufferers. The agitation caused by Alzheimer's is soothed by rocking. If you don't have a rocking chair, you may want to consider getting one.

A study in the *International Journal of Nursing Practice* found that looking in a mirror raised patient awareness regarding self-care in most individuals. For a small number of patients, looking into the mirror aroused feelings of anger or despair, but this was quickly followed by relief and calmness. Mirrors may be another household object you may want to use to help someone with Alzheimer's, but probably not during a period of agitation.

What to Do If Nursing Home Care Is Needed

If Alzheimer's progresses to a point of great memory loss and combativeness, nursing home care may be a distinct alternative. In these cases be sure to enlist the services of a gerontologic advanced practice nurse (GAPN), who can treat urinary incontinence, pressure ulcers, depression, and aggressive behavior, as well as help families adjust to the transition to the nursing home. A study published in *Gerontologist* showed that nursing home residents who worked with a GAPN showed significantly less deterioration than residents who didn't work with a GAPN.

Make a tape of the music your family member loves. Bring it to the nursing home and play it in the dining room at mealtimes. You also can show an aide or a nursing technician how to massage your loved one's back, feet, or hands, or have a nurse demonstrate it. Ask the nurse to supervise the aide or technician at least the first time and randomly at other times to make sure the massage is performed competently and safely. By making touch, exercise, and music part of daily care, you can bring a spark of energetic life to your loved one and also have a feeling of satisfaction that you have done something important.

Arthritis

Arthritis means joint inflammation. The word comes from two Greek words: *arthron*, for joint, and *itis*, for inflammation. The most common forms of this disorder are rheumatoid arthritis and osteoarthritis. Joint inflammation also occurs in ankylosing spondylitis (spinal arthritis), lupus, gout, juvenile rheumatoid arthritis, inflammatory bowel disorders, psoriasis, and many infections, from rheumatic fever to Lyme disease.

Osteoarthritis is a disease that causes the breakdown of cartilage in joints. This leads to pain and stiffness. It can affect any joint, but it usually occurs in the hips, knees, spine, fingers, and toes. When it affects the big toe it is called gout. It rarely affects the wrists, elbows, shoulders, ankles, or jaw except as a result of injury or high stress. In healthy joints, a rubbery material called cartilage covers and protects the ends of bones and acts as a cushion or shock absorber. Arthritic joints usually hurt the most after overuse or long periods of inactivity.

Almost everyone over sixty has some X-ray evidence of osteoarthritis, but only a third have symptoms. Rheumatoid or inflammatory arthritis causes more serious health and financial problems, similar to coronary heart disease in lifetime costs for treatment.

Rheumatoid arthritis is an autoimmune condition, which means the body attacks itself. This type of arthritis is also characterized by progressive joint pain, redness, and swelling, often leading to deformity. It is also characterized by long periods of remission, during which all symptoms subside.

Juvenile arthritis is a chronic condition that begins before age sixteen and persists for more than six weeks. It involves a daily or twice daily low-grade fever (104° to 106°) associated with a fleeting, salmon-colored rash. Fatigue, morning stiffness, and irritability also are common.

Ankylosing spondylitis (spinal arthritis) causes immobility of the back and often the shoulders and neck. It is an inflammatory form of arthritis. Systemic lupus erythematosus (SLE) is technically not an arthritis, but an immune-related form of arthralgia that often affects the hip joints.

One explanation for arthritis is that it's the result of long-term *dehydration and malnutrition* of the connective tissues that act as shock absorbers among bones, muscles, disks, ligaments, and tendons. This is aggravated by increasing limitation of movement, increasing limits of flexibility, and more stiffness.

Studies show that *stress* can precipitate the flare-up of rheumatoid symptoms. The important role of stress on immune function has become more evident in recent studies. In one research report, almost every female patient interviewed reported an emotionally stressful event, often a personal or family relationship problem, prior to the beginning of joint pain. A research report in *Annals of Behavioral Medicine* concluded that increases in the number of interpersonal stressors in the same week and one week prior were associated with increases in pain and joint tenderness. Another study, in the *Journal of Personality and Social Psychology*, found that individuals reporting major life stressors showed greater next-day pain and that those with less social support showed more next-day mood disturbance.

Lack of social support (from family and others) and a recent history of major life stressors also was correlated with inflammatory disease in a study in the *Journal of Personality and Social Psychology*. In another study, in the *Annals of Behavioral Medicine*, interpersonal stress was associated with increases in disease activity among rheumatoid arthritis patients.

Strong negative feelings have been correlated with arthritis and osteoarthritis in other studies. Depression especially is related to elevations in pain for people with rheumatoid arthritis and osteoarthritis, according to research reported in *Psychosomatic Medicine*. Helplessness and depression also were significantly related to joint counts in rheumatoid arthritis in a study in *Arthritis Care Research*. Even in juvenile arthritis, negative mood and stressful events significantly predicted increased reports of fatigue, stiffness, and cutting back on daily activities, according to research in *Arthritis Care Research*.

A related explanation is a metaphysical one. The theory is that feeling unloved and full of criticism and resentment leads to arthritis. It contends that thoughts held and words repeatedly used create our lives and experiences. If you change your thoughts, you can change the way you view your experience and eventually your experience itself.

In a large study of thirteen hundred elderly white middle-class study participants, arthritis was correlated for women with earlier sexual abuse. The study was reported in *Psychosomatic Medicine*.

Nutritional factors also may play into whether arthritis develops. Research in *Clinical and Experimental Rheumatology* found that children suffering from juvenile arthritis had reduced serum levels or beta-carotene, retinol, and zinc compared with healthy children. Another study, in *Epidemiology*, found that low selenium and vitamin E levels may be risk factors for rheumatoid arthritis. Even meat was implicated, in a study in the *British Journal of Nutrition*. The studymakers suggested that the fat, iron, and nitrite in meat probably contribute to inflammation.

Arthritis is rare in poorer countries, where fresh fruits, vegetables, whole grains, and legumes are staples. Research supports the connection between diet and arthritis, which for years was considered quackery. The Arthritis Foundation now considers a healthy diet an important factor.

Psoriatic arthritis is associated with an accumulation of arachidonic acid, a proinflammatory fatty acid. If you eat animal flesh, eggs, and/or milk, or certain oils, including corn, safflower, and sunflower, you may be inflaming your psoriasis.

Your Risk for Developing Arthritis

Risk factors for *osteoarthritis* include being overweight (it stresses the workload your joints must bear), injury, smoking, and repeated overuse of certain joints.

How the Doctor Diagnoses Arthritis

Your doctor will diagnose arthritis based on your medical history and physical examination, and may order some other tests and X rays.

What the Doctor Will Probably Prescribe

According to the Arthritis Foundation, a good treatment program includes medication, physical and/or occupational therapy, and weight control.

If you're in pain, your doctor will probably prescribe an NSAID (non-steroidal anti-inflammatory drug). Although many are available over-the-counter without a prescription, be careful—their side effects range from discomfort to deadly. The most common side effect is bleeding in the stomach and intestines, and can be caused by something as seemingly innocuous as aspirin and ibuprofen-type drugs. Nearly fifty thousand people are hospitalized from taking too many NSAIDs a year, and some 6,000 die from complications directly related to taking NSAIDs. Almost 90 percent of patients admitted for stomach or intestinal bleeding had consumed NSAIDs in one study reported in the *Journal of Clinical Gastroenterology*. Older adults in long-term care are at particular risk for hospitalization due to stomach or intestinal complications, according to a study reported in the *Journal of the American Geriatric Society*. Never combine aspirin or ibuprofen-type medications with alcohol, or you will be four times as apt to develop bleeding in your stomach or intestines.

Acetaminophen (Tylenol) is advertised as a safe alternative to NSAIDs, but it can damage your liver and kidneys. Thousands of people incur damage to their liver and kidneys from taking acetaminophen, according to *Nordic Medicine*. Children are especially at risk when their parents given them liquid acetaminophen at the least sign of discomfort.

Aspirin, ibuprofen (Motrin, Advil, Midol IB, Bayer Select Pain Relief, Nuprin, IBU), and acetaminophen are useful for short-term, one- or two-day use, but should never be taken for more than a few days a month. Collagen is the glue that holds your tissues together. In one study reported in the *British Journal of Pharmacology*, Aleve was found to decrease collagen deposition at wound sites. A chronic pain relief program should be building the collagen you need between your body tissues, not destroying it.

The European Agency for the Evaluation of Medicinal Products (EMEA) reported recently that twenty-eight people in North America and Europe developed tuberculosis soon after they were given the anti-inflammatory drug Remicade (infliximab). Remicade is used to treat rheumatoid arthritis. The EMEA recommended that Remicade treatment should be stopped if active TB is suspected.

If you have rheumatoid arthritis and your doctor prescribes *prednisone*, you may want to get a second opinion from another physician. Findings presented at the 2000 annual meeting of the American College of Chest Physicians warned that even at very low doses daily use of this commonly prescribed oral steroid can double your risk of hip fractures and cataracts.

Self-Care Measures You Can Take

If you want to get better or stay healthy, follow at least one of the self-care actions that follow. The more you change your lifestyle to a wellness regime, the healthier you will be.

Change Your Eating Patterns

- If you want to feel better, you may need to lose weight so your joints aren't stressed. To reduce pain, focus your meals around whole grains, fresh vegetables, and fruits, and on reducing the amount of sugar, refined carbohydrates (doughnuts, muffins, cakes, pies, candy, potato chips) and saturated fats (meat, hard cheese, ice cream, and other dairy products unless they are nonfat) you eat. A study reported in *Osteoarthritis Cartilage* found that soy and avocado also may help reduce pain, as they may rebuild cartilage.

- According to a research report in the *American Journal of Clinical Nutrition*, many people with rheumatoid arthritis can benefit from a fasting period followed by a vegetarian eating regime. For very bad symptoms, check with your healthcare practitioner first, and if you get the okay, try a vegetable/fruit juice fast for three or four days, using no nightshade foods or substances (tomatoes, potatoes, eggplant, peppers, paprika, strawberries, mushrooms, cayenne, and tobacco). Fasting followed by a vegetarian diet has been used in several research studies reported in the *Scandinavian Journal of Rheumatology*, and showed a significant long-term effect. You will need a juicer to do this, so if you don't have one, buy it at a local health food store. Use fresh, and if possible, organic vegetables and fruits. Cut the tops and bottoms off carrots and beets before you juice them.

- Have several glasses of one or more of the following to help heal your joints. Space them through the day, leaving at least an hour, preferably two hours, between each combination. Because all fiber is removed from the vegetables and fruits, they are easy to digest. Sip the juices slowly and enjoy their fresh taste: (a) celery juice, (b) 10 ounces of carrot and 2 ounces of celery combined, (c) 5 or 6 large carrots or enough to make 10 ounces of juice intermixed with juiced pieces of ½ fresh beets and 1 medium-size cucumber (take the skin off the cucumber if it's been waxed). Drink 2 glasses of fresh grapefruit juice daily in the morning.

- Even if you don't want to turn into a vegetarian, you may want to eat more fish, especially herring, salmon, and tuna. Adding fish oils to your diet can reduce pain and stiffness, according to studies reported in *Epidemiology* and the *Scandinavian Journal of Rheumatology*.

- You also may want to avoid foods from the nightshade family for a month. If you get no relief, reintroduce each one slowly to see if they affect your symptoms. Keep a food/symptom diary, writing down your reaction half an hour after you eat one of the nightshade family foods. See if you can spot a pattern.

- If you have rheumatoid arthritis, you also may be sensitive to wheat, corn, milk/dairy products, and beef. Use a food-symptom diary to find out and eliminate the foods that create or increase symptoms. You also may have low levels of vitamin B_6, according to a study by Tufts University researchers. They found among rheumatoid arthritis sufferers reports of pain, swelling, and stiffness correlated with low levels of the vitamin. Foods that contain this vitamin include sunflower seeds, toasted wheat germ, brown rice, soybeans, white beans, liver, chicken, mackerel, salmon, tuna, bananas, walnuts, peanuts, sweet potatoes, and cooked cabbage.

- Make sure you eat enough foods containing copper, because a deficiency of the mineral can exacerbate arthritic symptoms. Foods rich in copper are almonds, avocados, barley, beans, dandelion greens, and lentils.

- Pantothenic acid, a B vitamin, also can reduce arthritis symptoms. Foods rich in this vitamin include soy flour, sunflower seeds, dark buckwheat, sesame seeds, brewer's yeast, peanuts, lobster, wheat bran, broccoli, mushrooms, eggs, oysters, sweet potatoes, and cauliflower.

- Avoid the artificial sweetener Aspartame, found in many bottled or canned drinks and foods. It may make your arthritis worse.

- Eat as many "living foods" or uncooked fruits and vegetables as you can for the rest of your life. An uncooked vegan diet of fruits, berries, vegetables, and roots (carrots, beets, etc.), nuts, germinated seeds, and sprouts provides a rich source of carotenoids (vitamin A precursor), and vitamins C and E, all capable of reducing your arthritis symptoms, according to a recent report in *Toxicology*. Bioflavonoid-rich fruits (blueberries, cherries, and blackberries) also may help. Bioflavonoids bind and strengthen collagen structures needed to keep your connective tissue healthy. They inhibit inflammation by inhibiting the enzymes that destroy your collagen.

- Eat half a fresh pineapple daily for one to three weeks. The bromelain in the fruit can reduce pain and swelling, but it must be fresh pineapple to work.

- Foods containing sulfur (garlic, onions, Brussels sprouts, and cabbage) regenerate and rebuild cartilage cells and can reduce inflammation and relieve pain.

- Water makes up two-thirds of your body, but you lose up to two liters of water every day through perspiration and other body excretions. That is why you must drink at least eight glasses of water every day. Other fluids are good, too, but drink plain water to get properly hydrated. When human tissue gets dry, tough, shrunken, and brittle, it needs to be softened, filled, and gently flexed to rebuild. Pain is often due to dehydration, so when you have pain, drink two glasses of water to reduce symptoms.

- Certain oils can protect against inflammatory reactions of arthritis, according to a report in the *British Journal of Nutrition*. Oils that can be beneficial include fish oil, olive oil (use for cooking and in salads), and evening primrose oil.

Take Glucosamine Sulfate or SAMe Instead of NSAIDs for Pain Relief

SAMe is a supplement to look into for pain, healing, and depression. The main components of your cartilage are chondroitin sulfate, collagen, and proteoglycans. SAMe (S-adenosylmethionine) is synthesized from the amino acid methionine and is found throughout your body. SAMe protects your chondrocytes, the cells that manufacture the main components of cartilage against wear and tear on your joints. In taking SAMe, production of proteoglycans improves, and your cartilage can be better maintained and repaired, according to studies in the *American Journal of Medicine* and the *American Journal of Bone and Joint Surgery*.

In studies reported in the *International Journal of Clinical Pharmacology and Toxicology* and the *American Journal of Medicine*, SAMe worked just as well as naproxen, ibuprofen, and indomethacin but had fewer side effects. Studies in the *American Journal of Psychiatry* and *Neuroscience and Biobehavioral Review* show that SAMe works faster and with more significant improvements than antidepressants and with fewer reported adverse effects. No studies have shown any reason not to use SAMe, as long as the normal daily dose recommended by Murray (1,200 to 1,600 mg divided in several doses for twenty-one days, then reduced to 400 mg a day) is followed.

Glucosamine sulfate reduced pain as well as NSAIDs in a study reported in *Osteoarthritis Cartilage*, and also had fewer and less damaging side effects. Talk to your physician about taking glucosamine sulfate instead of possibly dangerous NSAIDs.

Massage Aching Spots with Penetrating Oils

The skin is a living, absorbing organ, and by gently massaging your aching joints, you can provide soothing concern. Massage your body daily with castor or olive oil. If you want something more soothing, try this recipe. To an ounce of sweet almond oil, jojoba oil, or olive oil, add 10 drops of rosemary essential oil, 10 drops of eucalyptus oil, 5 drops of ginger oil, and 5 drops of peppermint oil. (You can obtain all of these from your local health food store.) Put some of the oil mixture in the palm of your hand and gently and soothingly rub the spot where you ache the most. When that spot feels better, move to another area.

Spots that may be especially sore and that can even result in spasms in the rest of the body are the muscles on and below the bony shelf at the back of the head (suboccipital muscles), so pay particular attention to that area.

Get Rid of Negative Thinking to Reduce Pain

Because strong negative feelings and thoughts can worsen, or maybe even bring on, arthritis, it is important to fill your mind with positive thoughts. This can be easier said than done, unless you have a plan to do this. One measure that can help replace negative thoughts with more positive ones is the use of affirmations. Write down one or more of the sayings below on 3 × 5 cards and put them in prominent places around your home and workplace, including mirrors, desk drawers, or where you might see it and read it. Make a specific effort to read the card at least twenty times a day and believe in its message.

- I let others be themselves, and I am free.
- I am full of love and forgiveness.
- I see others through loving eyes.
- I feel love toward myself and others.
- My joints are healing, my body is well.
- I can picture all negative thoughts and feelings flowing out of me.

Exercise Every Day to Feel Better

Exercise for twenty minutes daily. Try yoga, swimming, and/or walking. Even dance can be beneficial, as it reduces pain, depression, anxiety, fatigue, and tension, according to a study in the *American Journal of Physical and Medical Rehabilitation*. Every day rotate clockwise and counterclockwise each toe, your ankles, your knees, your hips, your waist, your shoulders, your elbows, your wrists, and each finger. Squeeze your fingers together and hold, then expand them as open as you can. Repeat several times. Do the same with your toes.

The American Chiropractic Association suggests these exercises for fingers:

- With your palm flat on a table, raise and lower your fingers one by one.
- Make an "O" by touching your thumb to each of the other fingertips, one at a time.
- Crumple a sheet of newspaper into a small ball with one hand.
- Squeeze a small rubber ball or sponge.
- Pick up coins or buttons of assorted sizes.
- Keep time to music with each finger by drumming with extended fingers.

- Resting your hand on a table, spread your fingers wide and then bring them together.

- Flip balls of paper with your fingers or flip a lightweight book or a folded newspaper off of extended fingers.

If you can't do the exercises yourself, ask a friend or family member to bend and straighten the affected fingers gently. Never force movement. Whether doing these exercises alone or with an assistant, stop if any movement causes severe pain or if soreness persists for more than twenty minutes, and consult your doctor promptly.

Other exercises you can do to stretch and enhance comfort include:

- Sit in a chair and press your buttocks together. This will strengthen the muscles that help support your back and legs. Hold for five seconds, relax, and repeat. Work up gradually to twenty repetitions a day.

- Lie in bed and bend each knee to your chest. Gradually increase to ten repetitions each, then pull both knees to your chest and hold for six seconds. Repeat, increasing to ten repetitions.

- Lie on your back and move your feet and legs in the air as if you're riding a bicycle while counting to five. Relax and repeat, gradually increasing to ten repetitions a day.

- To stretch your hips, lie on your stomach in bed or on a padded floor. Raise your leg and leg and foot off the bed or floor, keeping your knee straight. Hold for five seconds. Repeat; work up to ten repetitions. Repeat with the other leg.

For more exercises, see D. Sobel and A. C. Klein, *Arthritis: What Exercises Work* (New York: St. Martin's Press, 1995).

Investigate taking hula or tai chi lessons. Both can increase flexibility, increase circulation, and reduce pain. Dancing also is helpful, according to studies reported in the *American Journal of Occupational Therapy and Arthritis Care Research*.

Find a Support Group

Find a support group that makes you feel good, and use it. Spend time with people who make you feel appreciated and loved. Stop spending time with people who don't.

Get Help If You've Been Sexually Abused

If you've been sexually abused, get help. If not, you have a two- to three-fold increased disease risk if you had multiple abuse episodes. Find a psychiatric/mental health nurse practitioner or psychologist you trust and start weekly sessions to help you resolve your feelings. It could be an important factor in preventing arthritis and/or reducing its effects.

Use Warm Packs to Relieve Pain

Soak a piece of unbleached and undyed flannel cloth in warmed castor oil and place it on noninflamed joints. Keep it on for fifteen to twenty minutes while lying down and relaxing.

Rub Common Foods on Inflamed Joints to Reduce Pain

Find an onion, some garlic, or an uncooked potato. Rub the grated onion, garlic, or potato into inflamed joints. These substances can draw out heat and reduce swelling. Experiment and see which of them works for you.

Take Steps to Relax

Soak in a warm tub or use moist heat for relief. Brush your skin all over with a body brush before taking alternate cold and warm showers. Take an afternoon nap to relax your body. Try acupuncture, acupressure, therapeutic touch, or massage to relax your body and help it use its own internal healing mechanism. A study reported in *Journal of Family Practice* found that therapeutic touch reduced pain and improved function in patients with osteoarthritis of the knee. To find a therapeutic touch practitioner, contact the American Holistic Nurses' Association online at www.ahna.org/home/home.html (click on Resource Directory), or the Nurse Healers–Professional Associates International online at www.therapeutic-touch.org. Use the relaxation exercise on pp. 88–89 every morning and evening.

Consider Supplements

A study published in the *Journal of Rheumatology* showed that rheumatoid arthritis patients eat too much total fat and too little fish and fiber. Their diets also are deficient in pyridoxine, zinc, and magnesium. This suggests that regular supplementation with multivitamins and trace elements may be needed. A deficiency of copper may exacerbate arthritic symptoms. If your vitamin/mineral supplement has no copper in it, and you can't or won't eat foods high in this mineral, take 2 mg daily with food.

Evening primrose and borage seed oils may help. A study in the *Annals of Internal Medicine* reported that tender and swollen joints were reduced in patients taking the gammalinolenic acid dose as opposed to a group taking a placebo (sugar pill). Blackcurrant seed oil also may reduce inflammation and joint tissue injury. The study was published in the *British Journal of Rheumatology*.

If you are taking medication for arthritic pain, you may wish to combine it with either vitamin E or C. A study reported in *Arzneimittelforschung* reported that combining antioxidants or vitamin E with indometacin, sulfasalazine, and/or indometacin controlled symptoms more effectively than drugs alone. The *British Journal of Nutrition* reported that vitamin C, betacarotene, selenium, and polyunsaturated fatty acids can ameliorate the symptoms of rheumatoid arthritis and related conditions.

A vitamin supplement of 6,400 mcg of folate and 20 mcg of cobalamin worked as well as NSAID, had fewer side effects (none), and cost less. The study was reported in the *Journal of the American College of Nutrition*.

Low intake of vitamin D appears to be associated with an increased risk for progression of osteoarthritis of the knee, according to a study in the *Annals of Internal Medicine*. To enhance your intake of this vitamin, spend at least twenty minutes in the sunshine every day, eat fish, take cod liver oil, or eat vitamin D-enriched foods.

Drink green tea. It is rich in antioxidants that offset arthritis symptoms, according to a study reported in the *Proceedings of the National Academy of Sciences*.

Use Writing to Heal Yourself

Writing about your stressful experiences can relieve arthritic symptoms, according to research reported in the *Journal of the American Medical Association*. Spend at least twenty minutes on three consecutive days writing about the most stressful events in your life to achieve benefits.

Try Yoga

A study reported in the *Journal of Rheumatology* provided evidence that a yoga program provided relief in osteoarthritis of the hands. The yoga group met for eight weeks with an instructor, while another group of patients with osteoarthritis of the hands received no yoga. The yoga group improved significantly more than the control group in pain during activity, tenderness, and finger range of motion.

Try Progressive Muscle Relaxation, Guided Imagery, and Meditative Breathing

Self-regulatory techniques such as progressive muscle relaxation, guided imagery, and meditative breathing can lead to substantial reduction of pain intensity for patients with juvenile rheumatoid arthritis (as reported in *Pediatrics*) and in adults with rheumatoid arthritis (as reported in *Health Psychology*).

You can use your mind to help heal yourself. For an example of guided imagery, picture your joints being soothed one by one, from your neck to your toes, by a cool, healing salve or liquid, or picture them healthy and relaxed. For an example of a combination of relaxation, guided imagery, and self-hypnosis you can record and use, see pp. 88–89.

Investigate Herbs

Some herbs that may help include *feverfew, lemon myrtle, aniseed myrtle, mountain pepper,* and w*ild rosella. White willow bark* is available in capsules and works as well as aspirin, but without the digestive and bleeding side effects. Consult a herbologist or healthcare practitioner with special knowledge of the use of herbs prior to trying these or any other herbs. Also, always inform your doctor or healthcare professional of any herbs or supplements you are taking or thinking about taking.

Cancer

Cancer is a many-step process, but its cause is not fully understood. We do know that it can take seven to ten alterations to convert a normal cell into a malignant one and that chemical carcinogens, viruses, and ionizing radiation may be involved, which may be why many cancers take up to twenty years or more to fully develop. Each of these cancer-initiating factors has the ability to damage your genetic material, or DNA, and can lead to cancer when free radicals are present and their damage is not repaired.

Your body maintains a variety of antioxidants to defend against free radical damage, but because the body is continually being bombarded by these unstable molecules, what you eat is very important. Your body must have vitamins, flavonoids, and other compounds found in fresh fruits and vegetables to fight off the damaging effects of these free radicals. Epidemiological studies continue to find that people who consume inadequate amounts of these foods are at a higher risk for cancer, heart disease, and other degenerative diseases such as arthritis.

Cancer is an unpredictable process. Some tumors are extremely fast-growing, while most are slow-growing, and your immune system is most effective against small tumors.

Remember that not all lumps or cysts will turn into cancer and that the rate of actual deaths from cancer has not changed since 1935. What has increased is the risk of having cancer diagnosed (but not the likelihood of dying from it).

There are two theories of cancer causation, surveillance theory and decreased inflammatory reaction theory, that bear mentioning. *Surveillance theory* suggests that everyone has cancer at some time in their lives, but that their immune system conducts "surveillance," finds the tumor cells, and eliminates them. Most people have strong enough immune systems to recover and not even know they had it. In this theory, tumors appears to be life-saving mechanisms, as toxins and poisons are walled off by the body when it is unable to eject the material from the body. Evidence backs up this theory. When autopsies are done randomly, a high percentage of cancerous tumors have been found, though no clear diagnosis was made while the individuals were alive, and the death occurred due to an altogether different and unrelated cause.

Goldberg's *decreased inflammatory reaction theory* posits that cancer patients have had an early loss of their mothers, either through death, separation, or emotional distance. This is experienced as overwhelmingly traumatic. As a result, resignation, despair, depression, giving up, grief, hopelessness, and helplessness develop. Chronic negative feelings have been shown to inhibit the immune system and can lead to an inhibition of the inflammatory response throughout life, and cancer is just another example.

This could mean that the first available line of defense against any intruder, an inflammatory response, is inadequate. Fever is the body's own chemotherapy; it burns out toxic materials. Proponents of this theory point to the fact that cancer patients may not have had the common childhood fevers (associated with measles, mumps, etc.) and may instead tend to "wall off" intruders and then to regenerate or proliferate cells, leading to metastasis. These are both thought to be more primitive responses to attack, indicating their immune system may not be operating to its full capacity. These individuals also show a very low tendency to anger, infections, or allergic responses, providing further evidence for the theory.

A related explanation is a metaphysical one. It appears in Louise Hay's *Heal Your Body*. The theory is that having a deep secret, grief, and long-standing hurts lead to cancer. It contends that the thoughts that are held and the words that are repeatedly used create our lives and experiences. If you change your thoughts, you can change the way you view your experience, and eventually your experience.

It is at the level of hormones that the mind and the body meet. Hormones can be thought of as physical representations of our emotions. A change in feeling leads to a change in hormone release. The process by which excess hormones result in cancer cell changes was discovered by Otto Warburg, for which he won a Nobel Prize. He found that a cancer cell is an oxygen-deficient cell. Stressors that could interfere with normal cell respiratory process are radiation and chemicals. Of the chemicals, the hormones produced by one's own body are most often the culprits that cause irreversible damage. Warburg concluded that the destruction of cell capacity is the result of small, repeated doses of stress. The stress that leads to cancer is the continuous application of noxious substances rather than a sudden, infrequent, explosive attack.

Your Risk for Developing Cancer

Each type of cancer has different risks. Read about the differences in this section.

Breast Cancer

If you are a woman, your risk for developing breast cancer is 10 percent, while your risk for dying from breast cancer is a little over 3.5 percent. Most of this risk occurs after you turn seventy-five. Studies cannot confirm that a family history has any effect on whether you develop cancer. You're at the highest risk for developing breast cancer if you've already developed it in the other breast. The risk of developing breast cancer following a mastectomy is 0.5 percent to 1 percent a year after surgery.

Other risk factors for developing breast cancer are starting to menstruate at an early age; late first pregnancy (after age thirty); bottle-feeding infants; late menopause; obesity after menopause; prolonged use (more than four years) of birth control pills; postmenopausal estrogen replacement therapy; radiation exposure before age thirty (including X rays, mammograms, air travel, and electronmagnetic exposure to home appliances, office equipment, and outside electric power lines); exposure to organochlorine compounds (p-chlorophenyl, ethylene, or DDE, hexachlorobenzene or HCB, mirex, and several polychlorinated biphenyls or PCBs); high calorie consumption; environmental and occupational exposures to chemical and ionizing radiation; alcohol consumption; and insulin resistance (due to overconsumption of refined carbohydrates such as breads, pastas, and sugary foods; saturated fat such as in beef, butter, cheeses, and chicken skin; and omega-6 fatty acids found in polyunsaturated vegetable oils). There is some evidence that constrictive clothing may be related to breast cancer (due to the restriction of lymph processes in the breast that filter out toxins). A study in *American Journal of Epidemiology* showed that lack of physical activity also is linked with an increased risk for breast cancer, as are high waist-to-hip ratios and high total caloric intake.

Colorectal Cancer

Risks for colorectal cancer include eating meat, dairy products (except low-fat yogurt), refined sugar-containing foods or white flour products, a diet low in fruits and vegetables, smoking, drinking alcohol, and consuming chlorinated drinking water.

Gliomas (Brain Tumors)

Nine of ten nervous system cancers occur in or around the brain. Most tumors develop from glial cells. *Glioma* is a general term that includes any tumor arising from glial cells.

Most brain tumors are probably due to environmental exposures to physical, chemical, or biological agents. These exposures include electromagnetic fields, smoking, alcohol, certain medications, cosmetics, and lotions as well as working in certain jobs (manufacture of synthetic rubber and exposure to polyvinyl chloride, refining of crude oil and production of petroleum-based chemicals, manufacture of nuclear fuels and weapons, farm work exposures to pesticides and other chemicals) and those in certain professional groups (embalmers, anatomists, pathologists, chemists, and professional artists). Some studies have linked elevated brain tumor risk with exposure to farm animals and pets among adults and children, raising the possibility that a virus may be involved. Severe head trauma and loud noise also have been implicated.

Hodgkin's Disease and Non-Hodgkin's Lymphomas

Hodgkin's disease is a form of cancer involving the lymphatic system. When abnormal lymphocytes (white blood cells) congregate in the lymph glands, they produce solid masses or lymphomas.

Two viruses have been linked most specifically to Hodgkin's disease:

Epstein-Barr virus (EBV) and herpesvirus-6 (HHV-6). Being a wood-worker or being exposed to phenoxyacetic herbicides may increase your risk.

Viruses have been linked to non-Hodgkin's lymphomas also, including EBV. Pesticides have been associated with non-Hodgkin's lymphomas in farmers, other pesticide applicators, manufacturing workers, and those applying commercial pesticide lawn treatments. Grain handlers have a fivefold risk of non-Hodgkin's lymphomas. Those in other occupations that increase risk include rubber workers, petroleum refining workers, vinyl chloride workers, dry cleaners, and aircraft maintenance workers.

Leukemias

Leukemias form in the blood and bone marrow, and the abnormal white blood cells produced there travel through the bloodstream, creating problems in the spleen and other tissues.

A 50-percent increase in childhood leukemia has been associated with pregnancy-related diagnostic X-ray exposure. Radiotherapy treatments have been associated with leukemia among patients with ankylosing spondylitis, women with cervical and uterine cancer, heavy menstrual bleeding, breast cancer, and Hodgkin's disease. Children receiving radiation treatment for fungal infection of the scalp or for large thymuses in infancy have an elevated risk. Childhood leukemia has been weakly linked with residential exposure to magnetic fields, and more strongly associated to environmental pesticide exposures after birth.

Electricians, power line workers, and electronics and other workers exposed to nonionizing electrical and magnetic fields may have an elevated risk, as may benzene-exposed shoe, leather, rubber, and chemical manufacturing workers. Rubber manufacturing, petroleum refinery, and chemical plant workers, and some pressmen and printers, painters, and those in various other occupational groups may have an increased risk. Farmers exposed to viruses in poultry and dairy cows, pesticides, and other agrichemicals may be at greater risk. Smoking also may increase the risk for leukemia.

Liver Cancer

Risks for developing liver cancer include cirrhosis or chronic liver injury due to alcohol abuse, chronic hepatitis, prolonged obstruction of the outflow of bile from the liver, some viral forms of autoimmune liver disease, and hemochromatosis (a disorder of iron metabolism that results in an excessive accumulation of iron in the body). Exposure to some chemicals and toxins can lead to cancer; the most extensively studied is *aflatoxin*, produced by a common mold that infests poorly stored peanuts and other foods.

Lung Cancer

According to the National Cancer Institute, lung cancer is second only to melanoma in rate of increase (263 percent) since the 1950s. This is due primarily to the effects of smoking cigarettes, especially by women.

Secondhand smoke has been implicated as a risk factor for lung cancer. Radon, an inert gas produced by the radioactive decay of radium and uranium, may cause lung cancer, as can exposure to airborne asbestos. The risk for developing some forms of lung cancer is substantially higher for workers in asbestos industries, including miners and millers, and for textile, insulation, shipyard, and cement workers.

Lung cancer also is one of the major effects of high doses of ionizing radiation from therapy. Exposure to mustard gas, chloromethyl ethers, chromium, nickel, and inorganic arsenic also increases risk.

Air pollution has been suspected as a cause of lung cancer, but it has been difficult to establish definite links. Of special concern are the effects of the by-products of the combustion of fossil fuels, especially hydrocarbons, and indoor air pollutants from the use of coal for heating and cooking.

Melanoma

According to the National Cancer Institute, melanoma, or skin cancer, has increased in incidence by 321 percent since the 1950s. Major contributing factors are increased exposure to the sun and use of artificial tanning devices.

Stomach Cancer

Since the 1950s, the incidence of stomach cancer has declined by 73 percent. The reasons for this may be due to increased access to refrigeration, decreased use of salt, and the addition of vitamin C to nitrite-containing food products such as hot dogs and processed meats.

How the Doctor Diagnoses Cancer

The doctor will use a number of tests to determine if you have cancer. Not all practitioners agree on the best way to diagnose cancer.

Mammograms for Breast Cancer

The early research on mammography reported a 30 percent reduction in death from breast cancer in women over fifty years of age. This led to strong professional and public demand for mammography screening. Subsequent research, which was not publicized, showed no significant benefit in any age group, and did not mention the possible harm and costs associated with the procedure. For example, about 5 percent of mammograms are positive or suspicious. Of these, 80 to 93 percent are *false positives* (show positive results when there actually is no disease). A study in the *New England Journal of Medicine* concluded that these false positive reactions cause unnecessary anxiety and further procedures including surgery, with follow-up biopsies indicating no cancer.

There are at least three potentially harmful consequences of having mammograms: radiation exposure, false positives, and overdiagnosis. Since the benefit achieved is marginal, the harm caused is substantial, and the costs are enormous, it has been suggested that public funding for breast cancer screening not continue.

It may even be that mammograms spread an existing mass of cancer cells! During the procedure, considerable pressure is placed on the breast while it is firmly squeezed between two flat surfaces. In a study of 110 women with an average age of thirty-nine, rupture of *in situ* cysts in the breast spread cancer cells into surrounding tissue. Since mammographic screening was introduced in 1983, the incidence of a form of breast cancer called ductal carcinoma *in situ* (DCIS), representing 12 percent of all breast cancer cases, has increased by 328 percent, and 200 percent of this increase may be due to the use of mammography (Spratt et al. 1986; Spratt et al. 1993; Wright and Mueller 1995). *If you do have a mammogram, be sure to request reduced compression if there is undue pain or intensity.*

Because there is no safe level of ionizing radiation, it is not clear if the benefits of mammograms outweigh the radiation-related risks (Wright and Mueller 1995). Also, at least one study found that the PET scan is the only noninvasive procedure that will detect tumors in the breast with high sensitivity, specificity, and accuracy.

If you do have a mammogram, try to remain calm if you receive a callback for another mammogram. Remember that 90 percent of these callbacks are because the first readings were not clear due to the density of female breast tissue. Even if a biopsy reveals a tumor, that doesn't mean you have cancer. It could be benign. Try not to overreact and respond to internal and external pressures to have immediate surgery and radiation. Increasingly, women are developing slow-growing breast tumors. A second opinion is always helpful, and don't forget to take a calm and supportive significant other with you when you go to see the physician. Writing down your questions in advance and reading them off also will help you stay calm and focused.

Antimalignin Antibody Screen Test

There is an accurate blood test for early cancer detection. It was unveiled in 1990 by Sam Bogoch, M.D., Ph.D., and is known as the *antimalignin antibody screen (AMAS)* test. It analyzes a small sample of blood to reveal whether antibodies to cancer are present. The test was approved by the Federal Drug Administration in 1977, but it wasn't until 1994 that clinical trials with 4,278 patients validated the procedure. The AMAS test is 95 percent accurate on the first test and 99 percent accurate when repeated. It can detect cancer up to nineteen months before other medical tests can. It also can monitor the degree of remission following treatment, so it provides an effective way to measure the effects of medical and complementary procedures. The AMAS test is more accurate than and costs a fraction of the cost and inconvenience of standard tests for cancer. It will not work if you're in end-stage cancer or if you have undergone extensive high-dose radiation and/or high-dose chemotherapy. In these conditions, you cannot produce enough antimalignin antibody to score a positive on the test. In these cases, cancer markers, biopsies, and various scans are suggested. Ultrasound also may be helpful, and unlike X rays or mammograms, no harmful radiation is used to possibly seed cancer or further its progression. Even ultrasound cannot pick up tiny tumors; only AMAS can do that.

This test is especially valuable for the early detection of breast cancer. Even if a tiny tumor is found in your milk ducts, ask for an AMAS, which can detect ductal carcinoma *in situ.* Mammography cannot detect this type of cancer, nor can it detect whether a tumor is malignant. The AMAS test can help you avoid unnecessary anxiety and unnecessary medical intervention.

Another test was developed by a nurse researcher, Dr. Chandice Covington, at Wayne State University's College of Nursing in Detroit. She found that by analyzing breast fluids, risk factors for breast cancer can be identified. Since 90 percent of all breast cancers begin in the breast ducts where the fluids reside, it has been known for some time that dietary and environmental substances are present in breast fluids. A plastic syringe and a specially developed suction cup are used to extract a minute amount of fluid that can be tested for cancer risk. It is not a painful procedure, like so many breast fluid collection methods. Removing breast fluid in this way mimics the process that occurs during breast feeding, cleansing the breast ducts of cancer-causing substances. The procedure is being tested and probably will be available in individual doctors' offices soon. This approach can significantly increase the chances for early detection and treatment of the disease. Very soon, Dr. Covington's *breast fluid aspirating device* may be available to be used at home regularly to decrease the level of cancer-causing chemicals.

Breast Self-Exams for Breast Cancer

Although the jury is still out, two trials have indicated that breast self-examination has no impact on surviving breast cancer. This is probably because breast tissue is so dense that it is difficult to detect small tumors. With practice, detection can be enhanced, so it is still a good idea to do a regular breast self-exam.

Look for anything unusual, including swelling, breast enlargement, dimpling, and skin or nipple changes. Remember that the majority of breast lumps are benign, not malignant. By avoiding caffeinated beverages and chocolate, the size of any benign breast lumps will be reduced and your self-exams will be more reliable.

HOW TO EXAMINE YOUR BREASTS

Do the exam first while lying on the bed, and do it again while in the shower. Both kinds of examination are important to be able to feel all of the breast tissue. When lying down, place your other arm above the head so your breast tissue is flattened against your chest wall. Firmly press the breast tissue against the chest wall with the fingers of your other hand. Use circular patterns, moving from the outer edges of the breast toward the nipple. Palpate gently at first, then go deeper. Examine the entire surface of both breasts, covering the area up to the collarbone and over to the shoulder and around the armpit. The best time to examine your breasts is five to seven days after you begin menstruating or shortly after your period ends, when the breast tissue is least likely to be swollen. If you are no longer menstruating and have completed menopause, choose a specific day of the month and make sure you do your exam at the same time each month. Even if you've had a mastectomy or a lumpectomy, it's important to examine the incision for nodules or skin changes. Learn to know your body and the way it looks and feels.

PSA Test for Prostate Cancer

PSA is an abbreviation for prostate-specific antigen. It is a protein secreted by the cells of the prostate gland. Elevated levels of this protein may be related to prostate cancer. Since small amounts of PSA leak into the bloodstream, doctors are able to use this blood test to measure the levels of PSA. If high PSA levels are found, doctors become suspicious that prostate cancer could be present.

Thirty percent of men age fifty or older have prostate cancer, but only 3 percent die from it. This means that most of the prostate cancers are latent and will never need surgery or any other treatment. The PSA test cannot detect cancer until it has been growing for ten years, which is about the same time that the physician can detect it through a digital rectal exam. If your doctor suggests the PSA test, you might want to ask the following questions: (1) Has the test been shown to save lives? (2) What are the long-range positive and negative consequences of taking the test? (3) What are the odds that the PSA test might find the latent kind of cancer that would never cause any harm? (4) Are there any proven methods of curing advanced prostate cancer that you know of?

Hemoccult Test for Colorectal Cancer

Colorectal cancer is the second most common cancer in the United States. If your doctor requests a sample of feces, a small amount is applied to a card imprinted with a solution of guaiac, a plant gum. In the laboratory, the presence of blood in the feces is indicated by a color change (usually to blue) on the card. The results are used to indicate if you have colorectal cancer.

The test can yield a false positive result if you've recently eaten fruits or vegetables, red meat, or taken certain quantities of iron tablets, aspirin, nonsteroidal inflammatory drugs (Tylenol, Advil, Midol, Nuprin, ibuprofen), or vitamin C, so avoid ingesting these substances for the amount of time as directed on the card before taking the test.

Tests for Lung Cancer

Testing procedures for lung cancer include a medical history and physical, a chest X ray, and a CT scan.

Tests for Lymphomas

Testing procedures include a medical history and physical, a chest X ray, and an abdominal CT scan.

Tests for Stomach and Intestinal Cancer

Testing procedures include a chest X ray, a CT scan, a barium swallow, and possibly a liver scan.

Tests for Cervical Cancer

The major screening tool is the Pap smear. The American Cancer Society recommends a Pap smear for women every three years between ages twenty and sixty-five.

Energy Diagnosis

The realm of energy is at the forefront of the alternative approach to cancer diagnosis. In this approach, subtle levels of bodily functioning are assessed. Many of the most sophisticated diagnostic systems use the principles of energy medicine, including electrocardiogram, electroencephalogram, and MRI (magnetic resonance imaging that pictures internal organs). Energy medicine employs diagnostic procedures and therapies that use an energy field—electrical, magnetic, sonic, acoustic, microwave, or infrared—to screen for health conditions, including cancer.

Most energy medicine devices are based on the acupuncture meridians that run through the body in energy channels or pathways. Therapeutic touch, acupuncture, acupressure, reflexology, and a host of other energy therapies are based on this energy field theory.

It is believed that the detection of energy imbalances in the body provides an early warning system for potential disruptions in biochemical balance and functioning. *Electrodermal screening (EDS)* is a diagnostic system that can allow you to see disease coming *before* it manifests. EDS also can provide proof that therapies are working and that no further traces of illness remain, since energy changes precede physical ones.

Research has established that ion flow and concentration are major factors in skin conductance. Organ inflammation (indicated by a reading above 55) increases ion concentrations and electron flow, leading to a drop in resistance and a rise in conductance. Organ degeneration (indicated by a reading lower than 45) decreases ion concentration, leading to a rise in resistance and a drop in conductance. Your reading on an EDS can help your doctor tell if you are at the very beginning of a cancerous process or if you are healing from one. EDS probably will be available to you only if your doctor practices alternative medicine.

What the Doctor Will Probably Prescribe

Basic treatments include radiation, chemotherapy and surgery. All have their risks and uses.

Radiation Therapy

Radiation is used before or after surgery to stop any cancer cells from dividing and reproducing. Unfortunately, it also may kill healthy cells, including portions of your immune system that protect you from cancer and other invasions.

Some types of radiation therapy have been associated with an increased risk of dying from heart attack. Use of radiation may be especially troublesome if you are taking hormones, including estrogens or progestin, because they promote tumors.

If you have radiation treatments, some symptoms you may experience include fatigue, a change in your skin so it looks sunburned or swollen, and soreness in the chest area either during the treatment or afterward. Measures you can take to offset these symptoms include eating a well-balanced diet and plenty of liquids (to help rebuild tissue damaged by radiation), and protecting the affected areas from tight clothing, heat, sunlight, and any irritation (avoid perfumed soaps and colognes, heat lamps, hot water bottles, and deodorants or talcum powder anywhere near the site of treatment). If your skin does get red, itchy, or flaky, try applying a light dusting of cornstarch or apply unscented olive oil or castor oil.

Chemotherapy

Chemotherapy is a drug treatment used to destroy cancer cells that may have spread from the original tumor. The drug circulates throughout the body, reaching these undetected cells and killing them.

Chemotherapy is not effective for all cancers or in all situations. For example, thyroid cancers do not respond well, according to a study reported in *Thyroid*. Some combinations of chemotherapy drugs (e.g., FEMTX regimen) lead to severe blood toxicities and toxic death, according to a study evaluating this combination in *Anticancer Research*. Other chemotherapy combinations cause secondary leukemias and death, according to reports of research in *Cancer Research* and *Clinical Oncology*. A report in the *British Journal of Haematology* found that other failures of chemotherapy approaches occur due to high doses of cytarabine chemotherapy. Other chemotherapy agents result in toxicity and progressive breast cancer disease, according to a report in the *British Journal of Cancer*.

Often, more than one drug is used because cells divide at different times and because different drugs are effective at different points. Chemotherapy is used after surgery and may be given in your doctor's office. Because chemotherapy lowers white blood cell counts and immunity to infection, a white blood cell count is taken before a treatment is given. If your count is too low, no treatment will be given that day. Chemotherapy can be given as a pill, or as an injection in your vein or into a port that is inserted into one of your major blood vessels. Since chemotherapy suppresses your immune system, it is given in three-week or four-week cycles to give your bone marrow a chance to recoup. Because chemotherapy suppresses your immune system, it may be hard for you to fight off illness or metastasis during this time.

New chemotherapy drugs are being discovered all the time, but in general, side effects of chemotherapy include fatigue, hair loss, nausea, loss of appetite, vomiting, mouth sores, skin burn, heart problems, hot flashes, breast tenderness, numbness and tingly feelings, vaginal dryness, cessation of menstruation, and suppression of your immune system that can lead to other cancers. Food also may taste different, due to the interaction of chemotherapy drugs and what you eat.

What can you do to cope with the side effects of chemotherapy if you do agree to undertake the treatment? Some things you can do include: Eat a nutritious well-balanced diet with at least five vegetables and fruits a day to strengthen your immune system, help maintain your current weight, combat fatigue, and minimize any digestive problems. Make nutritious drinks with protein powder and fruit juice or yogurt, bananas (or other fresh fruits), or powdered carob to provide many needed nutrients in a palatable form.

Buy a wig or cut your hair short prior to treatment. Attend a support group with others who are using chemotherapy. Regular attendance can lessen feelings of isolation, provide an outlet for feelings, and provide helpful information.

Like your immune system, chemotherapy is most effective against small tumors because cancer cells have not yet limited blood circulation within the tumor. It is also effective for childhood leukemias, Hodgkin's disease, lymphoma, ovarian cancer, testicular cancer, and a few other, more rare, cancers. Because chemotherapy is not a panacea, you may wish to explore natural agents.

Even when taking chemotherapy, you also can talk to your doctor about complementary treatments you may wish to use and why. Be sure to ask whether any of them could interfere with your medical treatment and just which kind of cancers the suggested chemotherapy works best with. Also ask how carcinogenic the chemotherapy drug is, and if it increases the risk of secondary tumors by suppressing your immune system.

Surgery

Whenever your physician suggests surgery, it is wise to obtain a second opinion. Find another doctor who is not affiliated with or recommended by your physician, and take your time. Take a supportive family member or a friend with you, and write down all your questions. Make sure you get them all answered. Ask the family member or friend to help you ask all your questions, and persevere until they're all answered. You have a right to complete information prior to deciding about treatment.

Remember, cancers usually take years to develop, so taking a few days to decide could be a wise investment. (It takes about a hundred days, more than three months, for the average solid tumor cell to double and become two cells.)

Although hearing that you may have cancer is frightening, remember that it is your body and your decision. Be sure to obtain all the necessary information you need to make a thoughtful decision, including what the side effects of surgery may be. For example, prostate surgery can cause impotence and urine incontinence, according to a summary of evidence in *American Family Physician*.

Think carefully before having silicon breast implants or silicon prostheses. They can cause an inflammatory state and a breakdown in your immune system so that a severe autoimmune disease such as scleroderma or lupus could be triggered, says a report in *Food and Chemical Toxicology*.

ACTIONS TO TAKE PRIOR
TO SURGERY

If you decide to have surgery, there are specific actions you can take to avoid infection, speed healing, and enhance your immune system. Be sure to take 15,000 IU of vitamin A (not beta-carotene) for several weeks before surgery and 50,000 IU for the two days before surgery, unless you're pregnant; then don't take more than 15,000 IU a day. Take 400 IU of vitamin E, an extra 1,000 to 2,000 mg of vitamin C (stop at the point of diarrhea), 200 mcg of selenium, and 15 mg extra of zinc. Drink lots of green tea to help speed wound healing. Gluta-mine (500 mg twice a day) between meals for a week before surgery and two weeks after surgery can speed healing, help detoxify your liver and kidneys, and keep your digestive system healthy.

Hormone Therapy

Hormone therapy is a treatment that is used either alone or combined with chemotherapy. The therapy is taken in pill form and usually occurs in your home. If cancerous tissue was removed during a biopsy, a test called hormone-receptor assay or estrogen-receptor assay probably was done to see if your breast tissue is sensitive to or influenced by estrogen. By lowering estrogen levels, hormone therapy is designed to slow the growth of this type of cancer. Tamoxifen (Nolvadex) is the drug most often used in hormone therapy. The most common side effects are hot flashes, nausea, vomiting, depression, vision problems, weight gain, inflammation of the veins, blood clots in the lungs, and vaginal discharge or dryness.

Tamoxifen therapy for breast cancer also can increase the risk of breast cancer in the other breast, according to the *Journal of the National Cancer Institute*. Recent studies (reported in *Prescrire International*) have shown that taking Tamoxifen for the prevention of breast cancer is too risky because it increases the risk of cancer of the uterus and of clots in the lungs and deep veins.

Your doctor may prescribe Megace to stop hot flashes, and various antinausea medication to lessen nausea and vomiting. To reduce weight gain, limit your salt intake and reduce or eliminate processed foods, which usually contain added salt.

Self-Care Measures You Can Take

There are many things you can do to prevent or treat the symptoms of cancer. Choose from the list below. *The more proactive you are in relation to your condition, the more likely you are to be successful, well, and healthy.*

If You're a Woman

• Have your first pregnancy before age thirty and breast-feed your infants to lower their risk for breast cancer.

- Limit your calories and keep your weight down; obesity, especially after menopause, is correlated with breast cancer.

- To give your lymph system every chance to filter out toxins, avoid wearing push-up bras, and never wear a bra for more than twelve hours a day. If you have red marks or indentations near the bra line, get a larger bra that does not constrict your tissues. Whenever possible, don't wear a bra, and never wear one that feels tight when you put it on.

- Sit on a soft mat, and cross your legs in front of you. Rub your hands together vigorously, feeling the heat and energy in your palms and fingers. Place your energized hands on your breasts and feel the heat entering your skin. Rub your breasts slowly in outward, circular motions. Your right hand will turn counterclockwise, and your left will massage clockwise. Rub in at least 36 circles to a maximum of 360 circles up to two times a day. This massage will increase circulation and cleansing of breast tissue (*The Complete System of Self-Healing Internal Exercises*).

- Avoid taking estrogen after you complete menopause; it increases your risk of breast cancer by 50 to 80 percent.

- Avoid taking oral contraceptives. They increase the risk of early-onset breast cancer before the age of forty-five.

- Eat lots of vegetables and fruits and take stress vitamins (vitamins B and C). Taking high levels of vitamin C and beta-carotene decreased the risk of death in women, especially those who ate a high-fat diet, according to a study in the *Journal of the National Cancer Institute*.

- Use only olive oil on salads and for cooking. A study reported in the *International Journal of Cancer* provided evidence that a high consumption of olive oil was significantly related to a lower risk of breast cancer, while eating saturated fats (meat and dairy products, fried foods, and products with cottonseed oil in them) prior to developing cancer is highly correlated with dying from the disease (*Journal of the National Cancer Institute*).

- Avoid polyunsaturated fats (fried foods, salad oils that aren't olive oil) and white wine. Both are associated with breast density, a significant risk factor for breast cancer, according to a study in *Cancer and Epidemiological Biomarkers and Prevention*. Eat plenty of omega-3 fatty acids, found in fish and fish oil. They can protect against breast cancer, according to a review in *Breast Cancer*.

- Obtain sufficient vitamin D (through food, supplements, or sunshine). This vitamin's metabolites may reduce breast cancer risk.

- Reduce exposure to magnetic fields. Avoid living or working close to power lines, or near radio, TV, or microwave transmitters (e.g., cellular phone towers) or radar units; restrict close exposure to computer screens (unless laptops), television sets, and microwave ovens; and avoid using electric blankets. (In a study of 1.1 million women published in the *American Journal of Industrial Medicine*, those who were exposed to a potential magnetic field had an increased risk of breast cancer.)

- Take coenzyme Q10, available in health food stores. A study reported in *Clinical Biochemistry* showed that women with breast cancer had lower levels of this enzyme. The researchers theorized that malignant cells may consume more coenzyme Q10, so taking this supplement may protect breast tissue.

- Avoid gaining weight, especially after menopause. Losing unneeded weight can contribute to the prevention of breast cancer, according to studies reported in the *Journal of the American Medical Association* and *Cancer Causes Control*.

- Remain physically active. It will help you lose weight and also is linked with a 30 percent risk reduction in breast cancer in postmenopausal women, according to a study in the *American Journal of Epidemiology*, and also 30 to 50 percent in younger women (*Journal of the National Cancer Institute*).

- Avoid powdering your genital area. Women who do use powder have an increased risk for ovarian cancer, researchers reported in the *International Journal of Cancer*. Using cornstarch may be okay, according to a study in the *American Journal of Obstetrics and Gynecology*.

- If you've been sexually abused, seek psychotherapy from a mental health nurse practitioner or psychologist. A study in *Psychosomatic Medicine* found that past sexual assault was associated with an increased risk of breast cancer.

If You're a Man

- Eat fish and/or take fish oil capsules. Numerous epidemiological studies and at least one study reported in *Urology* show that omega-3 fatty acids in fish oil prevent the development and progression of prostate cancer.

- Investigate herbs that can enhance prostate health: saw palmetto, pygeum, stinging nettle, zinc alanine, glycine, and glutamic acid. Before taking saw palmetto, have a PSA test, which examines the antibodies that accompany prostate cancer. Eat more tomatoes. The lycopene in tomatoes is good for the prostate. Drink more water. Dehydration is one of the greatest stresses on the prostate.

- This exercise is to strengthen and stimulate the prostate gland. Put on a loose robe and no underwear. Sit in a straight-back chair. Rub the palms of your hands together vigorously. Feel the heat and energy build. Cup your testicles with your right hand very gently and place the palm of your left hand one inch below your navel. Gently move your left hand in clockwise circles up to eighty times. Stop and rest, then rub your hands together again in a vigorous motion. Reverse hands and repeat the circular rubbing in the opposite direction up to eighty times. Concentrate only on feeling the warmth grow in your pubic area. Next, relax your hands and tighten the muscles around your anus as hard as you can, drawing them up and in, and holding them in for as long as you can, then stop and relax. Repeat. Concentrate on the feeling of a tingling sensation moving up your body. After a week of daily practice, urinate and try to stop the stream of urine entirely through anal muscle contraction. If you are successful, the exercise is working. *(The Complete System of Self-Healing)*

- Take zinc picolinate daily. Zinc regulates testosterone levels in the prostate and may prevent or suppress cancer of the prostate while surgery or radiation may not. A study in the *Journal of the American Medical Association* warned that surgery and radiation can damage the nerves leading to the penis and rectum and cause major heart and lung complications in some men who undergo these procedures.

- Eat more soy and soy products. Soy contains an antioxidant isoflavone called genistein, which may help fight prostate cancer, according to a study in the *International Journal of Epidemiology*.

- Eat more legumes (peanuts, chickpeas, black beans, kidney beans, lentils, mung beans, navy beans, peas, pinto beans, soybeans, split peas), yellow-orange vegetables, and cruciferous vegetables (broccoli, kale, cauliflower, Brussels sprouts). They can help to nourish and protect you.

If You're a Man or a Woman

- Lose weight if you are overweight, and limit your consumption of refined carbohydrates (breads, pastas, sugary foods, and candies). Eat less fat, especially saturated fat (animal food products, especially pork, red meat, and processed meats). Low-fat diets reduce estrogen production for women and testosterone production for men; these are the sex hormones that can stimulate tumor production. Toxic chemicals also collect in the fatty tissues in your body, so even if your tumor is not sex hormone–related or–stimulated, losing weight and eating low fat is a good plan.

- Change the way you eat. According to the U.S. Department of Health and Human Services, diet may affect risk for cancers of the colon and breast. As many as a third of cancer deaths are estimated to be related to diet. So:

  1. To fight free radicals and enhance your immune system, eat more fresh or frozen fruits and vegetables, fish, poultry, potatoes, green tea, olive oil, peanuts, and other legumes (baked or boiled beans), berries and seeds (especially flaxseed), and soybean products.

  2. Eat soy foods daily, such as 4 ounces of tofu or an 8-ounce glass of soy milk. Soy contains genistein, which prevents malignant angiogenesis, the development of blood vessels that promote cancer growth. Genistein also may encourage normal cell growth in some types of cancer cells. Soy and increased fiber consumption also can reduce the risk of endometrial cancer, according to the *American Journal of Epidemiology*, and ovarian and breast cancer, according to a study reported in the *Journal of Clinical Endocrinology and Metabolism*. Soybeans and peanuts also have decreased prostate, colon, breast, oral, pharyngeal, pancreatic, and stomach cancers.

  3. Choose fish (it contains omega-3 fatty acids that suppress the growth of tumor cells) over meat every time. Meat contains alpha-linolenic acid, which may increase the risk of invasive prostate cancer, according to a study by Edward Giovannuci, M.D., of Harvard Medical School, and lymphoma, according to a 1997 study reported in the *Journal of the American Medical Association*. Meat also is linked with colorectal cancer, adenocarcinoma, and ovarian and endometrial cancer. Even when eating fish, eat a

moderate amount, about the size of the palm of your hand, per meal. Too much protein just stresses your kidneys and liver.

4. Stop eating sugar. Adding sugar to coffee or tea and drinking nondiet carbonated soft drinks were associated with intestinal cancers in a study by Wu, Yu, and Mack. Sugar also is associated with biliary tract cancer and colon cancer risk. Eating highly processed foods, especially those containing a lot of sugar, is associated with breast cancer.

5. Eat more garlic. Rigg and other researchers found that garlic may protect against bladder cancer and found evidence that garlic may protect against prostate cancer. Sivam and colleagues found garlic protects against stomach cancer. If garlic is offensive to you or upsets your stomach, take Kyolic nonodor capsules, available at health food stores.

6. Citrus fruits and juices and citrus oils may protect against prostate cancer, concluded a study reported by Pienta.

7. A study reported in *Advances in Experimental and Medical Biology* found that foods containing lycopene can prevent or reduce the risk for developing cancer of the breast, cervix, colon, esophagus, mouth, pancreas, and rectum. These foods include tomatoes, watermelon, guava, apricots, and pink grapefruit. Even ketchup and tomato paste will help. Lutein, a carotenoid found in dark, leafy greens and broccoli, also protects against colon cancer.

8. Switch from corn and safflower oil (help mammary tumors grow) to olive oil, and take a fish oil supplement or eat a lot of fish to protect against breast cancer. Another oil that protects is sesame oil. A study conducted by Yo found it decreased risk of stomach cancer.

9. If you have trouble digesting your food or have undergone toxic treatments such as chemotherapy or radiation, or are taking powerful pain drugs, get a juicer and make vegetable juice, using carrot juice as a base. Be sure to wash the vegetables and cut the tops and ends off the carrots first. Such juice contains vitamins A, B, C, D, E, G, and K. It helps promote appetite and is an aid to digestion and healing. Add 1 to 2 ounces of raw spinach to the carrot juice to cleanse and regenerate body tissues. Drink several glasses of carrot or carrot and spinach juice a day. Carrot, beet, and

cucumber juice is a combination especially helpful for reducing fever and helping detoxify your body from the effects of cancer treatments or medications. Alternate the carrot juice drinks with nutritional fruit drinks. For example, make a smoothie in your blender. Combine plain yogurt with active acidophilus cultures, banana, pineapple juice, and cherries (frozen or fresh, preferably organically grown). Try a green drink several times a week: fill half a blender with fresh spinach, kale, and/or endive; add a cup of fresh parsley; fill the blender to the top with pineapple juice and add 1 to 2 teaspoons of cider vinegar; blend, and chew each mouthful carefully.

10. Use low-fat cooking methods such as steaming, broiling, or baking instead of frying, and don't eat fried foods.

11. Eat fresh pineapple or get bromelain tablets at a health food store. Bromelain can decrease metastasis of cancer cells, enhance the absorption of drugs, reduce inflammation, and reduce healing time, including that necessary for surgical wounds, according to reports in the *Journal of Cancer Research and Clinical Oncology*, the *Journal of Ethnopharmacology*, and *Alternative Medical Review*.

12. Sprinkle a little turmeric on your food. It is a spice that has strong anticarcinogenic effects for the skin, stomach, colon, small intestine, breast, and tongue, according to studies by Ren and Lien.

13. Eat yogurt with active cultures or take acidophilus; both have been shown to exhibit anti-tumor qualities by stimulating the immune system.

- Take a daily multivitamin to make sure you get enough folic acid every day. According to Harvard's long-running Nurses' Health Study, folic acid reduces the risk of colon cancer and birth defects. Additional calcium wouldn't hurt, either. Garland, Garland, and Gorham concluded that most cases of colon cancer can be prevented by taking 1,800 mg of calcium and 800 IU of vitamin D regularly. The importance of vitamin D as a prevention for breast cancer was also cited in the *British Journal of Cancer*.

- Investigate the use of natural agents that have been shown to defend against tumor cells (see *Cancer and Natural Medicine*), including marshmallow (the herb, not the candy!), turmeric, licorice (again, not the candy!), panax ginseng, psyllium seed, aloe vera gel, dang gui, astragalus, dan shen, pishen fang, shen xue tang, milk thistle, and *Echinacea purpurea*.

- Drink tea. A growing body of evidence suggests that moderate consumption of tea may protect against several forms of cancer. Green tea is good. Kombucha tea also may increase your life span, and it has potent antioxidant and immunopotentiating activities, according to a report in the *Journal of Ethnopharmacology*. Ask for it at your local health food store.

- Limit your radiation exposure as much as possible, and find alternative measures to all X rays, mammograms, frequent air travel, and electromagnetic exposure (home appliances; television screens; office equipment; and outside electric power lines, including using cellular phones or being within 1 meter of a cellular phone in the on position). Radiation is associated with an increased risk for cancer.

- Limit your exposure to environmental carcinogens: estrogens from plastics (containers, plastic wrap, etc.), herbicides, and pesticides. Use wax paper or glass containers, and natural insect repellents such as soapy water/garlic and vegetable oil (on plants to ward off insects), boric acid (either mixed with honey into a syrup and placed in anthills, or as a powder to eliminate roaches), and citronella or catnip oil (to ward off mosquitoes). Pesticides increase your risk for genetic and fetal damage, soft-tissue sarcomas, non-Hodgkin's lymphomas and Hodgkin's disease, according to studies reported in the *Journal of the American Medical Association*, *Epidemiology*, and *Environmental and Occupational Medicine*. Review the sections above for occupational and exposure risks and make an effort to avoid these situations.

- Stop using permanent or semipermanent hair dyes. Use henna, or natural coloring such as chamomile (for blond hair). Use highlighting mousses (available at health food stores), and natural coloring agents such as black tea and henna. Check out other natural products to color your hair, or keep your natural coloring. Researchers at the National Institute of Environmental Health Sciences showed that men and women who used these dyes for sixteen or more years had a 50 percent increased risk for leukemia. Another 1993 study reported that women who dyed their hair one to four times a year had a 70 percent risk for ovarian cancer. A 1992 study conducted at the National Cancer Institute and the University of Iowa revealed that 9 percent of the men diagnosed with myeloma used hair dyes. Another study, in the

International Journal of Cancer, found that women who used hair dyes had a 50 percent higher risk for developing lymphoma and an 80 percent higher risk of multiple myeloma than women who never dyed their hair.

- Avoid alcoholic drinks (a drink a day can increase breast cancer risk by 11 percent, according to Samuel S. Epstein, M.D.). Use filtered or distilled drinking water only. Exposure to chlorination by-products in drinking water is associated with increased risk of colon cancer, according to a study by Doyle and others.

- Avoid frequent air travel. In a study published in *Cancer Causes and Control*, flight attendants had significantly increased risk of cancer in general and breast cancer in particular.

- Avoid smoking and smoky places. Both are correlated with lung cancer and some other cancers. And think twice before using nicotine patches, sprays, or gum to quit smoking. Stanford University researchers have found that nicotine impairs the growth of new blood vessels and dramatically increases the number of times cells divide. The researchers found that when mice with certain types of human cancers were given nicotine, the tumors grew. Instead of using nicotine as a quit-smoking aid, find a psychologist or mental health nurse practitioner who uses behavioral methods such as hypnosis or affirmations. The nurse practitioner will probably also be able to help prevent weight gain and irritability after you stop smoking.

- Exercise regularly. It can exert a protective effect on your immune system and can enhance your body functioning and mood. It may even reduce the risk of endometrial cancer, according to a study in the *International Journal of Cancer*, and colon and breast cancer, according to a study in the *British Medical Journal*. Exercise also increases circulation (bringing nutrition to your cells and moving waste products out) and reduces stress, fatigue, anxiety, anger, fear, and depression. Be sure to check with your doctor before starting an exercise program, just in case there are specific instructions for your workouts.

  Set a regular time of day to exercise, and stick to it. In that way, it will become part of your daily activities. Start with some stretching exercises to ready your body. Find an exercise book or videotape to take you through the one that is right for your level of proficiency.

  You may want to start with walking a short distance, then build up gradually until you're walking twenty or thirty minutes a day. Slow down when you can't talk with comfort while walking. Always stop and consult an exercise specialist if you feel any pain, and be sure to report your symptoms to your doctor. Protect yourself by wearing walking sneakers and using good posture. Jogging and running put stress on your joints and may not be for you. You may want to consult a fitness coach to find the exercise that is right for you.

- Reduce your stress level. Stress encourages free radicals to form. This leads to a weakened immune system and increases your risk for at least one form of cancer, according to a *Science News* report. So:

1. If you have submerged anger and even positive feelings of joy, getting in touch with and expressing those feelings could be crucial. Pennebaker has completed the major research showing the healing power of expressing emotions by writing about them. As a start, purchase a blank journal that appeals to you and write about traumatic events or upsetting issues you've experienced. Be sure to put in all the details of what happened, how you felt, what you did, and the outcome. Research shows expressing your feelings in this way can enhance your immune system.

2. Join a support group. Be sure to provide and accept support from others undergoing the same procedures and experiences you are.

3. Discuss your thoughts and feelings about cancer with someone you trust.

4. Ask someone for help.

5. Improve your relationship with your spouse, partner, friend, or other family members. Choose one of the following, or do both:

   A. Ask the person to lunch for the express purpose of recounting every joyful time you've had together.

   B. Talk with a person who denies the seriousness of your condition. Plan and rehearse saying, "I know it's hard for you to think about my having cancer, but I need to be able to express my feelings. It would help me a lot if we could talk openly about my condition."

6. Express your feelings and thoughts more directly to your physician. If you don't understand a comment or disagree with a comment, speak up. You have a right to be heard. You are paying for a service.

7. Take an assertiveness or positive communication class, and practice what you learn.

8. Combine stress-reduction approaches.

Many relaxing and healing therapies, including relaxation, imagery, hypnosis, and deep breathing, work on the principle that if your body is relaxed, your mind is, too. The thought of cancer is scary, and treatments for the condition can be stressful. Relaxing complementary therapies can help you move through life with a calm and serene state of mind while improving the circulation to any stressed or diseased parts of your body. These are important actions because when you are relaxed, you do not resist treatment, and when your circulation is improved, nutrition and internally produced healing biochemicals flow more easily to where they're needed.

You may wish to purchase a relaxation or healing tape. Many large bookstores carry them. If you wish, devise your own script, or record the accompanying relaxation script onto an audiocassette and play it back for yourself. Also repeat the affirmations that follow them.

For relaxation therapy and imagery to work, you must find a quiet, restful spot, someplace where you will not be disturbed and can feel comfortable. If you are using a room, close the door and put a Do Not Disturb sign on it. Find a comfortable spot, and loosen your clothes. Remove shoes, glasses, and any restrictive clothes or jewelry.

RELAXATION SCRIPT

Speak slowly in a calm, monotone voice to enhance the positive effects of this script.

I am letting my body sink into the comfort and safety of this bed (chair, floor, etc.), feeling the sensations of the bed (chair, floor, etc.) against my body, breathing in comfort and relaxation, beginning to let go, to relax, to let my breathing move slowly and without effort to my center, my abdominal area, where I feel calm and serene. . . . I breathe in relaxation and comfort, as a soothing color, and breathe out whatever it's time to let go of, as another color (pause for a minute or two). . . . Each time I inhale, I am a hundred times more relaxed and comfortable than I was. It is so easy and effortless to be relaxed and comfortable . . . calm . . . serene . . . peaceful . . . (pause for a minute or two). . . . I am breathing in relaxation and comfort and breathing out whatever it is time to let go of (pause for a minute or two). . . . I am scanning my body now, looking for any areas that need more relaxation and comfort, and the next time I take a breath, I will send a wave of relaxation to them . . . (pause for three minutes). . . . I will continue to breathe in relaxation and comfort as a color and breathe out whatever it is time to let go of as a color until I am completely relaxed, knowing I am safe and relaxed, drifting or sinking, whatever feels right for me. . . . When I am ready, I will picture myself very small, small enough to go inside my ear or nose or some other way, taking a fantastic journey through the tissues of my body, maybe turning on a tiny flashlight so I can see very clearly what is going on in my tissues . . . picturing all the tissues healthy, pink, and functioning perfectly . . . continuing to breathe in relaxation and healing as a color . . . sending relaxation, healing, and health to my entire body (pause 3 to 4 minutes). . . . I am ready to come back through time and space now and return to the here and now, bringing with me everything I learned and all the healing and health-generating knowledge I've accumulated . . . knowing that I can return to this state of comfort, relaxation, and healing anytime I want to, simply by breathing in relaxation and comfort as a color and breathing out whatever it is time to let go of as another color. . . . In just a minute, this tape will end and I will either open my eyes and feel energized and healthy, ready to go about my day's activities, or I will continue to rest and fall into a peaceful sleep, whichever is right for me at this moment. . . . I will listen to this tape many times a day until I have put into action all the healing capabilities of my mind and body and have advanced to a higher level of being.

- Try healing affirmations. Affirmations are any thoughts you have or actions you take. They are based on the metaphysical theory discussed above. The more positive your thoughts and actions, the more your quality of life will be enhanced. Some affirmations you may wish to write on 3 × 5 cards and carry with you or post in important places in your home or office are:

  1. I am healing with each breath I take.
  2. It's getting easier and easier to be healthy and free.
  3. Nothing can harm me. I am safe and secure.
  4. It is okay to feel anger; I can use my anger constructively.

Carpal Tunnel Syndrome

Carpal tunnel syndrome (CTS) was almost unheard of a generation ago, but it has rapidly become the leading occupational hazard of the computer age. Any kind of repetitive action can lead to the problem. CTS includes a set of symptoms that occur when the median nerve in your wrist is compressed or damaged. This causes the tendons that connect your finger muscles to your wristbones to get irritated and inflamed. Once irritated, they swell. Within the narrow confines of the channel deep inside your wrist, the tissues press on the median nerve, and pain, tingling, and other symptoms result.

The median nerve controls your thumb muscles and also is responsible for the sensations you feel in your thumb, palm, and the first three fingers of your hand. Compression of the median nerve can occur due to swelling during pregnancy or water retention, from the pressure of bone spurs, from inflammatory arthritis (see the chapter "Arthritis" in this book), or even from tendinitis.

Most of the time, CTS is due to repetitive wrist motion and continuous rapid use of the fingers. It is a common affliction of people who earn a living using word processors or other computerized keyboards, supermarket checkout clerks, and bookkeepers. Those in other occupations linked to CTS include athletes, drivers, hair stylists, musicians, restaurant servers, writers, and assembly line workers. CTS also can be caused by steady, strong vibrations that shake the wrist for a long time, including using a jackhammer or chain saw, knitting, crocheting, playing tennis or racquetball, scrubbing or cleaning while leaning the full weight on one hand with the wrist bent backward, or hammering. Any activity during which you move your fingers or wrist in the same pattern for many hours can lead to CTS, even repeated flexing of your wrist during sleep.

Another explanation for CTS is a metaphysical one. It appears in *Heal Your Body.* The theory is that anger and frustration at life's seeming injustice lead to CTS. It contends that thoughts held and words repeatedly used create our lives and experiences. If you change your thoughts, you can change the way you view your experience, and eventually your experiences.

Women between ages twenty-nine and sixty-two are more afflicted with CTS than other segments of the population. Symptoms range from a mild numbness and a faint tingling to excruciating pain and a gradual weakening of the muscles in the thumb. To you, it may feel like "pins and needles" or like your fingers are "falling asleep."

At first you may feel this only once in a while, maybe at night or in the morning, when your circulation slows down. Symptoms get more persistent if you don't stop the action that caused the problem, and pain can spread to your forearm and even to your shoulder, although sometimes it affects only the dominant hand and then only the thumb and the first three fingers. You could damage your hand if you don't stop the repetitive movements. Fortunately, you don't have to let it advance to that stage. (See "Self-Care Measures You Can Take" in this chapter.)

Your Risk for Developing Carpal Tunnel Syndrome

If you engage in any repetitive activity that delivers a steady vibration to the wrist, you are at risk. Factors that increase the risk of CTS include pregnancy, diabetes (see the chapter "Diabetes" in this book), arthritis (see the chapter "Arthritis" in this book), thyroid problems, menopause, and Raynaud's disease. Each of these conditions can make your wrist swell more than usual, putting pressure on the median nerve. If pregnancy is behind the swelling, CTS should disappear after your baby is born and your hormone levels return to normal. Other factors that could damage nerves include toxic agents and a deficiency of B vitamins (due to alcoholism, pernicious anemia, malabsorption of nutrients, or chronic vomiting).

How the Doctor Diagnoses Carpal Tunnel Syndrome

Your doctor can tell if you have CTS by giving you an electromyographic test or EMG. The test transmits electrical impulses through your arm. Normal nerve impulses are transmitted at about 136 meters per second. If your nerves are damaged or entrapped, the speed of these impulses is slowed. If your neurotransmission rate is only 90 to 95 meters per second, your doctor will conclude that you have nerve damage or compression.

Although not foolproof, you can conduct a self-examination:

1. Hold your arms at shoulder height with your elbows bent, pointed out to the side.

2. Bend your hands so your hands point straight down and your wrists are at a ninety-degree angle.

3. With your hands in front of your chest, press the backs of your hands together and hold them there for one minute.

If you experienced tingling, numbness, or burning, chances are that you have CTS, but only your doctor can tell for sure.

What the Doctor Will Probably Prescribe

Your doctor will probably ask you to discontinue any tasks that require forceful flexing of your wrist. You may be given a cock-up splint to help relieve night pain and take pressure off the nerve. Local corticosteroid injections occasionally bring temporary relief. If the symptoms continue or progress, your doctor will probably recommend surgery. The operation includes decompressing the median nerve at the wrist.

Self-Care Measures You Can Take

There are a number of measures you can take to prevent or treat CTS. Experiment and see what works for you.

Watch What You Eat

Increasing your intake of B vitamins may be the best thing you can do to prevent and treat CTS. Foods rich in B vitamins are sunflower seeds, whole wheat flour, rolled oats, green peas, soybeans, lima beans, crabmeat, brown rice, asparagus, raisins, wheat germ, chicken, hazelnuts, peanuts, hickory nuts, spinach, kale, peas, salmon, prunes, lentils, tuna, turkey, rabbit, white beans, mackerel, bananas, walnuts, sweet potatoes, cooked cabbage, sardines, trout, herring, sea vegetables (kombu, dulse, kelp, and wakame) fermented soy products (tempeh, natto, miso), turnips, cantaloupe, buckwheat, lobster, broccoli, and cauliflower.

Eat more foods high in vitamin C. This vitamin is important in healing. Foods to concentrate on are green peppers, honeydew melons, Brussels sprouts, strawberries, papaya, watercress, raspberries, parsley, raw cabbage, blackberries, onions, sprouts, and tomatoes.

Magnesium also can be helpful. It can be found in figs, green leafy vegetables, citrus fruits, whole grain breads and cereal, brown rice, wheat germ, and soy flour.

Essential fatty acids also may help. You can increase your intake of them by eating fish (mackerel, salmon, herring, whitefish, and tuna), walnuts, Brazil nuts, sunflower and pumpkin seeds, canola, olive and flaxseed oil, and green leafy vegetables.

Vitamin A is important to healing. Foods high in vitamin A include carrots, broccoli, kale, turnip greens, watercress, beets, dandelion greens, spinach, eggs, papaya, parsley, red peppers, pumpkin, yellow squash, apricots, and cantaloupes.

Zinc enhances healing also. Some foods rich in zinc are pumpkin seeds, whole grains, oysters, herring, liver, eggs, nuts, and wheat germ.

Avoid foods high in oxalic acid because they can promote joint problems. Eat less asparagus, cooked beets, cooked beet greens, eggs, fish, rhubarb, cooked spinach, cooked Swiss chard, and cooked cabbage. Avoid salt and salty foods—they promote water retention and can aggravate the condition. Avoid caffeine and smoking; they both constrict blood vessels.

Eat half a fresh pineapple daily for one to three weeks. The bromelain in the fruit can reduce pain and swelling, but it must be fresh pineapple to work.

Some nutrients you may need to take in supplement form. All are available at your local health food store.

Lecithin supplies choline and inositol, both of which are important for nerve function and emulsifying fats. You can get lecithin in granular form (1 tablespoon three times a day before meals; follow directions on the bottle) or capsules (1,200 mg three times a day before meals). It is derived from soybeans.

Grapeseed extract is a powerful anti-inflammatory and a powerful antioxidant. Follow the directions on the label.

Kelp is a kind of seaweed that is beneficial to nerves. You can cut up kelp and put it in soups, salads, stews, and casseroles. There are many kinds; try them all.

Primrose oil contains essential fatty acids necessary for nerve function. Follow the directions on the bottle.

If you can't find fresh pineapple, you can take bromelain as a supplement. Take 250 to 500 mg three times a day before you eat.

Use Healing Affirmations

Choose one of the affirmations below to change your outlook. Say or write the phrase twenty times a day. Also, write the phrase on 3 × 5 cards and place them in places so you'll read often:

- I choose to create a life that is happy and peaceful.
- I forgive everyone who has harmed me in any way.
- I am calm.

Exercise

Compared to splinting, range-of-motion exercises were associated with less pain and fewer days to return to work in a study reported in the *American Journal of Industrial Medicine*. Some range-of-motion exercises follow. Choose one or two that sound good to you. Start small and gently. Work up to more repetitions and more exercises.

Do these exercises the first thing in the morning, and then hourly during the work day when engaged in repetitive wrist movements. If you're wearing a wrist splint, remove it to do the exercises, then replace it.

1. Rub the palms of your hands together gently. Let your palms face each other, an inch apart. Feel the energy between them.
2. Stretch your arms out in front of you and gently shake your wrists.
3. Stand with your arms outstretched in front of you and gently flex your wrists up and down in each direction for two minutes.
4. Rotate your wrists in circles for three minutes, moving first clockwise and then counterclockwise.

5. Bend your elbows, resting your hands on your shoulders as you breathe in. Then, exhaling, stretch your arms out in front of you. Repeat five times.

6. Bend your elbows out to the sides, resting your hands gently on the top of your shoulders as you breathe in. Exhaling, stretch your arms out to the side.

7. Hold both arms up toward the ceiling, letting your fingers stretch upward. Picture your ligaments and tissues relaxing and healing.

8. Keeping your elbows bent and your hands on your shoulders, inhale and draw your elbows up in front of your face and above your head. Exhale, lowering your elbows back down in a circular movement.

9. Hold your palms together, with your fingers touching but spread apart slightly. Exhale and press your palms and fingers against each other. Inhale and breathe in, relaxing your hands, but keeping them touching. Repeat up to five times.

10. Hold the palm of your right hand in front of you in a *stop* motion. Exhale and use your left fingers to gently pull your right fingers back gently. Inhale and release your fingers. Repeat several times. Repeat with the other hand.

11. Massage each finger, starting with your little finger and working your way in to the thumb. Start at the base of each finger and use your thumb and index finger; then pull out the end of the top of each finger.

12. Rest your little fingers lightly on a table or desk or on your thighs. Gently lower your hands to stretch the fingers. Repeat with each finger.

13. Rub your hands together and then gently shake your wrists out.

Try Yoga

If exercise doesn't seem to help, you might want to consider yoga. A report in the *Journal of the American Medical Association* found that the yoga group had significant improvements in grip strength and significant pain reduction compared to a control group that wore a splint or received no treatment.

Investigate Herbs

There are many herbs that could help you. Consult with a herb book and/or an expert in the use of herbs. Also let your doctor know about any herbs you are taking.

Perhaps the simplest thing you can do is to use turmeric as a spice on all your food. It is very mild, yet packs a wallop because its anti-inflammatory activity is comparable to using steroids. If you're taking aspirin or nonsteroidal anti-inflammatory drugs (Tylenol, Advil, and so on), don't mix them with turmeric.

Aloe vera, devil's claw, yarrow, and yucca can restore flexibility and reduce inflammation. Butcher's broom can relieve inflammation. *Capsicum* (cayenne pepper) relieves pain and is a catalyst for other herbs. Parsley is a natural diuretic. Put fresh parsley in your salads, soups, stews, and on your dinner plate. Be sure to chew it well at the end of your meal and it will provide you with many vitamins and minerals as well as freshen your breath!

Ginkgo biloba, as either a tea or a capsule, can improve your circulation and aid in nerve function. Marshmallow root soothes and softens tissues and promotes healing. Skullcap relieves muscle spasms and pain.

Before taking any herbs, consult with a doctor or nurse with herb knowledge. You might also want to buy a book on the use of herbs, one that tells you about interactions with drugs and foods.

Do Acupressure

There are several acupressure points that may bring relief, according to *Self-Massage* and *Blended Medicine*:

1. Press the point in the middle of your inner wrist, 2½ finger widths above the wrist crease. Apply steady penetrating finger pressure for two to three minutes every hour or every other hour.

2. Let your thumb slide around your wrist, and let your thumb come to rest on the acupoint on the upper side of your wrist in the depression between the tendons. Lift your thumb if you can't see these tendons, and they will be visible. Make several rotations into this point, pressing in the direction of your elbow.

Try Acupuncture

If acupressure doesn't help, you may want to consider acupuncture. A report in the *Journal of Alternative and Complementary Medicine* found that the hands that failed surgical release were successfully treated by laser acupuncture. The treatment may be performed by you at home under the supervision of an acupuncturist, and it is about a twelfth the cost of surgery ($12,000 vs. $1,000).

Do Aromatherapy/Massage

Worwood, a practicing aromatherapist, suggests using ice massage for any inflamed area. Fill styrofoam or heavy paper cups with water and freeze. Cut the cup down so the ice is protruding. Massage over sore areas in circular movements.

You can also massage your arms and hands for relief. Start at the top of your arms and work down with your fingers, being gentle with your wrist, hands, and fingers. Work down again, this time with a gentle movement, barely touching the skin. Work down and out the fingertips, going a few inches beyond the end of your fingers.

To enhance the effect, mix 10 drops of rosemary, 10 drops of lavender, and 10 drops of peppermint essential oil in 2 tablespoons of vegetable oil and massage the hands and wrists with the mixture.

Consider Environmental Approaches: If You Use a Computer

Computers are meant to make your life easier, but they're also associated with carpal tunnel syndrome. If you want to prevent CTS:

1. Keep your feet flat on the floor. Use an adjustable chair, and make sure you can easily rest your feet on the floor.
2. Avoid bending your wrists when you use your keyboard. Your arms should be bent at a ninety-degree angle before extending them to the keyboard. Adjust your seat or the level of your keyboard so you don't bend your wrists.
3. Make sure you are looking slightly down, not up, when you look at your computer screen.
4. Take a break from the keyboard every thirty minutes. If necessary, set a timer to make sure you stop; then get up, walk around, or do some stretches.
5. Avoid using a laptop as your main computer. It isn't designed for prolonged use and can exacerbate CTS.

6. Position the screen 19 to 28 inches away from your eyes, and angle it away from direct light sources to minimize glare.

7. Avoid extreme lighting between your computer monitor and papers or materials you're using.

8. Force yourself to blink every few minutes.

9. Perform eye exercises throughout the day.

   - Make figure eights with your eyes.

   - Trace diagonals with your eyes, from the upper left-hand corner of the screen to the lower right-hand corner, and from the upper right-hand corner to the lower left-hand corner.

   - Look out the window into the distance, then look at an object in front of you. Look back out into the distance. Repeat this several times, holding on the far and near vision points for a minute or so.

10. Palm your eyes at least twice a day. Put the palms of your hands over your eyes and close them. Hold your hands there until you see velvet black with no light spots. Breathe in your abdomen and enjoy the tranquillity.

11. When you get up to walk around, move your eyes up and down and from side to side. Use your peripheral vision. Let your eyes linger on pleasant shapes and colors. Give your eyes a vacation from the fixed stare of computer work.

12. Use a computer shield to reduce glare and EMF emissions.

13. Type with a soft touch. Pounding the keys can make CTS symptoms worse.

14. Try using a foam keyboard to minimize strain on your wrists.

Stop Smoking

Stop smoking. It constricts your blood vessels, and that in turn impedes blood flow to your wrists and hands.

Wear a Splint or Gloves

Wear a splint during the day or at night. You can find them in drugstores and medical supply stores. Make sure that your wrist is almost straight and in about the same position as when you're writing with a pen. Check with your nurse to make sure your splint fits properly. Be aware that doing range-of-motion exercises (see above) can reduce pain more effectively than a splint. And if your hands are cold, wear cotton gloves. They will warm your hands and improve your circulation. If they get in the way of typing, cut off the fingers.

Increase Your Circulation

To increase the circulation in your wrists, immerse your hands and wrists in hot water for 3 minutes, then in cold water for thirty seconds. Repeat three to five times once or twice a day.

Chronic Fatigue Syndrome

Chronic fatigue syndrome (CFS) is a group of symptoms that includes fatigue, reduced activity level, aching muscles and joints, back and head pain, coldness, weakness, tremors, fevers, sleep disturbance, sweats, secondary infections, yeast infections, allergies, constipation, nausea, urine retention, appetite disorders, light and sound sensitivity, swollen glands, heart palpitations, anxiety, depression, memory lapses, irritability, jaundice, sore throat, swollen glands, loss of balance, and mood swings.

The symptoms resemble the flu and other viral infections, so it is often mistaken for them. Because there are so many symptoms in the syndrome, sufferers often feel misunderstood by their doctors, according to a report in the *Journal of Social Medicine.*

Your Risk for Developing Chronic Fatigue Syndrome

The cause of this condition is not well understood. Some experts believe the syndrome is linked to the infection Epstein-Barr virus (EBV), a member of the herpes virus family that causes mononucleosis. This theory is based on the fact that many people with the CFS have high levels of EBV antibodies in their blood and date the beginning of their symptoms to a prolonged viral infection. No connection has been proved, and many people have high levels of EBV without any ill effects. Many cases of CFS develop without any known preceding infection. Many people with CFS also have fibromyalgia. (See the chapter "Fibromyalgia" in this book.)

Some research points to chemical and/or food sensitivities as the source of CFS. Other possible causes of CFS are immune system problems, defect in blood pressure regulating mechanisms, anemia, chronic mercury poisoning from amalgam dental fillings, infection with *Candida albicans*, sleep problems, low blood sugar, and/or an underactive thyroid gland. A report in the *Journal of the American College of Nutrition* confirmed that magnesium deficiency may lead to oxidative stress. Another explanation of extreme fatigue is iron deficiency.

A psychoanalytic explanation, as presented in the *Journal of Psychology*, includes the body as a battleground for the fight to separate from the mother. A metaphysical explanation appears in *Heal Your Body*. The theory is that thoughts held and the words that are repeatedly used create our life and experience. If you change your thoughts, you can change the way you view your experiences, and eventually your experiences. The specific theory for fatigue is that you may be full of resistance and boredom, and lack love for what you're doing.

How the Doctor Diagnoses Chronic Fatigue Syndrome

Two major criteria distinguish chronic fatigue syndrome from flu or fibromyalgia or other conditions:

1. Persistent fatigue that does not end with bed rest and that is severe enough to reduce daily activity by 50 percent for at least six months.

2. All other conditions, including psychiatric disorders, can be ruled out as the cause.

What the Doctor Will Probably Prescribe

CFS cannot be cured. Some individuals recover spontaneously, but it can recur at any time. Recurrences usually follow a bout with another illness or increased stress. Medications are usually prescribed depending on your symptoms.

Immunoglobulin and hydrocortisone have showed some limited effects, according to a review in the *Journal of the American Medical Association*, but the evidence was inconclusive.

Self-Care Measures You Can Take

There are nutritional, exercise, herbal, cognitive, and stress reduction measures you can take to prevent or treat CFS. You also may want to consult a massage therapist, reflexologist, acupuncturist, or a homeopathy or therapeutic touch practitioner. Each has something to offer. Ask your friends and healthcare professionals for recommendations, or consult your yellow pages, then ask for the names and numbers of clients who have used their services. Talk to the references and ask all your questions. Also, talk to your doctor about any benefits you notice.

Get Adequate Nutrition

A number of nutritional deficiencies may appear in CFS patients, although these deficiencies may be due to the illness process. These include deficiencies of various B vitamins, vitamin C, magnesium, sodium, zinc, iron, L-tryptophan, L-carnitine, coenzyme Q10, and essential fatty acids, according to a review of nutritional strategies for CFS published in *Alternative Medical Review*. You will probably want to get your L-tryptophan, L-carnitine, and coenzyme Q10 in capsule form. There may be enough of the other vitamins and minerals in the foods you eat, provided you eat plenty of the recommended sources that follow.

Foods rich in B vitamins include sunflower seeds, whole wheat flour, rolled oats, green peas, soybeans, lima beans, crabmeat, brown rice, asparagus, raisins, wheat germ, chicken, hazelnuts, peanuts, hickory nuts, spinach, kale, peas, salmon, prunes, lentils, tuna, turkey, rabbit, white beans, mackerel, bananas, walnuts, sweet potatoes, cooked cabbage, sardines, trout, herring, sea vegetables (kombu, dulse, kelp, and wakame), fermented soy products (tempeh, natto, and miso), turnips, cantaloupes, buckwheat, lobster, broccoli, and cauliflower.

Foods rich in C vitamins include green peppers, honeydew melon, Brussels sprouts, strawberries, papaya, watercress, raspberries, parsley, raw cabbage, blackberries, onions, sprouts, and tomatoes. Magnesium can be found in figs, green leafy vegetables, citrus fruits, whole grain breads and cereal, brown rice, wheat germ, and soy flour. Zinc is plentiful in oysters, nuts, wheat germ, and herring. Essential fatty acids appear in fish (mackerel, salmon, herring, whitefish and tuna), walnuts, Brazil nuts, sunflower and pumpkin seeds, canola, olive and flaxseed oil, and green leafy vegetables.

Foods rich in iron include kidney beans, molasses, whole grain breads and cereals, beets, cherries, red cabbage, spinach, cucumbers, tomato juice, fish, coconuts, blackberry juice, and green leafy vegetables.

If you have taken antibiotics, many of the "good" bacteria in your intestines have been killed. This is often the source of yeast infections. You need to replace the friendly flora. For a natural treatment, try *L. acidophilus*, *L. lactobacillus*, *L. bidfidobacteria*, or other capsules or powders of live "good" bacteria. Some plain yogurts contain active cultures that can overpower the candida and replace its colonies. Read package information carefully to make sure the cultures are active and the product does not contain sugar, which promotes candida growth.

A diet that starves yeast while supporting your immune system includes soy and fish protein, lots of fresh vegetables, olive oil, nuts (without oil), seeds (sunflower, pumpkin, sesame), legumes (dried beans and peanuts), whole grains (if tolerated), and small amounts of fruit (if tolerated). It avoids all saturated fats (meat, cheese, eggs), sweets, refined flours and cereals, caffeine (coffee, tea, chocolate), alcohol, dairy products (they contain tryptophan, an amino acid known for its sedative effects), salt (unless you have low blood pressure), any mold-containing foods if you are sensitive (e.g., MSG, food dyes, food colors, preservatives, mushrooms, and aged cheeses and wines), and allergic foods (that bloat, give you gas, make you feel tired, or give you a headache or other negative symptoms after you eat them).

The best way to identify foods you react to is to keep a food/reaction diary. Write down everything you eat for a week. In a column alongside the food, write down how you feel after you eat that food. You will soon notice patterns. Eliminate the foods to which you have a negative reaction, as you may be sensitive to them.

At the first sign of pain, drink one or two glasses of water. Dehydration is a common source of pain.

It's best to try to get your vitamins and minerals in your food, but if that is not sufficient, try taking 1,000 mg of vitamin C in either capsule or powder form (in juice or water). It can relieve pain. For pain that moves around, try 1,000 mg vitamin C and 50 mg of L-lysine. Both are available in your local health food store. Talk it over with your doctor first to see if there is any research-based reason why you should not take the vitamin C and/or L-lysine.

If you perspire a lot or are going through menopause, you may be losing minerals and vitamins in your sweat that can lead to feelings of weakness and nausea and bone and muscle pain. First try a mineral juice, such as V-8. Consider taking a multimineral if that doesn't do it. You also may want to consider taking a good multivitamin that contains at least 50 mg of the major B vitamins, selenium, and less than 15 mg of iron. You will have to take both, since no multivitamin will be large enough to contain sufficient amounts of the minerals you need.

Exercise

Graded aerobic exercise proved useful for patients with CFS when compared to participation in flexibility exercises and relaxation therapy. The results were published in the *British Medical Journal*. Exercise has been shown to be helpful, but first erroneous beliefs about avoiding exercise and activity, if you have CFS, must be changed.

Try Acupressure/Massage

There are some self-pressure/massage things you can do to relieve pain. Start by working with your hand. Gently massage it, working deep in the webbing between each finger. Use your thumb to work up the inside of your palm, and work out each finger with your thumb and index finger. Use your index finger nail to poke the end of each finger. End by pulling down and out the hand with your other hand and then shaking the hand you just worked on as if you are flicking water off it. Repeat with the other hand. You can do the same thing on your foot, only work in the depression underneath the ball of your foot a third of the way along the sole. This is a general tonic point that can revive your spirit and give you energy. If you can't do it, have your partner or a friend do it, or find a good massage therapist or reflexologist

For neck and head pain, work along, above, and below the bony ridge along the back of your head where it meets the neck. Search for sore spots and give them loving massage. Work your fingers up and through your scalp, too, again finding any sore spot and working with it gently until it releases and pain leaves. If pain increases, stop and consult with a massage therapist. If you find relief, work across your shoulders and down your arms, across your chest and abdomen, and down your legs and feet.

Investigate Herbal Treatments

Extracts of *Echinacea purpurea* and *Panax ginseng* significantly enhanced the immune system in individuals with CFS, according to a report in *Immunopharmacology*. Other herbs that have been suggested are kombucha tea (to offer renewed energy), and ginger, licorice root, and Siberian ginseng to decrease fatigue and weakness.

Grapefruit seed extract (GSE) can be very effective in killing off yeast. Three to five teaspoons in a quart of liquid is suggested by Landis. Echinacea root, garlic, Pau d'arco bark, oak bark, and astragalus also can kill yeast. If you are having trouble sleeping, have night sweats, are irritable and tired all the time, and are a woman between thirty-five and sixty years (perimenopausal), consider taking black cohosh.

Work with a healthcare practitioner skilled in the use of herbs, and be sure to discuss any herbs you are taking with your doctor. Although herbs have many fewer side effects than drugs, herbs must be used carefully and cannot be used if you are taking certain prescribed or over-the-counter drugs.

Use Cognitive Therapy to Reduce Symptoms

Cognitive behavior therapy is a structured approach that includes the client as an active participant. During sessions, you are asked to challenge your erroneous beliefs and work out a plan to use until the next session.

In a study reported in *Lancet*, cognitive behavior therapy was shown to be more effective in reducing fatigue as compared to a guided support group and the natural course. Cognitive behavior therapy was more effective changing beliefs than was relaxation therapy, according to the report of one study in the *Journal of Psychosomatic Research*. Based on these findings, it may be wise to find a nurse psychotherapist or psychologist you trust and obtain individual or group cognitive therapy.

Consider Aromatherapy Possibilities

Essential oils can stimulate or relax. A few drops of essential lavender oil in a warm bath can prepare you for a night of refreshing sleep. Oil of lemon can help you unwind. It also can prevent night sweats and fevers. If you mix lemon and lavender, the two scents combine to produce the aromatic equivalent of knockout drops. If you are having periods of unrefreshing sleep, you may wish to put a mixture of these two essential oils in an aromatic infuser. A few sniffs of oil of rosemary can snap you out of early-morning sluggishness. A sniff of oil of orange or oil of sweet orange can refresh and uplift you. Although the oils are safe, a few may irritate the skin and should be used in a carrier oil such as oil of sweet almond oil. Some shouldn't be used if you're pregnant or breast-feeding. If you plan to use essential oils, purchase a textbook and follow it, or find a healthcare practitioner knowledgeable in their use.

Reduce Stress

There are many methods of reducing your stress. One way is to use the exercise on pages 88–89. You also may wish to find a healthcare provider skilled in acupressure, reflexology, massage, homeopathy, and/or hypnosis.

Use Affirmations to Relieve Boredom

Affirmations are based on metaphysical explanations for fatigue. Choose one or more of the following statements as your antidote. Say or write it twenty times a day to remove boredom. Write the saying on 3 × 5 cards and place them in prominent spots around you.

- I am enthusiastic about my life.
- I love my life and what I do.
- I am filled with positive energy.

Depression

According to the National Institute of Mental Health, depression is the leading mental health problem in America.

Postpartum depression can occur any time within a year after giving birth. This kind of depression lasts six to nine months, but may precipitate a chronic condition if it is not treated *(The American Journal for Nurse Practitioners)*.

A *major depressive episode* includes sleep disturbances, loss of interest in everything, withdrawal from normal daily activities, guilt or poor self-worth, loss of energy, lack of concentration, appetite loss, agitation or slow movements, and thoughts of suicide *(The American Journal for Nurse Practitioners)*. Children may be more irritable, not show the usual developmental weight gains, and look sad. Adolescents may stay up all right watching TV, sleep during the day, fail in school, take drugs, appear bored, wear black clothes, and write poetry with morbid themes *(Advance for Nurse Practitioners)*.

A *bipolar disorder* is a combination of depression alternating with manic behavior such as wearing flamboyant clothing, distributing gifts of money, talking quickly and as if feeling pressured, fleeting ideas, buying sprees, sexual indiscretion, school or work failure, substance abuse, decreased need for sleep, and engaging in risky and impulsive behaviors.

While you might not always recognize that you are depressed, you may realize that something is bothering you and go to see your doctor about it. Sometimes you may develop physical symptoms, possibly because you're not eating or your immune system has been depressed by your mood. These may be the symptoms you tell your doctor about, but you may also notice that you have trouble sleeping, that you've lost a lot of weight (or gained a lot) and feel so tired you barely can get out of bed. You also may feel worthless and guilty about everything. You probably have trouble concentrating on simple things such as reading the newspaper or watching TV because negative thoughts about you and your life keep intruding. Underneath it all, you may be extremely angry, but those feelings may be hidden under guilt and low self-esteem. You may even have thoughts about ending your life and how you'd do it.

All of these symptoms must be reported immediately to your doctor. Depression can cause a severe impairment in your life, can depress your immune system so that you're not able to fight off infections, and can lead to suicide, so it's important that you get treatment right away.

Your Risk for Developing Depression

If you lose someone or something, it's normal to feel depressed, but this is usually fleeting. Loss of a parent, a favorite pet, or even major success can result in a prolonged grieving period, but daily activities are gradually resumed. Recently widowed older adults can have a complicated grief reaction that consists of disbelief, feeling stunned, prolonged crying, yearning for the deceased, and preoccupation with thoughts of the lost partner. This can continue for two years or more (*American Journal of Psychiatry*).

It is at the point that the loss interferes with your ability to function for a prolonged period of time, you feel life isn't worth living, you are riddled with guilt, and you don't want to get up in the morning that a manageable loss becomes depression. Psychological makeup plays a role in vulnerability to depression. If you have low self-esteem, view the world with pessimism, or are easily overwhelmed by stress, you are probably prone to depression (*Plain Talk about Depression*).

A metaphysical explanation for depression examines how what we think about ourselves and our lives affects our body and mind. This theory is described in *Heal Your Body*. In this format, if you feel anger you think you do not have a right to have and/or hopelessness, depression will result.

If you feel pressure to be feminine, you may be at greater risk for depression. A study reported in *Nursing Dimensions* found that pressure to be "ladylike" and conform to society's image of femininity may cause depression in some women. This finding may help explain why women suffer depression more frequently than men. Women are raised to squelch their anger. This strong feeling must go somewhere, and if it can't be expressed in aggressive games, physical fights, or verbal sparring, it can fester inside and be turned against the self, eventually developing into depression.

If you smoke, you are at risk for depression, according to a study in the *Archives of General Psychiatry*. Not only did smoking seem to lead to depression, depression, in turn, led to more smoking.

If you have a chronic disease or chronic vitamin deficiencies *(American Journal for Nurse Practitioners)* or if you have few people near you who support and nurture you and few personal coping resources *(Health Psychology)*, your risk for being depressed increases.

Drugs can bring on depression. If you are taking any of the following drugs, your risk for depression increases: alcohol, Valium, Librium, Cortone, Premarin, Ogen, Estradiol, Estroderm, Provera, Depo-Provera, Norlutate, Norplant, Progestasert, Sinemet, Dupar, Larodopa Symmetrel, Serpasil, Ineral, Aldomet, Ismelinsulfate, Catapres, or presoline hydrochloride *(American Journal of Nurse Practitioners)*.

If you were abused as a child *(American Journal of Psychiatry)*, you may be at greater risk for suicide as an adult. If you don't have social support, frequent social interaction, or don't perceive that there are people around you who support and care about you, you are at risk for a decline rather than a recovery from depression *(American Journal of Psychiatry)*. If you have just had a baby, the risk for postpartum depression increases with any of the following predictors: prenatal depression, prenatal anxiety, previous history of depression, lack of perceived emotional and physical support from family members or friends, dissatisfaction with marital relationship, presence of stressful life events, temperament problems with the infant, or mood swings or periods of tearfulness during the first week after delivery *(Journal of Obstetric, Gynecologic, and Neonatal Nursing)*.

If you have a family history of recurrent major depressive disorder, emotional reliance, or conflict with your parents (for girls), you are more apt to have recurrent depression in young adulthood. Smoking may cause depression in adolescents, too *(American Journal of Nursing)*. If you have low self-esteem, a sense of having little control over life events, and a predisposition to excessive worrying and pessimism, this combination can foster the development of depression.

If you are separated or divorced, your risk for depression rises, but the highest rates are seen in women who are unhappily married. Widowhood, the winter season, and hormones also may precipitate depression.

If you've been diagnosed with a heart attack or cancer, depression may follow, especially for women. Depression and cigarette smoking can be a particularly dangerous combination, especially for men. If you smoke, there is more bad news: there is an immune pathway by which depression and smoking together might promote cancer *(Science News)*.

Once depressed, heart complications, a second heart attack, the need for bypass surgery, and death are more frequent. An explanation is that depression leads to eating improperly or becoming more sedentary, and more likelihood of smoking and skipping or abusing medications *(Health & Stress)*.

The level of polyunsaturated essential fatty acids in the body is also a potential risk factor because it is correlated with aggression and depression. Differences in the prevalence of major depression have been linked to dietary intake of omega-3 fatty acids in epidemiological and double-blind placebo controlled trials. Countries that consume large amount of fish (high in essential fatty acids), such as Japan, Taiwan, and South Korea, have a lower prevalence of depression and violence than countries with a lower intake of fish *(Pufa Newsletter)*.

How the Doctor Diagnoses Depression

Your doctor will probably ask you questions or piece together from observing you and hearing what you say that you might be depressed. Some questions you may be asked include when your symptoms first started, how long they have lasted, how severe they are, whether you've had them before, what treatment you've had for them, what alcohol and drugs you use, if you have thoughts about death or suicide, if any family members have had a depressive illness, and which treatments they had that worked. You may be given a mental status exam to see if your speech or thought patterns or memory have been affected, as is often the case in depressive or manic-depressive illness.

It may not be easy to diagnose depression because of the many underlying conditions that have similar symptoms. Weakness and fatigue can be symptoms of anemia or hypothyroidism. Weight loss can be due to hyperthyroidism or diabetes. For women, the inability to think clearly or concentrate on a task can be related to menopause. Older adults who appear depressed may have vitamin B deficiencies or infection. Because drugs also can cause depression, your doctor will ask you about the prescription, nonprescription, and recreational drugs you take.

Your physician may order a complete blood count, urinalysis, chemistry profile, thyroid-stimulating hormone, serum B_{12} level, and drug levels for the medications you're taking to rule out any chronic illness. When your laboratory tests don't correlate with your complaints or if you don't seem to be responding to treatment, your doctor may ask you questions about whether you're having trouble sleeping (a classic symptom of depression) or are waking up early in the morning and can't go back to sleep.

If you or a family member is a resident in a nursing home, the doctor may use the Yesavage Geriatric Depression Scale (GDS). This is a fifteen-item survey that is administered by the provider, takes about five minutes to complete, and requires only a simple "yes" or "no" response from the interviewee. The Yale Depression Scale is a test that asks for a response to the single question "Do you often feel sad or depressed?" A "yes" should be followed by the GDS test.

What the Doctor Will Probably Prescribe

Your physician will probably suggest that you stop drinking coffee or tea or having anything with caffeine in it because it is known to destroy sleep. So do alcohol, minor tranquilizers, chronic pain, and sleep apnea. You will probably receive a prescription for an antidepressant and be given a referral for psychotherapy, although counseling is something used by itself *(Depression in Primary Care.)*

A number of drugs are prescribed for depression. Bupropion (Wellbutrin, Zyban) inhibits the reuptake of serotonin and dopamine, the neurotransmitters that help determine your mood. The most common adverse effects are rashes, agitation and mental status changes, seizures, headache and sleep disturbances, nausea and vomiting, constipation, weight loss, increased appetite, stomach discomfort, menstrual problems, dry mouth, excessive sweating, tremors, insomnia, hearing disturbances, blurred vision, taste disturbances, dizziness, heart arrhythmias, high blood pressure, palpitations, agitation, confusion, fainting, decreased sex drive, hostility, anxiety, fever, and chills. This drug should not be used if you have a seizure disorder, bulimia, anorexia, are manic-depressive (it can bring on manic episodes), are taking other antidepressants or antipsychotic drugs, have had head trauma, recently had a heart attack, or have liver or kidney conditions (it is toxic to the liver). Extreme restlessness, agitation, anxiety, or inability to sleep is a signal to discontinue it because delusions, hallucinations, psychosis, confusion, or paranoia can occur. Taking this drug with alcohol can cause seizures. Taking this drug with L-dopa makes adverse effects more likely. Taking this drug with MAO inhibitors such as phenelzine can bring on deadly toxicity.

Venlafaxine (Effexor) inhibits the reuptake of the neurotransmitters serotonin, norepinephrin and dopamine. Adverse effects of this drug include nausea, insomnia, dizziness, sleepiness, abnormal ejaculation, nervousness, headache, dry mouth, anxiety, excessive sweating, weakness, loss of appetite, decreased body weight, mania, seizures, and elevated heart rate. Allow at least two weeks between stopping MAO inhibitors and starting venlafaxine. Be cautious using this drug if you have high blood pressure (it may raise it more), or kidney or liver impairment (it can be toxic to them), if you take it for more than six weeks (it has not been tested for use beyond this), or if you have another illness that affects your blood pressure.

Selective serotonin reuptake inhibitors (SSRIs) can play a role in improving mood, but they also can create a false sense of emotional detachment. This means that the source of the depression is never uncovered or treated. Adverse effects include nervousness, insomnia, drowsiness, fatigue, weakness, tremor, increased sweating, dizziness, anxiety (especially with Prozac), headache (especially with Paxil), dry mouth (for Paxil and Zoloft), male sexual dysfunction (especially for Zoloft, but also for Paxil), loss of appetite, nausea, diarrhea, stomach discomfort (for Prozac and Zoloft), altered appetite and weight, constipation (with Paxil), rash, fever, joint pain, abnormal changes in blood cell counts, swelling, and liver or kidney damage (with Prozac). Fifteen to 21 percent of people taking these drugs in clinical trials stopped taking them due to unpleasant side effects. A new syndrome called "serotonin syndrome" is caused by an overdose or an interaction with other drugs. It can be fatal and includes hallucinations, confusion, agitation, fluctuating blood pressure, fever, seizures, irregular heartbeats, and stiffness. Withdrawal from SSRIs can be difficult, and symptoms include dizziness, nausea, headaches, poor concentration, fatigue, moodiness, and mental fogginess. It is best to withdraw from any drug, especially SSRIs, over a period of two weeks using natural alternatives and under the supervision of a healthcare professional. The long-term effects of these drugs have not been studied systematically, so don't take them if you are diabetic (it makes blood sugar low until withdrawal and then makes blood sugar high), have impaired liver function, if you're manic (they can make you more so), if you are taking diuretics to lower blood pressure (they can cause heart dysrhythmias), or if you are taking MAO inhibitors.

Tricyclic antidepressants (TCAs) (amitryptyline or Elavil) also are used to treat mood. The list of adverse effects fills a page and runs from blurred vision to hallucinations to tremors and black tongue. As with the other drugs mentioned, ability to drive and perform other hazardous tasks may be impaired. Symptoms of schizophrenia and manic depression can be worsened by taking this drug. Developing a sore throat or a fever can be a sign of a serious drug reaction. Stop taking Elavil prior to elective surgery. Work with your doctor to withdraw from the drug. Do not attempt to withdraw on your own.

Studies have shown that TCAs have an effectiveness range from 8 to 45 percent, while a placebo (or sugar pill) has an effectiveness range from 17 to 68 percent. Also, TCA side effects can be problems, especially in children, because they include potentially dangerous heart changes. Based on a review of the literature on the use of these drugs, asking the following questions is recommended if the drugs are suggested for your child (*Professional Psychology: Research and Practice*): Is the youth depressed despite the absence of family conflict or divorce? Do the depressive symptoms include sleep disturbance, physical complaints, and/or appetite change? Is there no positive change after ten to fifteen sessions of psychotherapy? Does the youth express a clear preference for drugs over psychotherapy? If the answer is "yes" to all these questions, then this medication may be suggested as an adjunct to psychotherapy.

Self-Care Measures You Can Take

General ways to help yourself feel less depressed include:

- Avoid taking on additional responsibility.
- Set small goals, and reward yourself when you achieve them.
- Lower your expectations until your depression has faded.
- Be with other people as much as possible, even when you don't feel like it.

- Do at least one activity every day that makes you feel good.

- Don't overdo, and get plenty of rest.

- Refuse to get upset if you don't improve as quickly as you'd like; feeling better takes time.

Even though you may not feel like it, push yourself and try each of these specific actions:

- *Exercise.* You don't have to run or even jog to feel the effects of exercise. Gardening, walking, line dancing, swimming, and more will help raise your mood. Even if you don't feel like it, exercise every day. You'll feel much better after you do. In fact, exercise works better than Zoloft for treating depression (*American Journal of Nursing*).

- *Avoid drugs that make you depressed.* According to *Prescription Alternatives*, there are many common prescription drugs that can lower your mood and make you feel depressed: amphetamines (to lose weight and stay awake, including antihistamines), antibiotics, anticonvulsants, antidepressants (that's right, antidepressants!), barbiturates, high blood pressure drugs (diuretics and beta-blockers), hormones (estrogen, Premarin, Provera), narcotics, painkillers, sleeping pills, steroids (cortisone, prednisone), Tagamet, Zantac, and tranquilizers (Librium, Xanax, Restoril, Halcion).

- *Be in touch with your depressed children.* A study of teens who commit suicide found they often showed signs of depression and alcohol abuse that parents missed. Parents seriously underestimated the frequency or extent of use, could not understand the depth of feelings their children were going through, did not know the extreme pessimism about the future and life in general their children held, and didn't know their children had been intoxicated at least once in the past six months before the suicide (*Ball State University News*).

- *Use massage.* When swollen membranes around the sinus openings swell shut and pressure builds, infections and depression, among other conditions, can result. Massage above and below the band of bone at the back of your head, working gently, but more intensely wherever you feel pain.

- *Take Saint-John's-wort.* This herb can alleviate mild to moderate depression. The usual dose of Saint-John's-wort is 300 to 450 mg twice a day of the standardized extract (*Archives of General Medicine*). It should not be taken with nasal decongestants or hay fever and

asthma medications. Amino acid supplements that contain phenylala-
nine and/or tyrosine can cause hypertension, so should be avoided.

- *Take Acetyl-L-carnitine (ALCAR).* Many major well-designed studies
have shown ALCAR to be beneficial in the treatment of major depression *(Molecular Psychiatry).*

- *Volunteer to help someone else.* Volunteering is one of the best ways to
reduce depression. It removes you from your worries and makes you
concentrate on helping someone else. The good feelings and boost to
your self-esteem that result can help jog you out of your depression.
Contact Volunteers of America, 1-800-988-0089, or National Senior
Service Corps, 1-800-424-8867, or look in your local paper for volunteer opportunities.

- *Find a therapist who conducts cognitive behavior therapy groups.* In studies reported in *Psychotherapy Psychosomatics* and *Archives of General Psychiatry,* patients who were depressed and participated in cognitive
behavior therapy groups improved to a considerable degree.

- *Stay active.* A study reported in *Psychology and Aging* found that staying active in leisure and productive activities has a positive effect on
depression.

- *Get a massage and learn relaxation therapy.* A study reported in *Adolescence* found that both massage and relaxation exercises reduced anxiety and depression.

- *Try SAMe.* S-adenosyl-methionine is a popular supplement synthesized from the amino acid methionine and is found throughout the
body. In a study reported in the *American Journal of Psychiatry,* by the
end of the second week in a small trial, 66 percent of the SAMe participants had a reduction in depression versus 22 percent of participants taking imipramine (Tofranil). SAMe had no side effects, while
Tofranil had the following adverse effects: drowsiness, heart arrhythmias, low or high blood pressure, fatigue, nausea, rash, increased perspiration, headache, changes in blood sugar, sensitivity to light/sun,
water retention, jaundice, muscle spasticity and uncontrollable movements, and blood cell disturbances, and must be taken with caution by
many people (those with glaucoma, psychosis, diabetes, hyperthyroidism, kidney or liver disorders, asthma, women who are pregnant
or nursing, and people who have epilepsy, heart or blood vessel disease, epilepsy, or urine retention). In sum, SAMe works better and has

fewer adverse effects. If you are depressed and on an antidepressant, talk to your doctor about SAMe.

- *Take fish oil.* A study reported in *Science News* reported that fish oil helps stabilize the volatile moods of people suffering from manic depression.

- *Use guided imagery while listening to music.* A study reported in *Health Psychology* found depression, fatigue, and total mood disturbance significantly decreased during guided imagery with music sessions.

- *Music by itself is also effective.* A study reported in *Issues in Mental Health Nursing* found that depressed women who listened to music reported more tranquil mood states.

- *Try ginkgo biloba.* A study reported in *Geriatric Forsch* found that ginkgo biloba may offer a significant benefit as an antidepressant on its own or in combination with standard antidepressants.

- *Get assertiveness training.* A study report in the *Journal of Clinical Psychology* found that depressed outpatients reported more self-reported assertiveness and less depression than outpatients in traditional psychotherapy.

- *Change what you say.* When things go wrong, do you think negative thoughts about yourself or chide yourself for being at fault? A study published in *Psychological Reports* found that learning to restructure these negative thoughts can improve self-esteem and reduce depression. Say one or more of the following affirmations to balance the negative messages you may be giving yourself:

  1. I go beyond my fears and limitations.
  2. I create a joyous life.
  3. I release all anger.
  4. I forgive others; I forgive myself.

- *Quit smoking.* Major depression has been linked to smoking in a study published in *Archives of General Psychiatry.* A history of daily smoking significantly increased the risk of depression. Find a mental health nurse specialist or psychologist skilled in hypnosis, or join a quit smoking group (many are sponsored by the American Lung Association; check your white pages).

- *Take additional vitamin B$_{12}$.* A study published in the *American Journal of Psychiatry* found that after adjusting for sociodemographic characteristics and health status, participants with a vitamin B_{12} deficiency were 2.05 times as likely to be severely depressed as were participants who had sufficient vitamin B_{12}. Foods you might want to eat to ensure that you have a sufficient amount of this vitamin include liver, clams, oysters, sardines, mackerel, trout, herring, and eggs. You also may want to find nutritional yeast, sea vegetables (kombu, dulse, and wakame), fermented soyfoods (tempeh, natto, and miso), and kelp, found at your health food store.

- *More toward vegetarianism.* In a study published in the *Bulletin of the Medical Association of Puerto Rico*, depression was more likely to occur in nonvegetarians than in vegetarians. The researchers suggest that vegetables provide more antioxidants, and they may protect vegetarians.

- *Take additional magnesium.* A study of women in the United Kingdom published in the *Journal of Women's Health and Gender-Based Medicine* found that mood swings and depressive symptoms were reduced by taking 200 mg of magnesium (as MgO) and 50 mg a day of vitamin B_6. The researchers also concluded that this form of magnesium was poorly absorbed, so try eating more absorbable forms of the mineral (citrate). Also eat foods high in magnesium and vitamin B_6: whole grain breads and cereals, fresh peas, figs, soy flour, brown rice, wheat germ, nuts, Swiss chard, green leafy vegetables, citrus fruits, sunflower seeds, chicken, mackerel, salmon, tuna, bananas, peanuts, and sweet potatoes.

- *Find a nursing service that offers a home visiting program.* If you're at home with young children and feel depressed, look in the yellow pages for nursing services. Find one that makes home visits. A study in the *Journal of Clinical and Child Psychology* found that depression lifted in mothers who were visited at home by nurses who showed mothers how to deal with their children, taught parenting skills, and reinforced maternal competence. The nurses also suggested resources and positive ways to cope.

- *Get involved in a weight-lifting program.* A study reported in the *Journal of Gerontology Biological Science and Medical Science* found that resistance training had a significant effect by lowering depression and improving strength, morale, and quality of life.

- *Investigate acupuncture.* A study in the *Journal of Traditional Chinese Medicine* reported that acupuncture was more effective than an antidepressant (Elavil) in reducing depression.

- *Try meditation.* In a study reported in *General Hospital Psychiatry*, meditation reduced depression, anxiety, and physical symptoms in participants who met for eight-weeks to learn and use the technique.
- *Read cognitive therapy books.* In a study reported in the *Journal of Consulting and Clinical Psychology*, cognitive bibliotherapy worked well to reduce depression (when combined with traditional treatment), and treatment gains were maintained over a three-year period.
- *Explore phototherapy.* High levels of illumination have been shown to be helpful in reducing depression due to seasonal light changes. A study reported in *Acta Psychiatry Scandinavia* found that high levels of illumination combined with antidepressant medication reduced depression. The higher the level of illumination, the greater the decrease in depression.
- *Get a pet.* At least one study has shown that pets can erase the stress of the death of a spouse *(Delta Society International)* and help you deal with other losses, too. Other studies have shown that a pet can give you a sense of belonging and of being needed. Even a stuffed toy animal or a plant that you water can improve your well-being.

Diabetes

In countries where people eat a diet low in fat and sugar and high in whole grains and fresh fruits and vegetables, diabetes is almost nonexistent. As Western processed and fast foods and soft drinks are introduced into Third World countries, the rate of diabetes rises rapidly.

Type 2 diabetes is the fastest-growing health problem in the United States. Sixteen million Americans suffer from it, including many youngsters as young as age ten. It is characterized by abnormally high levels of blood sugar (glucose) and insulin levels that increase your risk of heart disease; stroke; nerve disorders; blindness; kidney stones; cancer; and in men, impotence.

In the United States, diabetes is the leading cause of blindness, amputation, kidney failure, and use of dialysis. Diabetes kills more than 178,000 people every year and is the second leading cause of childhood death by disease. It kills three times more women than breast cancer and eight times more people than AIDS.

Diabetes is the major cause of stroke and causes a third of all heart disease in America. The condition has increased 50 percent in the past ten years. Hispanics are two to four times more likely to have diabetes. African Americans are more than twice as likely to have Type 2 diabetes. Forty to 45 percent of individuals sixty-five years or older have diabetes. Thirty-five percent of all Medicare costs are driven by diabetes.

There are two main kinds of diabetes. Type 1 usually occurs during childhood and adolescence and is due to antibodies destroying the cells in the pancreas that make insulin. Type 2 used to be thought to occur after age forty-five, although with a nationwide switch to junk food, soda and juice drinks, and couch potato behavior, more and more children are being affected. In this condition there may be plenty of insulin being made, but the body cannot use it properly. The condition afflicts fifteen million Americans; a third of them are unaware that they have the condition. Are you or one of your family members one of them?

Both glucose and insulin are essential for life, but too much of either can derail health. Glucose, a simple sugar, fuels your cells. Without glucose your brain would not think and your heart would not beat, or when paired with too little or too much insulin, glucose remains in the blood and creates biochemical mischief.

High levels of glucose generate large numbers of free radicals, unbalanced molecules known to promote aging and to damage your cells. Normally, when you eat and your food digests, glucose levels rise and signal your pancreas to secrete insulin, which helps move glucose into cells to be burned or stored as fat.

Throughout most of history, humans consumed protein (meat) and unrefined, fiber-rich carbohydrates found in vegetables and seeds. These foods are digested slowly and result in gradual increases in glucose and insulin.

Diabetes has many complications. One of them is neuropathy, which causes pain, burning feelings, and numbness. The most common form is peripheral neuropathy. The feet and lower part of the legs are affected, then the hands. The heart also can become involved, leading to light-headedness and fainting. Neuropathy also can affect the digestive tract and cause loss of appetite, bloating, nausea, vomiting, and indigestion. Weakening of the thigh muscles also can occur, making it difficult to climb stairs or stand up from a sitting position. Carpal tunnel syndrome is more than twice as likely to develop in individuals with diabetes as in those without it.

A form of bone diabetes affects one in every seven hundred people with the condition. It is probably triggered by small trauma, so be careful with your feet. Don't cut or bruise them or let anyone else hurt or cut your feet. A misstep or twist of your foot also could damage the ligaments supporting the arch, causing the bones to begin to grind against each other. A small bone fracture could go unnoticed. The result is a loss of bone density. As the bones disintegrate, the arch can collapse. This alters the way weight is distributed on your feet and causes irritation, which can lead to blistering, ulceration, and infection.

The foot becomes deformed in a condition called Charcot foot. The most common is a "rocker bottom" appearance of the foot. The foot also may appear swollen and warm to the touch, and there may be signs of inflammation.

Your Risk for Developing Diabetes

If you eat the wrong foods, get little or no exercise, are overweight, and don't get adequate nutrients, you're at risk for diabetes. Let's take a look at the particulars.

For the past hundred years, Americans have increased their consumption of highly refined grains in the form of breads, rolls, muffins, pastries, and packaged foods, and refined sugars in candy, pies, cakes, and so on. Because these foods are digested so fast, glucose levels shoot up and so does insulin.

This shocks the body and rocks your biochemistry. After several years of this, your body's cells become "insulin-resistant," so the pancreas secretes even more insulin. Eventually your body is overwhelmed by too much insulin and starts ignoring the hormone. At that point both glucose and insulin levels remain high, and diabetes results.

Some people bypass diabetes and go directly to other conditions, such as high cholesterol and blood pressure, triglycerides, and thickening of the arteries. All of these happenings increase the risk of heart disease.

Insulin also promotes the storage of body fat and sets the stage for overweight and obesity. In addition, extra insulin increases your risk for diabetes and heart disease and levels of cortisol, a stress hormone, associated with heightened risk for Alzheimer's and heart disease. Finally, since insulin promotes cell proliferation, it can increase your risk for cancer.

Another contributing factor may be cow's milk. Finnish researchers monitored babies in diabetes-prone families and found that infants getting formula that included cow's milk were more likely to develop the immune reactions associated with juvenile-onset type 1 diabetes than babies getting a substitute. Their findings were reported in *Science News*. The precise cause of this form of diabetes is not known, but the children in the study were genetically predisposed to it. Most may never get it. Something in the environment or diet may trigger it.

Chromium is an important mineral. Glucose intolerance, which may be the primary sign of chromium deficiency, is the key problem in type 2 diabetes. A research report in *Nutrition Review* showed that chromium has an insulin-signaling mechanism. This mineral helps improve insulin binding, according to *Clinician Reviews*.

The good news is that nine out of ten cases of type 2 diabetes can be prevented by exercising more, eating better, not smoking, and adopting other healthy behaviors, according to a report in the *New England Journal of Medicine*.

How the Doctor Diagnoses Diabetes

Your doctor may ask you questions that show you are at risk for diabetes. Some of those questions are:

- Are you overweight? (He may weigh you and compare what you weigh to weight charts.)

- How old are you? (Type 2 diabetes can now appear from age ten, but adult-onset diabetes often appears between forty-five and sixty years of age, and your risk increases even more after age sixty-five.)

- How much exercise do you get each day? (If you get little or no exercise each day, and are overweight, you are at risk for diabetes.)

- Does anyone in your family have diabetes? (Your risk for diabetes rises greatly if you have a parent or brother or sister with diabetes.)

- If you are a woman: Did you ever have a baby weighing more than nine pounds at birth? (A baby weighing more than nine pounds usually indicates gestational diabetes, a carbohydrate intolerance in the mother, with first recognition occuring during pregnancy.)

Your doctor will probably also order a fasting plasma glucose test to confirm that you have diabetes. That means you won't be able to eat before the test. The doctor will draw a small amount of blood from your arm and measure the plasma glucose concentration. A fasting plasma glucose value of 126 mg/dL indicates diabetes.

Researchers at the National Institute of Diabetes and Digestive and

Kidney Disease reviewed results of fasting plasma glucose tests given to 12,800 adults and found that afternoon tests showed significantly lower blood glucose levels than morning tests. If you're scheduled for a diabetes check, ask for a morning appointment to ensure a more reliable test result.

If you already have symptoms of diabetes, a confirmed nonfasting plasma glucose value of 200 mg/dL indicates diabetes. In certain circumstances your doctor may order a fasting oral glucose tolerance test. In this case he will ask you to drink a glucose and water solution. Two hours later he will measure the concentration of glucose in your blood by drawing a small amount from a vein in your arm.

What the Doctor Will Probably Prescribe

Your doctor will probably ask you to follow a carefully calculated diet, planned physical activity, home blood glucose testing several times a day, and in some cases, daily oral medication or insulin injections.

One type of diabetes drug your doctor may order for you is Acarbose (Precose). It works by slowing the digestion of carbohydrates in your small intestine. It blocks enzymes that normally break down carbohydrates. Unpleasant side effects are abdominal pain, cramps, gas, and diarrhea. This drug can impair kidney function and has caused cancerous kidney tumors in animals. Be sure to have an available source of sugar on hand, because it also can lower your blood sugar. Be careful if you have kidney problems, intestinal problems, or are exposed to stress such as fever, trauma, infection, or surgery. This drug can increase the action of insulin and sulfonylurea drugs and reduce or throw out of balance your vitamin B_{12} levels. If you do decide to take this drug, be sure to take a vitamin B_{12} supplement in a form that is activated under your tongue.

Insulin is another diabetes drug. Usually it is taken as an injection. It used to be thought that insulin would be a cure-all for diabetes, but most people with the condition have enough insulin. Their main problem is insulin resistance, a situation where cells resist using the available insulin. Even if insulin does help lower blood sugar, it can create its own problems, including high blood pressure and poor cholesterol levels, increasing the risk of complications as the diabetes progresses. This is why it's important to use diet, supplements, and exercise to lower your blood sugar.

If you do take insulin, there are allergic reactions you need to be aware of, including rashes, shortness of breath, fast pulse, sweating, a drop in blood pressure resulting in light-headedness or dizziness, and insulin shock. Insulin also lowers the available vitamin B_{12} in your body, so if you do take insulin, be sure to replace this vitamin. Coffee decreases the amount of insulin and the length of time it is in your system, so it is not a good idea to drink coffee and take insulin, even if not at the same time.

Sulfonylurea drugs also may be prescribed by your doctor. If you take any of these drugs, also take extra vitamin B_{12}, because they all lower levels of that vitamin in your body. The names of these drugs are Acetohexamide (Dymelor), Chlorpropamide (Diabinese), Glimepiride (Amaryl), Glipizide (Glucotrol), Glyburide (Blyburide), Tolazamide (Tolinase), and Tolbutamide (Orinase). These drugs are taken by mouth and lower the amount of sugar in your bloodstream by stimulating your pancreas to make more insulin. They also increase the risk of dying of heart disease, and tend to cause weight gain, one of the causes of diabetes. In addition, they can lead to hypoglycemia or low blood sugar by removing too much sugar. Other side effects include vomiting, nausea, gas, heartburn, diarrhea, and constipation. Over time, the effects of these drugs lessen. Also, if you have heart problems and take these drugs, you are 2.5 times more likely to die from heart problems. If you are pregnant or have liver, kidney, pituitary, or adrenal problems or are an older adult, debilitated, or malnourished, you may not want to take these drugs. Do not drink alcohol when taking any of these drugs or you may suffer from dizziness, weakness, mental confusion, collapse, or coma.

Another diabetes drug is called metformin (Glucophage). Like all of the other diabetes drugs you take by mouth, it can cause digestive discomfort, impair kidney and liver function, and should never be taken if you drink alcohol. Troglitazone (Rezulin) is another antidiabetic agent. Heart failure and liver failure are possible side effects of taking this drug.

Your doctor also may order medication for you if you have pain. All pain medications have adverse effects. Some of the most commonly ordered pain agents and their negative effects were recently listed in *Clinician Reviews*.

Pain Agent	Negative Effects
Amitriptyline	dry mouth, light sensitivity, urine retention, drowsiness, weight gain, fast heartbeat, delirium, bone marrow depression, severe heart effects
Capsaicin cream	local redness, burning, itching, cough
Carbamazepine	rash, drowsiness, blurred and double vision, headache, nausea, anemia, cardiac toxicity, bleeding, reeling gait
Gabapentin	sleepiness, reeling gait, fatigue, dizziness, eye problems, movement disorders, behavioral changes in children
Ibuprofen or Naproxen	drowsiness, nausea, diarrhea, dizziness, indigestion, stomach/intestinal ulcers, liver toxicity
Lidocaine	drowsiness, agitation, ringing in the ears, slurred speech, disorientation, coma, seizures, heart disorders, strange skin sensations
Mexiletine	stomach and intestinal upset, fatigue, nervousness, fever, tremor, sleep upset, psychosis, liver inflammation, visual disturbances, seizures, blood disorders
Phenytoin	double vision, drowsiness, rash, anemia, liver toxicity, kidney inflammation
Tramadol	nausea, vomiting headache, constipation, dizziness, seizures

If you have Charcot foot, rest is the primary treatment. No weight should be placed on the foot for eight to twelve weeks or longer. Once healing has occurred, you may be asked to use a walking brace, followed by a permanent foot orthosis. Once you develop Charcot foot in one foot you are at risk for developing it in the other foot. Protect your unaffected foot with a soft orthosis and a soft supportive shoe.

Self-Care Measures You Can Take

Specific foods and herbs, supplements, foot care, and exercise can reduce your risk for diabetes. Being overweight is an important risk factor for diabetes. If you're overweight, make sure you lose weight. Smoking also is a risk factor for heart and blood vessel complications, so you must quit.

Watch What You Eat

Cut down on salt, refined carbohydrates including white bread, pastries, candies and cake, fish oil capsules, and supplements containing large amounts of paraaminobenzoic acid (PABA). Consumption of these products can result in elevated blood sugar. A study in the *American Journal of Clinical Nutrition* found that it's important to eat whole grains to reduce risk for adult diabetes and to limit intake of white bread, white rice, and potatoes. Add good fats, including olive oil and fish, and chicken and turkey without skin to your regular eating fare.

Eat whole fruits and stop drinking fruit juices. Drinking fruit juice causes blood sugar to rise more rapidly than eating the fruit itself.

Prepare more spinach and beef, or take alpha lipoic acid as a supplement (50 to 200 mg a day). It greatly improves insulin function and protects against nerve damage, a complication of diabetes.

Eat green peppers, strawberries, citrus fruit, honeydew melons, cooked broccoli, Brussels sprouts or kale, cantaloupes, papayas, cooked cauliflower, raspberries, parsley, raw cabbage, blackberries, onions, and spinach. All are full of vitamin C, which may correct insulin resistance and the inflexible blood vessels characteristic of diabetes.

Eat more onions and garlic. Studies in the *Indian Journal of Experimental Biology* and the *American Journal of Natural Medicine* provided evidence for the ability of onions and garlic to lower blood sugar levels, and to lower blood pressure and cholesterol in people with diabetes.

Foods that help normalize blood sugar including spirulina, berries, cheese, fish, garlic, kelp, sauerkraut, soybeans, and vegetables. Make sure you eat plenty of them.

Breast-Feed

To protect your children from diabetes, breast-feed them. Studies reported in *Diabetes Metabolism and Research Review* and *Diabetes* provide evidence that cow's milk can trigger diabetes in children.

Use Herbs to Heal

Investigate the use of herbs. Use them in consultation with a herbologist. Ginseng root can lower glucose levels, according to a study in *Journal of the American College of Nutrition*. **Caution:** Do not use this herb if you have high blood pressure.

Try fenugreek seeds as a tea or powder. A study in the *European Journal of Clinical Nutrition* found that fenugreek seeds show significant antidiabetic effects.

Take milk thistle (silymarin), an antioxidant that enhances the function of your liver, an organ that works with the pancreas to regulate your level of glucose. A study in the *Journal of Heptology* found that 600 mg of silymarin daily reduced glucose by 9.5 to 15 percent over twelve months, lowered the level of sugar in the urine, required less insulin, and showed less glucose damage to the cells.

Some other herbs that may be helpful are huckleberry (promotes insulin production), bilberry, dandelion, and uva ursi. Talk to a herbalist or a healthcare practitioner who is knowledgeable prior to taking any herbs.

Investigate Vitamins and Supplements

Try some vitamins and supplements; avoid others. A study in the *American Journal of Clinical Nutrition* found that high doses of vitamin E (1,200 IU per day) reduced the risk for hardening of the arteries (atherosclerosis) in people with diabetes.

Another study in the *American Journal of Clinical Nutrition* found that vitamin A helped insulin control blood sugar, while a 1996 study in the *Journal of Clinical Investigation* reported that vitamin C helps blood vessel changes in diabetes. Other research is investigating the use of vitamin C supplements to inhibit the process of glycosylation, the binding of glucose (sugar) onto proteins in the blood, nerve cells, and lenses of the eyes that may be responsible for many of the long-term effects of diabetes. Vitamin C supplements may slow it.

You may want to take a vitamin E supplement. This powerful antioxidant reduces the risk of heart disease, stroke, cancer, and Alzheimer's, all strongly associated with diabetes. Some research provides evidence that vitamin E can improve insulin function and reduce blood sugar. Take 400 IU only in the form of natural d-alpha tocopherol vitamin E.

Avoid taking supplements containing the amino acid cysteine (interferes with insulin absorption), and large amounts of vitamin B_1 (thiamine). Excessive amounts can inactivate insulin.

Take chromium picolinate daily. A study published in *Diabetes* found that people with type 2 diabetes who took chromium picolinate daily brought glucose and insulin levels back to normal after four months. Although there are no known contraindications to chromium use and no documented studies show that chromium interacts with other drugs, be sure to have your doctor monitor your glucose levels carefully and reduce your diabetes medication as chromium begins to enhance your body's insulin sensitivity. A usual daily dose is 200 micrograms a day, but if you have severe glucose impairments it may take 400 to 600 mcg a day. Do not exceed 1,000 mcg a day. **Caution:** According to *Clinician Reviews*, there have been reports of single instances of kidney impairment at 1,200 to 2,400 mcg a day.

Vitamin D is associated with type 1 diabetes, according to a study in *Clinical Endocrinology*. Until definitive studies are completed, make sure either to obtain sufficient protected sunlight or take a multivitamin that contains vitamin D.

Zinc supplements can protect against type 1 diabetes, according to a study in *Experimental Biological Medicine* and *Journal of the American College of Nutrition*.

According to a study in *Lik Sprava*, people with diabetes may have low levels of iron, manganese, and zinc. As a precaution, you may want to take a multivitamin that contains these minerals.

A study in *Archives of Medical Research* showed that magnesium depletion is present in patients with foot ulcers. If you have foot ulcers, or want to protect against them, you may want to take a multivitamin that contains magnesium.

Curcumin (turmeric), a common spice, may protect you from diabetic nephropathy through its ability to lower blood cholesterol levels, according to a study in *Molecular Cell Biochemistry*.

Take Care of Your Feet

Take good care of your feet. Loss of pain, pressure, and temperature sensitivity in the feet due to blood vessel changes put you at a high risk for foot problems, including ulcers and amputation. Here's what you can do:

- Inspect your feet, toes, and between your toes every day for cuts and blisters.

- Wash your feet daily in lukewarm water. Use a thermometer to check water temperature so it's 80 degrees Fahrenheit.

- Dry your feet thoroughly and apply moisturizer, but not petroleum jelly. Castor oil is very good for dry skin. Avoid applying anything between your toes.

- If your feet perspire a lot, apply foot powder, but don't let it accumulate between your toes.

- Don't walk around barefoot.

- Make sure your shoes fit properly. Break in a new pair of shoes over several days.

- Always wear 100 percent cotton socks without seams with shoes. Avoid nylon knee-high stockings and constrictive clothing. Change your socks and shoes every three to four hours while you're awake or whenever your feet are damp or wet. All shoes begin to allow the foot to slide parallel to the length of the sole of the shoe after three to four hours of continuous use.

- File your toenails straight across. Do not cut them.

- Do not cut or use chemical removers on corns or calluses. See a podiatrist.

- See a healthcare provider regularly for a thorough foot examination.

- Avoid using antiseptics and strong adhesives on your feet.

- Avoid exposure to cold. If your feet feel cold, put on another pair of socks. Don't use heating pads, electric blankets, or hot water bottles, or soak your feet in water.

- Notify your healthcare provider if you notice unexplained swelling, change in color, throbbing pain, new wounds or an increase in wound draining in your lower legs or feet, or fever.

Exercise Daily

Exercise daily. Studies in *Journal of the American Medical Association* and *Stroke* showed that exercise reduces the development of diabetes.

Check the Drugs You're Taking

Be sure you are not taking prescription drugs that can cause high blood sugar, including drugs to lower blood pressure (clonidine, diazoxide); diuretics; drugs to treat tuberculosis (rifampin, isoniazid); calcium channel blockers (nifedipine, nicardipine, diltiazem, verapamil corticosteroids [prednisone; diuretics; bronchodilators and decongestants containing epinephrine]); blood thinners (heparin); H2 blockers (Tagamet, Zantac); hypothyroid drugs (Levoxine, Synthroid); painkillers (morphine); oral contraceptives; and drugs to treat seizures (Phenytoin [Dilantin]).

If you are diabetic and having trouble controlling your blood sugar, be aware that taking any of the following substances can lower your blood sugar: alcohol, allopurinol (Lopurin, Zyloprim), ampicillin, Bromocriptine, Chloramphenicol (Chloromycetin), Clofibrate (Abitrate, Atromid-S), Fenfluramine (Pondimin), Indomethacin, lithium, Mebendazole, monoamine oxidase (MAO) inhibitors, phenylbutazone (Butatab, Butazolidin), probenecid (Benemid, Probalan), salicylates (aspirin), tetracycline, and theophylline.

Use Affirmations

Another explanation for diabetes is a metaphysical one. It appears in *Heal Your Body*. The theory is that longing for what might have been, a great need to control, and deep sorrow without sweetness lead to diabetes. It contends that thoughts held and words repeatedly used create our lives and experiences. If you change your thoughts, you can change the way you view your experiences, and eventually your experiences.

To begin to reverse negative thoughts that could be damaging, choose one of the following statements and write or say it twenty times a day. Also write it on 3 × 5 cards and place them in prominent places around you:

- I fill all my moments with joy and sweetness.
- I choose to experience the wonder and sweetness of this day.

Digestive Problems

Digestive problems range all the way from constipation, diarrhea, and flatulence to Crohn's disease, colitis, diverticular disease, gastro-esophageal reflux disease, irritable bowel syndrome, ulcers, and leaky gut syndrome. Many digestive conditions have similar symptoms.

Constipation is the inability to have regular bowel movements. As few as two to three bowel movements a week should be considered normal if you have limited activity and low fluid intake. *Diarrhea* is a signal that not all is well. It is your body's way of getting rid of offending toxins. It could be spicy foods, dairy products, old leftovers, or a virus that causes the symptom. *Flatulence*, or gassiness, is created by bacteria in your large intestine feeding upon carbohydrates that your body cannot digest. Fermentation produces gas. Most people pass gas an average of fourteen times a day.

Crohn's disease is a condition of ulcerating lesions that can occur anywhere in the gastrointestinal tract, but most often in the small intestine. *Colitis* is an inflammation of primarily the large intestine or colon. *Diverticular disease* is a distinctly Western condition that causes herniations, mostly in the lining of the colon or large intestine. It affects about half of the U.S. population over age sixty. Diet, especially eating many low-fiber foods, is a strong contributing factor.

Gastroesophageal reflux disease (GERD), also called severe heartburn, is a chronic condition. It occurs when the food in your stomach enters and remains in the impaired lower esophagus. Usually the muscle between the esophagus and the stomach, the lower esophageal sphincter (LES), clamps tight, keeping acid and partly digested food in the stomach, where they belong. It relaxes temporarily when you swallow to let food into your stomach. When this muscle becomes loose, lazy, or otherwise weak, the muscle relaxes and stomach acid can splash up your gullet. This hurts, and if it happens often enough, it can damage the lining of your esophagus. It is most apt to happen in people who are overweight, pregnant, have a hiatal hernia, use foods or drugs that relax the sphincter, or are stressed. Pyrosis, the classic symptom, is perceived as a burning pain in the sternum area, above the stomach, neck, throat, or back. It usually occurs after a meal and is heightened by bending over or lying down. It is relieved by standing up and swallowing saliva, water, or antacids. Other symptoms include difficulty swallowing (dysphagia), belching, regurgitation of food, pain during swallowing (odynophagia), and feeling full without eating much (early satiety).

Irritable bowel syndrome (IBS) is a disorder of the upper and lower gastrointestinal tract. The likely symptoms include abdominal pain, constipation or diarrhea, and distention or bloating after meals. Women are more often afflicted than men, and there is no known anatomical cause. Emotional factors, diet, drugs, or hormones may precipitate or aggravate it. Stress and emotional conflict that result in depression often coincide with the beginning or recurrence of IBS. One study found a relationship between IBS and emotional abuse. Self-blame and self-silencing are apt to be responses of a person feeling responsible for the abuse but being unable to express their feelings about it. This in turn could stop them from seeking help and raise their stress levels. Both could exacerbate IBS symptoms, according to a study in *Psychosomatic Medicine*.

Ulcers were once thought to be caused by nerves and were treated with milk and cream. It is now believed that a bacterium named *Helicobacter pylori (H. pylori)* is a cause of stomach ulcers. Doctors are still puzzled about why some people catch this bug and others don't. Only 75 percent of those with stomach ulcers have this bacterium. Although it runs in families, it can't be spread from one person to another. Nearly all the medicine currently used to ease joint pain and stiffness can create bleeding ulcers, including aspirin and ibuprofen. Many drugs also can mask the condition.

Leaky gut syndrome, or intestinal permeability, is an inflammation of the intestinal wall. The condition allows bacteria, partially digested food particles, and toxins to leak into spaces in your gut wall. Experts believe that a number of digestion-related ailments either cause or result from it, including irritable bowel syndrome, fatigue, and malnutrition. The syndrome also may be caused by the use of nonsteroidal anti-inflammatory drugs such as ibuprofen and aspirin. Other causes include consumption of hard liquor, sugar, caffeine, antacids, and antibiotics, as well as other prescription drugs.

Inflammatory damage to your gut wall can compromise the carrier proteins that attach to nutrients and carry them through the gut wall into the bloodstream, where your body puts them to use. Without carrier proteins, you are at risk for vitamin and mineral deficiencies.

Your Risk for Developing Digestive Problems

If you eat a low-fiber, highly-processed-food diet, including refined flour, sugar, and canned foods, your risk for digestive diseases increases. Dietary habits usually are set in our youth, when we can get away with eating poorly because our own enzymes compensate and we have abundant gastric juices and a strong liver to get rid of toxic wastes. In middle age you produce less hydrochloric acid in your stomach, and digestive problems can occur. Other sources of digestive problems are stress and prescribed or over-the-counter drugs.

How the Doctor Diagnoses Digestive Problems

In many cases, the symptoms you tell your doctor about will be enough to help him or her decide which digestive condition you have. Your doctor may order a barium enema (you'll be asked to swallow some barium, and X rays will be taken that show how it moves through your digestive system) or a colonoscopy (a scope is passed up to your colon through your anus, and changes in your large intestine can be viewed).

If bleeding is suspected, the doctor may order a tagged red blood cell bleeding scan. An occult blood test also could be used. In this case the doctor or nurse practitioner will perform a rectal exam to obtain a sample, which is placed on a test card. You also can send a stool sample, on the card, to the doctor. Developer is then placed on the card. The appearance of blue on or at the edge of the test sample within sixty seconds indicates the presence of occult blood—blood that may not be visible to the eye—according to the *American Journal of Nursing*.

Early signs of a silent ulcer include weight loss, a feeling of fullness before you finish your meal, anemia, and fatigue. If you experience these symptoms, seek medical care immediately.

What the Doctor Will Probably Prescribe

Antacids and acid-blocking drugs such as Tagamet and Zantac are often used for heartburn or ulcers. H2 blockers block the stomach's response to acid stimulators such as food, caffeine, insulin, and histamine. Since ulcers aren't caused by excess stomach acid but by bacteria, these drugs will not help with ulcers. They also can cause calcium, phosphorus, and magnesium level imbalances in the body, according to *Prescription Alternatives*, and vitamin B_{12} may not be very well absorbed if you are taking Tagamet, Pepcid, Axid, or Zantac. The valve that must open to allow food to pass from the stomach into the small intestine is triggered by the acid in your stomach. If you take acid-blocking H2 blocker drugs, your body may not be able to absorb nutrients properly. Antacids also deplete your body of calcium and phosphate, resulting in weakened bones and muscles and making it hard for you to absorb vitamins A and D and thiamin. Since antacids block stomach acid, it will be hard for your body to absorb necessary nutrients from your food.

Possible side effects from Zantac include reduction in your liver's ability to detoxify other drugs you may be taking, rash, severe headache, sleepiness or fatigue, diarrhea, jaundice, stomach pain, and itching, decrease in the number of your blood cells, dizziness, blurred vision, hepatitis and changes in liver function. This drug shouldn't be used if you have porphyria, kidney or liver problems, or if you are under sixteen. Zantac prolongs the effects of sulfonylureas (used by adult diabetes), theophyllines (for asthma, shortness of breath, and water retention), blood thinners (warfarin), alcohol, and procanbid (for heartbeat irregularity). If you have any of the adverse effects listed, report them to your doctor.

Pepcid and Pepcid AC are used for ulcers, heartburn, acid indigestion, and Zollinger-Ellison syndrome (which causes oversecretion of stomach acid). If you have kidney or liver problems, use these medications with caution.

Axid is used for ulcers, acid indigestion, heartburn, gastroesophageal reflux disease, and prevention of bleeding in the stomach and intestine. Adverse reactions include dizziness, anemia, sweating, and itching. Axid also can increase blood levels of aspirin and can make the effects of alcohol stronger.

Tagament is used for ulcers in the stomach or small intestine, GERD, and prevention of bleeding in the stomach and intestine. Take this drug with caution if you have a liver or kidney condition. Tagament can potentiate blood thinners, lidocaine, phenytoin, and other drugs. It can cause diarrhea, dizziness, sleepiness, heartbeat irregularities, low blood pressure, nervous system disturbances, kidney inflammation, pancreas inflammation, rash, joint swelling, headache, muscle pain and stiffness, blood cell changes, and enlargement of male breasts.

Antacids don't treat underlying problems and can make symptoms worse because they inhibit pepsin, the enzyme that helps you break down proteins.

Antacids also can cause rebound acid production and make your acid levels rise above normal once the antacid wears off. If you use an antacid or antacids with high levels of calcium carbonate and sodium bicarbonate at the same time, you can develop *milk-alkali syndrome*, which includes headache, nausea, irritability, kidney damage, and weakness.

Long-term use of aluminum-containing antacids can lead to phosphate depletion and loss of appetite, exhaustion, weakness, and bone problems. Using Tums as a source of calcium will only replace what the antacid is blocking. It does not provide sufficient calcium to enhance healing and strengthen bones.

Avoid antacids if you have high blood pressure, kidney failure, congestive heart failure, or are on a low-sodium diet, until you use a low-sodium version. If you are undergoing or have had a recent stomach or intestinal hemorrhage, avoid aluminum-containing antacids.

Antacids can reduce the potency of or decrease the amount of time they are effective for many drugs. Consult your pharmacist.

Antidiarrhea drugs have constipating effects, making feces more solid. Don't use Motofen if you've been taking antibiotics, if your diarrhea is caused by bacteria, or if you have colitis, jaundice, glaucoma, a heart condition, urinary problems, myasthenia gravis, angina, or liver or kidney disease.

Logen, Lomotil, Lonox, and Lomanate also are prescribed for diarrhea. If you have colitis, have been taking a broad-spectrum antibiotic, or have liver or kidney disease, use caution in taking this drug. Consult your pharmacist and also ask about possible interactions with other drugs you're taking.

Diar-Aid, Imodium A-D, Kaopectate, Maalox, Neo-Diaral, and

Pepto Diarrhea Control are all medications used to slow the water and electrolyte transfer into the bowel. Never use these drugs if you are taking a broad-spectrum antibiotic, have a kidney problem, have ulcerative colitis, have blood diarrhea or a fever above 101 degrees Fahrenheit, you may have a bacterial infection or you have any other disease that could be worsened by constipation.

Other drugs for diarrhea include Bismatrol and Pepto-Bismol. Adverse effects include severe constipation, especially in debilitated people and infants. Stools may be temporarily gray or black. Never use these drugs if you have a high fever, rectal bleeding, muscle cramps, weakness or dizziness, are on a low-salt diet (find a low-sodium version), or have congestive heart failure or kidney disease.

Drugs for constipation include laxatives, stimulants/irritants, lubricants, and surfactants. All of these can alter your body's fluid and mineral balance. If you take any of them, be sure to drink eight to ten glasses of water a day and take a mineral supplement that includes magnesium and potassium.

Irritants include Ex-Lax, Espotabs, Feen-a-mint, Modane, Evac-U-Gen, Medilax, Senokot, Dulcagen, Dulcolax, Fleet Laxative, Bisco-Lux, and Senexon. If you take any of these regularly, you may become dehydrated and low in potassium. Your large intestine will lose its ability to contract on its own, and some of these products can discolor your stools.

Bulk-producing laxatives are full of fiber. They hold water and make your stools softer and easier to evacuate. These agents are the safest products to use, but be sure you take them with plenty of water. Psyllium is useful for irritable bowel syndrome, spastic colon, and hemorrhoids. It lowers LDL (bad) cholesterol, too and has no adverse effects.

Lubricants such as castor oil and mineral oil are sold under the brand names of Fleet Flavored Castor Oil, Purge, Neoloid, Neo-Cuetol, and Milkinol. Large doses of any of these produces can cause discomfort, leakage from the anus, irritation, hemorrhoids, and itching. They also make it difficult for you to absorb needed nutrients, including vitamins A, D, and E.

Self-Care Measures You Can Take

Be active in preventing digestive disorders. It is always more difficult to treat a disorder once it occurs. Remember, if you are taking medications to treat digestive symptoms, you are only *treating the symptoms, not the underlying cause or causes.*

Affirmations for All Digestive Conditions

Optimism and positive thinking have been shown to affect disease progression. Being chronically hostile, depressed, or apathetic can lead to disease. Friedman has found that hardy people have self-healing personalities that make them resilient and healthy.

Consider using one or more of the following affirmations. Be sure to write or speak them at least twenty times a day to replace the negative thoughts that may be holding back your self-healing personality. Put the ones you like best on 3 × 5 cards and place them in prominent spots where you'll read them every day.

For colitis:

- I am part of the perfect flow of life.
- Everything in my life is orderly and clear.
- Life flows through me in perfect rhythm.

For constipation:

- I release the past and new and fresh life flows through me.
- I allow joyous life to flow through me.
- I give of myself to others.

For Crohn's disease:

- I relinquish the past.
- I live in the joyous present.
- I am free.

For diarrhea:

- I am at complete peace.
- I live in calm and serenity.
- My digestion and elimination are ordered and perfect.

For diverticular disease:

- Everything flows through me in an even and calm way.
- I easily eliminate whatever is nonuseful.

- My life is calm and peaceful.

For heartburn:

- I am calm and safe.
- I trust my life processes.
- I breathe calmly and fully.

For irritable bowel syndrome:

- I absorb precious nutrients.
- I release only what is not useful to me.
- My body uses whatever I eat for its greatest good.

For ulcers:

- I am healthy and calm.
- I am at peace in my world.
- I believe in myself.

Nutrition for All Digestive Conditions

No matter what your digestive condition, a few principles will prove beneficial. Digestion begins in the mouth, so be sure to chew your food well before swallowing. This will trigger acid in your stomach and enzymes that aid in digestion. This action also will put less stress on the rest of your digestive system.

Consider changing to a vegetarian diet. Vegetarians have lower cholesterol and also may have a lower risk for constipation, diverticular disease, appendicitis, and gallstones.

Another thing you can do to aid your digestive system is to eat foods high in zinc, magnesium, B vitamins, pantothenic acid, biotin, molybdenum, manganese, copper, iron, and selenium. Each plays the role of digestive enzyme cofactor. To have healthy digestive enzymes you need to eat foods rich in B vitamins: sunflower seeds, whole wheat flour, rolled oats, green peas, soybeans, lima beans, crabmeat, brown rice, asparagus, raisins, wheat germ, chicken, hazelnuts, peanuts, hickory nuts, spinach, kale, peas, salmon, prunes, lentils, tuna, turkey, rabbit, white beans, mackerel, bananas, walnuts, sweet potatoes, cooked cabbage, sardines, trout, herring, sea vegetables (kombu, dulse, kelp, and wakame), fermented soy products (tempeh, natto, and miso), turnips, cantaloupes, buckwheat, lobster, broccoli, and cauliflower.

Magnesium also can be helpful. It can be found in figs, green leafy vegetables, citrus fruits, whole grain breads and cereal, brown rice, wheat germ, and soy flour. Zinc enhances healing also. Some foods rich in zinc are pumpkin seeds, whole grains, oysters, herring, liver, eggs, nuts, and wheat germ.

Eat more biotin-rich foods, including nutritional yeast, liver, eggs, mushrooms, lima beans, yogurt, and a variety of nuts, fish, and grains. You can increase your supply of molybdenum by eating more beans, cereal grains, legumes, peas, and dark green leafy vegetables.

Other foods to focus on that are rich in manganese, copper, iron, or selenium are almonds, avocados, barley, beans, dandelion greens, lentils, sea vegetables, kelp, kidney beans, egg yolks, whole grain breads and cereals, seafood, brewer's yeast, asparagus, garlic, and mushrooms.

Don't drink fluids, especially cold ones, when you're eating. They can suppress stomach acid, according to *Prescription Alternatives*. A large percentage of people over fifty make too little stomach acid, so they aren't able to thoroughly digest their food. Taking antacids, Tagamet, and Zantac can alleviate symptoms for a while, but they can aggravate the underlying problem, which is usually too little stomach acid. Long-term use of these drugs can compromise digestion and decrease the uptake of needed vitamins and minerals.

Because you have indigestion and discomfort after you eat, you may think it's because of too much stomach acid, so you pop an antacid. Doing this further suppresses your stomach's ability to generate hydrochloric acid (HCL) and can aggravate the problem if your problem is that you have too *little* HCL!

How can you tell if you have too little HCL? Take a tablespoon of apple cider vinegar or lemon juice when you have heartburn. If the heartburn goes away, you need more acid, not less. If your symptoms worsen, take enzyme products or supplements that contain HCL. You can find them at any health food store.

The Web site of Andrew Weil, M.D., "Ask Doctor Weil," suggests other actions to take to promote healing of your intestines and leaky gut syndrome. Take an amino acid, l-glutamine, take extra vitamin A (drink 12 ounces of carrot juice and 2 ounces of kale, watercress, beet, spinach, or dandelion greens juice; eat papayas, fish, sweet potatoes, pumpkin, yellow squash, apricots, cantaloupes, parsley, broccoli, or turnip greens); eat foods high in B vitamins, folic acid, and zinc (see the foods just recommended); drink 2 to 3 ounces of aloe vera juice (do not use an aloe plant; buy the juice from a health food store) after each meal; and take probiotics such as acidophilus and bifidus ("good" bacteria) to restore the normal flora of your intestinal tract.

If you use oil for salad or cooking, choose extra virgin olive oil. A review of studies of olive oil in the *European Journal of Cancer* reported that patients with ulcerative colitis and Crohn's disease generate high quantities of reactive oxygen species. Antioxident compounds present in olive oil inhibit this free-radical generation and enhance healthy tissue.

Massage Your Ileocecal Valve Points

A lazy ileocecal valve can make it difficult for your body to process your food properly, resulting in food backing up or moving too quickly through your body. Massaging some points on the body could help. These points may be extremely sore at first. If you are too weak, have a trusted friend firmly massage the points, or use a vibrator (available in health food and department stores).

The next time you have flulike symptoms, fatigue, sore throat, constipation, or diarrhea, try rubbing these points. Massage with firm pressure, for no longer ten to twenty seconds, the inside and outside of your thighs, angling across the top of the left arm, right beneath the bony ridge that runs across the back of the head on the right side, and outside of the right calf about a third of the way down from the knee. According to *Alternatives*, massaging longer than twenty seconds is not beneficial and could negate the effect. If you have been "backed up," detoxify your body by taking chlorophyll tablets or liquid; eliminating spicy foods for a week or ten days; and totally eliminating alcohol, cocoa, chocolate, and caffeine products.

For Colitis

- Take acidophilus (from a health food store) daily to restore the overgrowth of *Clostridia difficile*, an organism that can cause relentless colitis.

- Eliminate sweets, alcohol, and caffeine. All can irritate your intestinal lining.

- If you have a lactase deficiency, don't eat dairy products. These can trigger an inflammation of your intestine.

- Eat foods high in essential fatty acids. These substances can prevent ulcerative colitis and are found in green leafy vegetables, flaxseed, rapeseed, and walnuts (*American Journal of Clinical Nutrition*).

For Constipation

- Slowly move to a vegetarian eating style. Vegetarians have been found to have a lower incidence of constipation, according to *Digestive Diseases*.

- Drink at least ten glasses of water every day. You could be dehyrated. Water is used by many digestive processes, and for them to work correctly, you must supply water daily.

- Avoid aluminum-containing antacids. They cause constipation, intestinal blockage, and dangerously high levels of aluminum.

- Try psyllium (a teaspoonful in a full glass of water before breakfast, and drink it down before it gels).

- Eat more fresh vegetables, fruits, legumes (dry beans, peas, and peanuts) and nibble on prunes. Eating guava, plum, mango, and quince also can prevent *Escherichia coli* infections according to a study in the *Archives of Medical Research*.

- Exercise every day, even if you only take a walk. Gradually build up to walking twenty minutes a day at a brisk clip. Your digestive system will be massaged, and it will work better.

- Find alternatives to medicines that cause constipation (diuretics, painkillers, tranquilizers, antihistamines, narcotics, decongestants, antidepressants, and the overuse of laxatives).

- Acidophilus culture taken with a little milk (for better absorption) or as plain yogurt with active cultures also may help. It builds up "good" bacteria, which help digest stagnating food and increase the movement of the intestine in a day or two.

- Explore taking the herb silymarin (milk thistle). A study in *Planta Medica* showed silymarin reduces colon damage and has anti-inflammatory activity.

- Consider biofeedback. A study reported in *Gut* found that patients with constipation showed significant improvement after biofeedback treatment. Ask your doctor for a referral, or find a practitioner in the yellow pages.

- Acupuncture works for children with constipation, according to a study reported in *Digestive Diseases and Science*.

For Crohn's Disease

- Fatty acids have been shown to be helpful in Crohn's disease, according to a report in the *American Journal of Nutrition*. Make sure you eat plenty of fish, green leafy vegetables, flaxseed, and walnuts to get sufficient fatty acids.

- A study reported in the *Scandinavian Journal of Gastroenterology* found that participants with Crohn's disease had lower levels of certain antioxidants. The authors suggested taking beta-carotene, vitamin E, and gluthathione peroxidase for Crohn's disease.

- Another study, this time reported in the *European Journal of Gastroenterology and Hepatology*, found that a vegetable, soy, and lactose (milk)-free diet improved the nutritional status of participants. If you have this condition, consider adding more vegetables and soy products and eliminating milk and cheese.

- Another supplement to consider taking is zinc. In a study reported in *Inflammatory Bowel Disease*, zinc helped heal the gut in patients with Crohn's disease and could help reduce the risk of relapse.

For Diarrhea

- Drink at least ten glasses of water every day so you don't get dehydrated.

- If diarrhea goes on for more than five days, see your doctor. Severe diarrhea in infants, children, or older adults needs medical attention within three days.

- Mix 1 heaping teaspoonful of carob powder (from a health food store) with water one to three times a day.

- Avoid magnesium-containing antacids (check the label). These antacids can worsen diarrhea.

- *Prescription Alternatives* recommends a number of natural alternatives to drugs. Let the diarrhea run its course for a day or two; you should drink at least eight glasses of water a day. Avoid caffeine, soft drinks, and sugary foods, which exacerbate the condition. See which foods seem to irritate the condition. Try to eat rice, cereal, bananas, and potatoes—they are rich in carbohydrates and gentle to your stomach. Fill up on acidophilus or plain yogurt to restore the good bacteria you've lost through diarrhea. Take a mineral supplement that has potassium and magnesium to restore lost electrolytes.

- A report in the *British Journal of Nutrition* found that large doses of vitamin A is recommended in cases of persistent diarrhea and even dysentery.

- If you have fecal incontinence, take dietary fiber found in psyllium. It was associated with a decrease in the percentage of incontinent stools, according to *Nursing Research*.

For Diverticular Disease

- Avoid nuts, seeds, corn, and popcorn if they seem to bother you. Also avoid meat. A study published in *Disease of the Colon and Rectum* found that frequent meat consumption was correlated with diverticulosis.

- Gradually eat more fruits, vegetables, and whole grains. A high-fiber diet seems to completely relieve symptoms and may prevent further diverticular formation, according to *The Clinical Advisor.* In fact, a total vegetarian diet may be best. Vegetarians were found to have a lower incidence of diverticular disease, according to *Digestive Diseases.*

- Take one to three teaspoonfuls of psyllium in a glass of water an hour before breakfast.

- Avoid antibiotics unless you have an infection (diverticulitis) as diagnosed by your doctor.

- Exercise. A study reported in *Gut* found that physical activity, especially jogging and running, along with a high-fiber diet, can prevent the symptoms of diverticular disease. If you can't jog or run, start walking, building up gradually to a brisk rhythm.

For Flatulence and Upset Stomach

- Take three to four charcoal capsules after meals for one to two days. **Caution:** Don't take it for more than three days in a row because it will retard your body's ability to absorb needed nutrients. Do not take charcoal with other medicines or nutritional supplements. Charcoal can turn your stools black.

- Avoid eating melons with other foods. Eat them separately at least two hours between other foods.

- Start a food/gas diary. See what foods and what combinations of foods and at what time of day result in gas. Avoid eating those foods and those combinations. Foods that often cause gas are oat bran, high-fiber cereals, beans, onions, apples, and broccoli, but you may have your own foods that create gas for you. Consider trying Beano (for gas from beans, or add cider vinegar to beans). Lactaid may reduce gas from milk and dairy products.

- Peppermint tea has been used for centuries in Europe to quell stomach and liver ailments. King Henry VIII, well known for gluttony, supposedly was advised by his court physician to drink a goblet of hot mint tea with heavy meals. Both peppermint, and to a lesser extent, spearmint tea help to neutralize excess hydrochloric acid that accompanies a previous meal.

- Chamomile tea is made from the dried flowerheads of Roman chamomile, so if you are allergic to those flowers, don't use this tea. The tea releases an almost hypnotic odor that may work on your brain and nervous system to calm you. A cup of it can neutralize gas and reduce muscle spasms.

- Try eating more papaya. The unripe fruit, leaves, and trunk yield a milky substance rich in papain, a digestive enzyme. You also can take it in tablet form, but many of the products have a lot of sugar and other nonbeneficial substances in them, so read the label carefully. Consider eating a slice of ripe papaya or drinking a glass of papaya juice with your meals.

For Severe Heartburn (GERD)

- Eliminate the following foods to see if your symptoms abate: caffeinated food or drink (coffee, tea, cola, and chocolate), esophageal irritants (citrus fruits, vinegar, spicy foods, tomatoes), lower esophageal sphincter relaxants (onions, garlic, mint, alcoholic beverages), high-fat foods (including fried foods, cheese, meat, cakes, pies, and processed foods that contain oil and have a high fat content).

- Change the way you eat. Don't drink fluids while you're eating—drink before you eat or two hours later. Stop eating big meals, and don't eat a meal within three hours of bedtime.

- Eat a dark green salad or raw vegetables at least once a day. Add sprouted beans, peanuts, and seeds.

- Chew your food thoroughly.

- Try chewing gum for half an hour after you eat. A study in *Psychology & Health Update* found that chewing sugarless gum (Peelu and Sylifresh NF are both all-natural and sugar-free) after meals increases saliva production, which helps clear away the gastric acids that cause heartburn.

- If you're low on stomach acid, which you may be if you're over fifty, add from a teaspoonful to a tablespoonful of cider vinegar to a glass of water and drink it half an hour before meals. Try deglycyrrizinated licorice, or a glass of raw cabbage or potato juice. Herbal teas that can help include fenugreek, slippery elm, and licorice. Fresh papayas or bananas can help, too. Eat several small meals a day, and don't overeat, or eat on the run or right before you exercise.

- Never lie down after you eat. Since stress may be a factor, try meditation and exercise to reduce it.

- Here are some of the drugs that can cause heartburn: antacids, antibiotics, antidepressants, antihistamines, aspirin (take the herb white willow instead; it is the basis of aspirin but doesn't upset your digestion), transdermal nicotine (to stop smoking), anticholinergics, adrenergic antagonists, benzodiazepines, calcium channel blockers, cholecystokinin, levodopa, narcotics, nitrates, ibuprofen, asthma drugs, chemotherapy drugs, prednisone, beta-blockers, cholesterol-lowering and blood-pressure-lowering drugs, painkillers/narcotics, Premarin, Provera, tranquilizers/barbiturates, and ulcer drugs (sulfasalazine, sucralfate, misoprostol). Stop taking the over-the-counter drugs and find alternatives. If you're not sure if you're taking any of these drugs, ask your pharmacist. Talk to your doctor about alternatives to the prescription drugs that may be irritating you.

- Eat artichokes or take artichoke-leaf extract. Artichokes stimulate the formation and flow of bile to and from the liver. They help you break down and eliminate fats, including cholesterol, ease digestive discomfort, and protect your liver.

- Learn stress reduction techniques such as relaxation therapy, guided imagery, self-hypnosis, and meditation. You also may want to use the relaxation script on pages 88–89. Purchase a relaxation tape and listen to it at least twice a day. Let it play softly in the background the rest of the day. Your subconscious mind will hear it and relax. A study in *Gastroenterology* found that relaxation training reduced the symptom reports of patients with GERD, including gas production.

- Avoid wearing tight-fitting clothing.

- Stop smoking.

- A herbal preparation that is popular in Germany has been shown to improve symptoms of upset stomach (functional dyspepsia), according to a study reported in *Clinician Reviews*. The preparation included chamomile, peppermint, and licorice root.

- Avoid alcohol.

- Elevate the head of your bed.

- Begin an exercise program.

- Lose weight if you're overweight.

For Irritable Bowel Syndrome and Crohn's Disease

- For irritable bowel syndrome and Crohn's disease, identify the food allergies that may be contributing to bowel irritability. Start a food diary, and notice what foods seem to make your bowel act up. Digestive disturbances, minor aches and pains, rashes, and vague health complaints are often due to food allergies. Common triggers of food allergies are wheat, corn, dairy products, soy, citrus fruit, tomatoes, potatoes, eggplant, red and green peppers, cayenne pepper, peanuts (especially if not organically grown), eggs, beef, and coffee. Almost any food can create a sensitivity if you eat it every day. Food additives and colorings such as BHT, BHA, MSG, benzoates, nitrates, red and yellow food dyes, sulfites, antibiotics, and aspirin and ibuprofen also can cause reactions. If you can't identify the food, try not eating the same food more often than once every four days. That will give your body time to clear the irritating substance.

If that doesn't work, try eliminating for two weeks all the foods you were eating every day and more than five times in ten days. Read the labels on all cans and bottles. Many allergens such as corn, dairy products, and eggs are hidden in the foods you eat. Make sure you eliminate those, too. Avoid getting into the habit of eating new foods every day. Keep drinking eight to ten glasses of water every day, and take a good multivitamin and multimineral supplement daily.

At the end of two weeks, reintroduce the restricted foods one at a time. Continue keeping your food diary, writing down your reactions/symptoms to everything you eat. The lining of your intestine is shed and regenerated every three days, so you can heal yourself quite rapidly as long as you don't ingest irritating substances.

When you reintroduce the foods you're sensitive to, you might have extreme reactions of disturbed heart rhythms, sleepiness, stomach cramps, bloating, gas, diarrhea, constipation, chills, sweats, headaches, flushing, and aches. If you have symptoms, stop eating that food and wait two months before reintroducing it. If the symptoms return when you try to eat that food again, wait six months before trying to eat it again. Eventually you will probably be able to eat those foods again, but not every day, and only occasionally.

- Some experts suggest taking a third to a half cup of aloe vera juice two to three times a day after eating. Chamomile or peppermint tea also may feel soothing after you eat.

- Hypnosis may be the answer. One study found that symptoms of abdominal pain, constipation, and gas improved significantly when patients were treated with hypnosis, according to a report in *Applied Psychophysiology and Biofeedback.*

- Seek counseling assistance to help you learn how to express your feelings instead of turning them into physical symptoms.

- Use enteric-coated peppermint capsules to reduce symptoms. A study reported in the *Journal of Gastroenterology* found that participants who took the capsules reported less flatulence, reduced stool frequency, reduced bloating, and were pain-free. Try taking peppermint capsules unless you have gallstones, severe liver damage, gallbladder inflammation, or GERD.

- Avoid using laxatives.

- Drink plenty of water, and add fiber to your diet by eating bran cereal or taking psyllium supplements.

- Exercise daily. Start with a short walk and work up to a longer, more brisk rate.

- Get relaxation training to learn how to manage your stress. In a study reported in *Behavior Research and Therapy*, a group of participants who attended a six-week relaxation response meditation class showed significant improvement in reducing gas, belching, bloating, diarrhea, and constipation.

- Group therapy may be helpful, too. A study reported in *Psychosomatic Medicine* found that focused cognitive-behavioral therapy can have long-term benefits in alleviating complaints and reducing medical care costs for a variety of medical disorders.

For Ulcers

- Try licorice extract (deglycyrrizinated licorice). It increases the production of protective mucus in your stomach. Other substances to try include unripe bananas (buy the extract and take 150 mg four to six times a day), the herbs slippery elm (200 mg four to six times a day) and marshmallow root (200 mg four to six times a day), and the juice of raw cabbage. A review of *Phytotherapy Research* discussed the anti-ulcer properties of herbs, including licorice extract, aloe gel, and capsicum (chili).

- Use garlic and onions. The antibacterial effect of garlic juice and onions has been known for a long time. Allium vegetables, particularly garlic, exhibit a broad antibiotic spectrum against all kinds of bacteria. A study reported in the *Journal of Nutrition* found that both onion and garlic have an antibacterial effect, and some strains of *H. pylori* bacteria are susceptible to garlic. Use both onions and garlic in your cooking and salads.

- In a study reported in the *Annals of Nutrition and Metabolism*, older adults in a geriatric center were tested. Two-thirds of them had low serum values of vitamin C, folate, zinc, and selenium. Participants who received zinc and selenium alone or associated with vitamins A, C and B had significantly fewer infectious events. You may want to consider adding them to your daily intake.

- Try this flaxseed ulcer recipe: Place 3 cups of cold water and 3 table-spoonsful of flaxseed (available at a health food store) in a pot and heat on the stove until the water bubbles. Let simmer for ten minutes, then let it cool for seven to ten minutes. Strain and put the thick liquid in the refrigerator. Thirty minutes before each meal, pour ¼ cup of liquid in a cup, add ¼ cup of water, and drink. Drink this tea between meals if your stomach feels uncomfortable.

Fibromyalgia

Fibromyalgia is a chronic disorder characterized by widespread pain in the muscles and bones, fatigue, and multiple tender points in the neck, spine, shoulders, and hips. If you have this condition, you also might have morning stiffness, anxiety, irritable bowel syndrome, sleep disturbances, malabsorption problems, and even depression.

Your Risk for Developing Fibromyalgia

The cause of fibromyalgia is unknown. There are several theories about what causes or triggers the condition. Some scientists believe that the syndrome could be caused by a trauma or injury that affects the central nervous system. Fibromyalgia may be associated with changes in muscle metabolism, including decreased blood flow that results in fatigue and decreased strength. Altered sensory processing may result in the interpretation of nonoxious stimuli as painful in fibromyalgia. Another explanation is that the syndrome can be triggered by an infectious agent such as a virus, but no such agent has ever been found. The thyroid may also be to blame.

Intestinal health is thought by some experts to be related to FMS. This theory posits that permeability across the intestinal surface is often increased in fibromyalgia, creating a leaky gut syndrome that begins with a disruption of intestinal flora that can result in inflammatory immune reactions that bring on symptoms. Individuals with FMS may not have the normal liver's capacity to detoxify what gets across the intestinal lining. FMS also is associated with high levels of stress. During stress, the body produces large quantities of powerful toxic chemicals called free radicals, which can cause inflammation and cell destruction. NSAIDS or nonsteroidal anti-inflammatory drugs, from ibuprofen to aspirin and countless others, can lead to leaky gut syndrome, pain, and body aches.

When cases of FMS seemed untreatable improved, there has been a common thread: hidden food and chemical sensitivities were at the root. Excitotoxins also may stimulate fibromyalgia symptoms in a portion of the population that has the condition, according to a report in *The American Journal for Nurse Practitioners*. Excitotoxins are molecules such as MSG (found in Chinese and other oriental foods, soups, and many other canned foods) and aspartate (found in many foods, beverages, and drugs), which excite neurotransmitters and can lead to neurotoxicity when used in excess. The elimination of MSG and other excitotoxins from the diets of patients with fibromyalgia resulted in a dramatic reduction of symptoms for them.

How the Doctor Diagnoses Fibromyalgia

Fibromyalgia is difficult to diagnose because many of the symptoms mimic those of other diseases (e.g., chronic fatigue syndrome). A diagnosis is made based on your medical history, widespread pain that persists for more than three months, and tenderness in at least eleven of eighteen specific tender point sites.

Your doctor also may want to do some laboratory tests to make sure you don't have rheumatoid arthritis or chronic fatigue syndrome or some other condition. The doctor will probably order a blood cell count, thyroid function, and blood sedimentation rate (to see if you have a body disorder). While most people with FMS have no significant lab abnormalities, the tests can be used to make sure you don't have another condition.

What the Doctor Will Probably Prescribe

Your doctor may suggest an antidepressant. Amitriptyline (Elavil) has been the most thoroughly studied in FMS patients. Adverse affects include dry mouth, dizziness, weight gain, and drowsiness. Doxepin, imipramine, nortriptyline, and desipramine also have been used. Over time, the benefit of using any of these drugs decreases, so that after six months they provide no more benefit than that of a placebo (sugar pill).

Cyclobenzaprine, a muscle relaxant, is sometimes used, too, either alone or in combination with ibuprofen. After six months its effects are no greater than those of a placebo.

Acetaminophen is an inexpensive treatment for FMS, but it is no more effective than the other drugs. It also can cause liver damage.

Tramadol has also been used to treat FMS pain. Potential bad effects include dizziness, headache, nausea, constipation and seizures. If you experience seizures, this would not be the drug for you.

Naproxen is sometimes used in combination with amitriptyline. Ibuprofen (Motrin, Advil, Midol IB, Bayer Select Pain Relief, Nuprin, IBU) has been combined with alprazolam (Xanax), but studies in *Arthritis and Rheumatism* and the *Journal of Rheumatism* show mixed results. For the most part these nonsteroidal anti-inflammatory drugs or NSAIDs do not provide relief, yet according to a study in *Arthritis and Rheumatism*, 91 percent of patients with FMS reported using NSAIDs, even though they didn't work. Not only don't they work, they also have bad side effects, including increased blood pressure and bleeding, pain and ulcers in the stomach, and/or intestinal tract. They also have a destructive effect on cartilage, according to the *American Journal of Medicine* and the *Journal of Rheumatology*, and can accelerate the breakdown of already damaged cartilage because it absorbs greater amounts of the drugs, according to the *British Journal of Pharmacology*.

Selective serotonin reuptake inhibitors or SSRIs such as fluoxetine (Prozac) do not show positive results according to a report in the *Scandianavian Journal of Rheumatology*, although a study published in *Arthritis and Rheumatism* did find that combining fluoxetine with amitriptyline (Elavil) had better effects than that of a placebo.

Other pain medications that have been tried include narcotics, but the body soon develops a tolerance, and bigger and bigger doses are needed to relieve pain. Also, dependence or addiction to such drugs develops. Lidocaine injections into tender points offer temporary relief; if you have nonspecific pain, frequent injections of Lidocaine are discouraged. Steroids are ineffective in the treatment of FMS, and any benefits are outweighed by the risks, according to a report in *Internal Medicine*.

Self-Care Measures You Can Take

Since medications are for the most part ineffective, it will be up to you to take steps to deal with the symptoms of FMS. Possibilities include nutritional and cognitive-behavioral approaches, moderate exercise, and other approaches.

Find the Cause of Your Fibromyalgia

Factors that are unique to you *may* be at the root of your pain and fatigue. Keep a food/stress diary for at least two weeks. Write down everything you put in your mouth and all environmental dust, mold, and pollen you are exposed to. For all note when, and how you feel thirty minutes later. You will begin to notice patterns. If you don't, keep the diary for another two weeks. Once you find which foods and environmental factors make you feel worse, eliminate them.

Change What and How You Eat

- Read labels of all foods, drinks, and drugs, and make sure they do not contain aspartate or monosodium glutamate (MSG). Glutamic acid, the main component of MSG, can be found listed by any of the following names: autolyzed yeast, calcium caseinate, hydrolyzed protein, hydrolyzed oat flour, hydrolyzed plant protein, hydrolyzed vegetable protein, monosodium glutamate, plant protein extract, sodium caseinate, textured protein, yeast extract, bouillon, broth, flavoring, malt extract, malt flavoring, natural beef flavoring, natural chicken flavoring, natural flavoring, seasoning, spices, carrageenan, enzymes, soy protein concentrate, soy protein isolate, or whey protein concentrate. Try eliminating all products with any of these ingredients for two months to see if your symptoms are relieved. To be sure you aren't ingesting any of these ingredients, you will have to forgo eating in restaurants during this time.

- Eat a diet rich in whole, fresh foods, including fresh fruits and vegetables, raw nuts and seeds, whole grains (if tolerated), dry beans and peas, soy products, and fish. Once in a while, eat turkey or chicken, but never eat the skin. This kind of regime will help your body neutralize dangerous free radicals. Try to eat 50 percent raw foods and fresh juices. Buy a juicer and drink at least 12 ounces of carrot juice a day.

If you like, add the carrot juice to 2 ounces of spinach juice and/or 2 ounces of beet juice or 2 ounces of cucumber juice.

- Avoid green peppers, eggplant, tomatoes, and white potatoes. These foods contain solanine, which interferes with enzymes in your muscles and may cause pain and discomfort.

- Avoid meat, dairy products, or any other foods high in saturated fats that can raise cholesterol levels and interfere with circulation. They also can promote inflammation and pain. Avoid fried foods, processed foods (in cans, bottles, bakeries, and fast-food restaurants), shellfish, and white flour products such as bread and pasta. Avoid caffeine, alcohol, and sugar. Sugar in candy, cake, pies, ice cream, and even yogurt promotes fatigue, increases pain, and can disturb sleep. If you've eaten a lot of these foods, gradually withdraw from them, as your symptoms may get worse at first as your body "withdraws" from them. Avoid wheat and brewer's yeast at least until your symptoms improve. Eggs, sardines, tuna, liver, and brewer's yeast can tune up your thyroid.

- Eat four to five small meals daily to keep a steady supply of protein and carbohydrates available to your body. Never skip breakfast, and never eat after 7:00 P.M. (in that way you'll be hungry by breakfast). Don't eat junk foods, but carry a small bag of fresh nuts and raisins to snack on if you get hungry.

- Investigate the use of acidophilus and related "good" bacteria that can balance the flora in your intestine. Some plain yogurts have active cultures that can help. You also can find other sources of "good" bacteria at health food stores.

- Drink at least ten glasses of distilled water a day, or purchase a reverse osmosis water filtration system to ensure that you are not taking in parasites. Infection by these creatures can mimic fibromyalgia symptoms.

Investigate Supplements

SAMe is a supplement to look into to alleviate depression and pain and to promote healing. SAMe (S-adenosylmethionine) is synthesized from the amino acid methionine and is found throughout your body. SAMe protects your chondrocytes, the cells that manufacture the main components of cartilage, against wear and tear on your joints, according to studies in the *American Journal of Medicine* and the *American Journal of Bone and Joint Surgery*.

In studies reported in the *International Journal of Clinical Pharmacology and Toxicology* and the *American Journal of Medicine*, SAMe worked just as well as naproxen (Naprosyn), ibuprofen (Motrin, Advil, Midol IB, Bayer Select Pain Relief, Nuprin, and IBU) and indomethacin (Indocin) for pain relief but had fewer side effects. Studies in the *American Journal of Psychiatry* and *Neuroscience and Biobehavioral Review* all show that SAMe worked faster and produced more significant improvements than antidepressants and had fewer reported adverse effects. No studies have shown any reason not to use SAMe as long as the normal daily dose recommended (1,200 to 1,600 mg divided in several doses for twenty-one days, then reduced to 400 mg a day) is followed.

Other supplements that have been reported to be helpful include magnesium malate (300 to 900 mg per day), pycnogenol (25 mg twice a day), chromium picolinate, vitamin C (until you get gas), CoQ10 (50 to 100 mg three times a day), vitamin E (400 to 800 IU a day), glutathione (150 mg three times a day), and acetyl carnitine (250 mg three times a day). These supplements can reduce oxidative stress due to free radicals that cause severe inflammation and destruction. Borage oil or evening primrose oil capsules may help with inflammation and pain. Vitamin A (10,000 IU daily) and B-complex (100 mg daily) can help tune up the thyroid.

Try Herbs

Investigate the use of herbs. Buy a book with research-based references, or find a health care professional with expertise in the use of herbs. Some herbs that have provided relief from fibromyalgia include the Chinese herb combination Tuo Li Xiao and Gui Pi Tang. Saint-John's-wort taken with Bach Rescue Remedy at the first sign of a FMS flare-up can provide emergency relief.

Devil's claw is a muscle and joint anti-inflammatory. Saint-John's-wort decreases pain and is an antidepressant and a muscle relaxer. Scullcap decreases pain and is a nerve sedative and muscle relaxer.

Milk thistle can help protect your liver. Skullcap and valerian root improve sleep, and ginkgo biloba improves circulation and brain function. Topical applications of 1 part cayenne powder mixed with 3 parts wintergreen oil can help relieve muscle pain. Teas brewed from dandelion and red clover can promote healing by cleansing the bloodstream and enhancing immune function. Parasites can be a problem in fibromyalgia. Black walnut and garlic can help remove them.

Choose which herbs to use in consultation with your doctor. Bring along your herb reference book or any information you have about the use, action, and side effects of the herbs you choose for your doctor to read.

Try Homeopathic Remedies

Pulsatilla is a homeopathic remedy used to decrease tension, anxiety, and emotional agitation. Arnica removes blood; is an analgesic, muscle relaxer, and warmer; and can reduce stress.

Start to Exercise

FMS patients are generally at a lower fitness level than the average population. Pain and fatigue encourage physical inactivity. This can fuel a hopeless cycle of pain, physical inactivity, and more pain.

Low-level aerobic exercise such as swimming, walking, low-impact aerobic dancing, or bicycling can reduce FMS pain and reduce stress. You may have to begin with just five minutes a day if you have been inactive for quite a while. Warm water pool exercises may be the easiest way to begin. You also can try walking up a single flight of stairs instead of taking the elevator.

Use Cognitive Behavioral Therapy to Reduce Stress

Cognitive behavioral therapy can help you learn to prioritize your time and activities so you can include meaningful work and pleasurable leisure activities in your day, change your self-critical attitudes when tasks take longer than they used to, learn ways to deal with daily hassles without feeling stressed, and reduce attention spent on your symptoms while increasing focus on your accomplishments. You will probably need cognitive behavioral therapy if you hold any myths that are keeping you from changing your exercise and eating patterns.

Relaxation strategies, meditation-based stress reduction techniques, self-hypnosis, and guided imagery techniques may help you restructure negative thoughts that have left you feeling helpless and hopeless. It may be beneficial to do this work in a group with other FMS patients so that you see others like yourself master situations. Also, it probably will be easier to listen to your peers' ideas than it will be to take advice from a therapist.

FMS patients also tend to catastrophize (make situations sound worse than they really are) and make depressive self-statements. Both of these behaviors may have a role in your pain, according to a study reported in *Arthritis and Rheumatism*. A cognitive-behavioral therapist also can help you bring your self-statements to a more positive level, which in turn can brighten your outlook by focusing on positive outcomes.

People who develop chronic fatigue syndrome and fibromyalgia are more apt to come from a life of neglect and physical abuse; a considerable subgroup will have experienced lifelong victimization. Family and/or a current partner were the most frequent abusers, according to a study in *Psychosomatics*. If this is you, be sure to get individual psychotherapy from either a mental health nurse practitioner or a psychologist to overcome your victim role. You cannot hope to conquer your FMS symptoms without tackling this important area of your life.

Relax More

Purchase a relaxation, hypnosis, and/or fibromyalgia healing tape, and listen to it twice a day. When your body is relaxed, you will feel much less pain. Tight, tense muscles ache and hurt. Try listening to the tape when you first wake up, to relax you and give you energy. Listen to it before you go to sleep to get a good night's sleep. If your muscles are tense, it will be difficult to rest.

Start Postural Retraining

Common postural distortions in individuals with chronic pain conditions such as FMS include a forward-positioned head, rounded shoulders with a locked chest, and inefficient mouth breathing. Postural retraining can help you learn how to correct improper use of your muscles for long-term relief. Two easy exercises follow, which prove more effective if you listen to a relaxation tape first.

• Stand against a wall with your hands at your sides and with your buttocks, head and back touching the wall. While inhaling from your abdomen, slowly raise your arms up along the wall until they touch over your head. While exhaling, slide your arms down the wall until they are at your sides again. Repeat several times, building up to ten times a day.

- Stand against a wall with your arms bent and your knuckles touching each other at nipple level. Slowly inhale from your abdomen while pulling your hands apart and letting your elbows move toward the wall until they touch it. Hold your breath for several seconds, then slowly exhale, returning your bent arms to nipple level. Repeat several times, building up to ten times a day.

Here are some other things you can do to improve your posture:

- Avoid staying in the same position for long periods of time. Shuffle your feet, slowly reach out in front of you with your arms, slowly stretch your arms over your head, or touch your knees and then your buttocks several times. If you're driving, pull over every hour, get out, walk around the car, stretch up to the sky, take a deep breath, and find at least one little thing to enjoy in your surroundings.

- Sit in a rocker when watching television or sitting and relaxing. This will prevent the muscles in your back from locking and build up strength in your knees and ankles.

- When you stand, lean forward and let gravity help you. Don't just push yourself up with your arms.

- Sleep with a small, soft pillow between your knees to keep your back in alignment. Never sleep on your stomach. When turning in bed, roll with your head down and use your arms to help turn. Relieve stress on your neck by not lifting your head or leading with it to roll over.

- Avoid sitting in drafts or cold rooms. Both can tighten your muscles, especially in your neck and shoulders, and increase pain. Put a small towel or scarf around your shoulders and neck to keep them warm.

Try Magnets

A report in the *Journal of Italian Medical Laboratory Ergonomics* presented the results of a study of the effect of magnets on the prevention of musculoskeletal disorders. The results showed that the magnets prevented muscle contractures that arose due to sitting in one position for a prolonged time.

Another report, published in *Newsletter of the American Institute of Stress*, found that two-thirds of participants who slept on mattresses with magnets reported substantial pain relief, decreased fatigue, and an improved sense of well-being.

Engage in Meditation

A study reported in *General Hospital Psychiatry* found that participants with fibromyalgia in a meditation-based stress reduction program showed moderate to marked improvement. Another study, presented at a meeting of the American Psychosomatic Society, found that women with fibromyalgia who meditated six days a week slept better, improved their quality of life, and alleviated their depressive symptoms. These two studies provide strong evidence that joining a meditation-based stress reduction program could help.

Use Affirmations to Reprogram Negative Thinking

Affirmations can replace negative thinking with more positive thoughts. Say or write one or more of the following sayings on 3 × 5 cards and place them in prominent spots around you.

- I lovingly release the past.
- I am free and so is everyone else.
- My heart is healed.
- I can hear and accept other people's viewpoints.
- I am safe and secure.

Also see the chapters "Arthritis," "Chronic Fatigue Syndrome," and "Digestive Problems" in this book for more ideas.

Heart and Blood Vessel Disorders

Conditions affecting your heart and blood vessels can include a myocardial infarction (heart attack or blood clot to the heart) or stroke (blood clot), rheumatic heart disease (inflammation of the heart and damage to the heart valves as a result of having rheumatic fever), high blood pressure (due to too much table salt, overweight, stress, or anger), congestive heart failure (due to impairment of the left ventricle of the heart, leading to increased back pressure in the lung circulation and reduced blood flow through the lungs), mitral valve prolapse (low blood volume due to a faulty feedback mechanism in the brain), atherosclerosis (deposits in the walls of the major blood vessels that slow down blood circulation and are hardened or sclerosed by deposits of calcium), coronary artery disease (hardening of the arteries of the muscle from the heart), and hemorrhoids and varicose veins (due to pressure on the veins, poor diet, or insufficient movement).

Your Risk for Developing Heart and Blood Vessel Disorders

The controllable risk factors for heart and blood vessel disorders include cigarette smoking, high blood pressure, overweight/obesity, diabetes, type A personality (have suffered early heartbreak through the emotional or physical loss of a loved one, perfectionism, denial of feelings, belief that success brings love, urgency due to the passing of time, rigid chest, and/or shallow breathing), stress, and lack of exercise. If you have any of these risk factors, you may be more likely to end up with heart and/or blood vessel disorders unless you commit to changing your lifestyle.

Pain, difficulty breathing, sweating, or lightheadedness are all messages from your body to pay attention, slow down, eat better, and enjoy life. If you don't pay attention to the messages, your body will give you stronger and stronger messages as the stress continues to build. The last message will be a fatal heart attack or stroke. Please take action before that happens to you. Direct the anger and resentment you feel, but may be denying, into healing yourself.

Stress, including negative feelings you're holding on to, can raise your blood cholesterol levels and blood pressure. You may have very high readings when you go to the doctor to have your blood pressure taken, but very low blood pressure when you take it at home. This is due to the stress of going to see the doctor. While stress can raise your blood pressure, loving contact from a significant other person in your life can lower both your cholesterol and blood pressure, as touch confers a "protective effect" on your heart and blood vessels.

The typical American diet is overloaded with foods high in saturated (animal) fats that overwhelm the vascular system, which is why we have a higher rate of heart disease than the Japanese or Mediterraneans, who eat little fat and few animal and dairy products, or the African Bantu, who eat mostly beans, grains, vegetables, and fruits. The soy foods and vegetables eaten and the green tea drunk by the Japanese and the olive oil and pasta eaten by the Italians help protect them from heart disease. If you eat a lot of meat, burgers, French fries, other fried foods, potato chips, pies, cakes, and cheese, you are putting yourself at risk for heart and blood vessel disease.

Many heart and blood vessel conditions are closely linked to diet and lifestyle, but there are other explanations for what happens. The metaphysical basis for heart problems includes the theory that there are serious emotional problems of a long-standing nature, lack of joy, rejection of life, and the belief that life is full of strain and pressure.

Research in the *Journal of the American Medical Association* has provided support that mental stress can affect heart and blood vessel conditions. Other research published in the same journal has shown that a sense of hopelessness can be a predictor of heart attack. Researchers at the University of Florida linked emotions to heart disease, too. They found that people who internalize their hostility and anger, suppressing their feelings and not experiencing them, are more apt to develop heart disease.

In the Chinese medicine system, the heart is associated with the nervous system and the spirit. It is believed that when the heart system is strong, the mind is clear, the emotions are positive and calm, and the spirit is strong. Joy is the main emotion associated with the heart. Lack of love and guidance during the formative years, traumatic experiences or illness, or lack of joy can all promote heart and vascular disease. Just as there can be too little joy, so can there be too much. Either situation can damage the heart, adrenal, and nervous systems.

According to psychoanalytic theory (as promulgated in *Deceits of the Mind*), heart disease, like cancer, begins as a natural healing process gone wild. Heart disease may begin early in life as an overly responsive heart responds to either the loss of a father or intense conflicts with a father. Heart disease in a person with type A personality develops as an attempt to deal with an environment that feels dangerous and threatening. Although the heart disease patient may look invulnerable on the outside, that only hides an inner self that has been exposed to more aggression from self and others than can be managed, and a desperate need for love. The discrepancy between these two opposite stances creates the greatest danger for a heart attack.

If you had or have a bad relationship with your father, can't remember the last time you felt real joy, aren't in touch with your body or your emotions, breathe in the upper part of your chest rather than in your abdominal area, and push yourself all the time, you also may be at risk for heart disease and blood vessel disorders.

If you are resentful of someone or something—even an early wounding by a parent or family member—and don't acknowledge the feelings or forgive the perpetrator, this can negatively affect your whole life. According to Stephen Sinatra, M.D., you can literally experience heartbreak from holding on to hostility and anger. A resentful heart traps negative energy in that area of your body and begins the process of forming a disease. Beneath this anger, layers of sadness and sorrow reside. Sharing your sorrow and allowing yourself to shed tears can be two of the most therapeutic things you can do to heal your heart. Harnessing those feelings and using them to nurture your heart is the best way to be healthy. (See "Self-Care Measures You Can Take" in this chapter for specific suggestions.)

How the Doctor Diagnoses Heart and Blood Vessel Disorders

From 10 to 40 percent of the time, the first recognized symptom of heart disease is a fatal heart attack. Some individuals may have chest discomfort, shortness of breath, sweating, or light-headedness, but frequently there are no signs or warnings. You could have heart disease and experience no symptoms, especially if you are out of touch with your feelings and your body. You may be putting too much strain on your body but just don't know how much stress you're under because you're not paying attention. You're too busy thinking and acting.

More than thirty years ago, George Engel studied 275 cases of sudden death due to fatal heart attack. He found that 20 percent of the individuals dying from sudden heart attack had recently experienced bad news about a loved one, another 20 percent were experiencing acute grief at the time of their sudden death, and another 27 percent had a fear of personal injury or damage. *In almost every case, some psychological stress occurred before the unexpected, sudden cardiac death.*

You may not even have any symptoms to let you know that your blood pressure is high. Your doctor or nurse can tell if you have high blood pressure by taking a reading of it using a monitoring device that is placed around your arm and inflated. When a blood pressure device deflates, the first sound heard via the stethoscope is your systolic pressure, the pressure exerted when your heart contracts and suddenly ejects a large volume of blood into your arteries. The second sound heard via the stethoscope is the diastolic pressure, or the resistance of the arteries, capillaries, and veins to the blood passing across them. Normally, the interplay between the pumping action of your heart and your blood vessels leads to an average systolic pressure of 120 mm Hg and an average diastolic pressure of 80 mm Hg. These values are recorded by the doctor or nurse as 120/80. The accepted normal range of blood pressure is below 140/90 in all patients and below 130/85 in patients with diabetes according to the National Heart, Lung, and Blood Institute (NHLBI).

The diagnosis of high blood pressure or hypertension is made when the diastolic is at or above 90 mm Hg. The major complication of chronic high blood pressure is hypertensive heart disease, a weakening of the heart caused by the overwork of pumping blood against the high pressures in the circulation. The strain of sustained hypertension on the blood vessels (due to stress, excitement, anger, or as a consequence of atherosclerosis) can cause them to rupture, much like pressure against a weakened water pipe can cause it to burst. The rupture of a blood vessel can cause a heart attack if the blood vessels around the heart (coronary blood vessels) are involved, and a stroke if the brain arteries become affected. Orthostatic hypotension is an excessive fall in blood pressure on assuming the upright posture, typically 20/10 mm Hg, and can lead to shock or fainting when the blood flow to the brain is diminished.

Be aware that your blood pressure varies significantly throughout the day. Exercise or agitation can make it rise, and sleeping and relaxation can make it drop. The level at which your doctor decides that blood pressure requires medication is somewhat arbitrary and may be different from one doctor to another. "White-coat hypertension" is the medical term for a reaction you may have when you see a nurse or a doctor coming toward you with a blood pressure cuff. Your pulse may quicken and your blood pressure can soar 20 or more points. Some experts estimate that 15 to 30 percent of patients diagnosed with high blood pressure may have a problem only in the doctor's office. Older adults may be most vulnerable to this reaction.

Your doctor may order an electrocardiogram (ECG) to determine if you have damage to your heart muscle. This diagnostic procedure is risk-free and painless. It examines your heart's electrical patterns while at rest. Electrodes are attached to your chest, wrists, and ankles while you are lying down. The electrical patterns your heart produces are recorded and can be read by your doctor to determine whether there is any deviation from normal.

A stress test measures the electrical patterns of your heart during exertion. You may be asked to walk or jog on a treadmill or ride a stationary bicycle. This test will reveal if there is any blockage to the blood flow when your heart is stressed through exercise. If the results of either the stress test or the ECG appear unusual, your doctor may order a thallium scan to provide a dynamic visual picture of your heart muscle. Radioactive materials are injected into your arm. Although this test is more accurate than the stress test, it does require radioactive substances and is much more expensive. The nuclear waste materials also must be specially handled to avoid environmental and personal danger.

According to Dr. Siegfried Kra, a Yale School of Medicine cardiologist, here are some instances when you should not have a stress test, or when it should be discontinued immediately:

1. You experience shortness of breath, chest pain, or irregular heartbeat.

2. Your blood pressure falls.

There are a number of reasons why stress tests are not effective. A positive stress test can be difficult to interpret, especially in women. Changes that dip below the baseline on the recording of your heart action may be a false positive change, meaning it looks like your test is abnormal, but it really isn't. In many of these cases the physician cannot tell if an artery is blocked, and different tests may be needed.

Mitral valve prolapse, rapid breathing, or a low potassium level in the blood also can produce false positive results. Taking diuretics (to lose weight, reduce swelling in the ankles or bloating), bulimia (forced gorging and purging with enemas), and excessive sweating also can lead to low potassium blood levels. Taking the drug Digitalis also can produce false positive stress test results.

An echocardiogram, also called a sonogram, uses ultrasound (extremely-high-frequency sound waves) to produce an image of your heart. It can give a clear picture of your heart, its size, how it is functioning, and if there are any valve or other changes in its structure before, during, and after walking on a treadmill or riding a stationary bicycle.

An arteriogram lights up the coronary blood vessels and shows life-threatening blockages that could require emergency surgery. A heart scan, also called electronic beam computerized tomography (EBCT), is a screening tool that allows the doctor to find out if you're at risk of a heart attack.

The equilibrium radionuclide angiocardiogram shows how well your heart is contracting and ejecting oxygenated blood to the rest of your body.

Magnetic resonance imaging (MRI) uses magnets to create a three-dimensional image of your heart.

Coronary angiography may be suggested if you have heart disease and your physician believes you've suffered serious damage to your heart muscle, if you've had a heart attack, or if heart surgery is being contemplated. The surgical procedure involved is called a cardiac catheterization, and it can indicate the location and degree of blockage to blood flow. You are given a local anesthetic in the right groin region; then a tube is inserted into the femoral artery in your groin. A dye is injected through the tube, and an X ray (angiogram) is taken.

A recent study from Boston estimated that 50 percent of these procedures are unnecessary, or at least should be postponed. In rare instances the procedure can cause strokes, hemorrhages, heart attacks, kidney failure ,or death. If you are obese, diabetic, or over age seventy, you are at greatest risk from the test. If you have kidney disease, the dye can cause your kidneys to shut down completely, necessitating renal dialysis for months.

Also, seek a second opinion before having a cardiac catheterization from a cardiologist who does not usually perform catheterizations. Even if your cardiologist is well known as an expert, make sure he or she takes the time to explain everything to you so you understand perfectly.

A new, noninvasive method to visualize the coronary arteries without having to resort to catheterization is now available. This painless procedure uses an ultrafast scanner that produces a CAT scan of your heart's arteries.

There is some risk involved in stress tests and stress echocardiograms, too, and none of the tests is 100% accurate, according to studies published in the *Journal of the American Society of Echocardiography*, the *American Journal of Cardiology*, and the *American Journal of Medicine*.

If you have a stroke, your doctor may not have a chance to ask you about your symptoms. All you will experience is a sudden and dramatic loss of consciousness, and loss of movement and sensory function on one side of your body. Long-term high blood pressure is the most important risk factor of stroke. Other factors that are correlated with stroke are cigarette smoking, high total cholesterol, diabetes and glucose metabolism, alcohol use, illicit drug use, obesity, physical inactivity, poor diet, oral contraceptives, and an elevated homocysteine level. Homocysteine is a naturally occurring amino acid that, when elevated, can induce adverse pathological change in your artery walls, leading to premature hardening of the arteries.

If you complain of pain in your calf muscles after walking a short distance (a hundred yards or less) that is relieved when you stop, your doctor may conclude that you have peripheral arterial disease, or poor circulation in your legs and arms. If you complain of pain in your abdomen or lower back and are sixty years or older, the doctor may take an X ray to see if there is an enlargement of the artery wall in that spot, which could indicate the possibility of rupture. If you smoke, have high total cholesterol, and had a stroke in the past, he will likely conclude you have an aortic aneurysm.

If you have fatigue and shortness of breath with only minimal exertion, trouble sleeping, coughing at night, swelling of your ankles, and a fast pulse, your doctor may perform some tests to see if you might be suffering from congestive heart failure. He might take a chest X ray, listen to your lungs, and order some laboratory tests.

You probably make your own diagnosis of varicose veins, but their extent is usually greater than you can determine by simple inspection and can be judged only by the doctor checking the pulse at the ankle and ruling out other possible diagnoses.

The Cholesterol Controversy

Although blood cholesterol is a proven predictor of coronary heart disease, lowering blood cholesterol levels does not necessarily save lives. There are no data to suggest that your life will be extended by lowering your serum cholesterol.

Avoid basing your risk of heart disease solely on one figure: a cholesterol reading above 200 mg means risk, but below 200 mg means no risk. There are just too many other factors involved.

More specific values, such as HDL (high-density, or "good" cholesterol) or LDL (low-density or "bad" cholesterol) carry a 15 to 20 percent margin of error, enough to matter.

Other risk factors for heart disease are the ratio between HDL and LDL. The more HDL ("good" cholesterol) you have, the better. For example, 65 mg/dl HDL to 160 mg/dl LDL would be better than 30 mg/dl HDL to 140 mg/dl LDL.

Cholesterol oxidation is another factor. Oxidized (free-radical-damaged) LDL may be more dangerous than cholesterol per se. Though testing for oxidized LDL is not common, you can protect yourself against free radicals by eating more fruits and vegetables.

Triglycerides are another class of blood fats that some doctors believe are more important than cholesterol. They can be controlled by eating fewer fatty and sugary products, especially those that are made with processed flour and sugars.

Homocysteine is also an important factor. High levels of this substance have been linked to heart disease. Ideal blood levels are under 8 micromoles per liter; 13 or higher is considered dangerous.

What does this controversy mean to you? Changing your eating, exercise, and stress management measures can lead to health and wellness. Worrying about cholesterol levels won't.

What the Doctor Will Probably Prescribe

Many of the less serious heart and blood vessel disorders—mitral valve prolapse, varicose veins, and peripheral vascular disease— can be treated in their early stages by self-care treatments including stop smoking, stop taking birth control pills, change the diet, and increase exercise. Other treatments your doctor may prescribe include drugs and surgery.

High-Blood-Pressure Drugs

Diuretics or "water pills" are the most commonly prescribed medications for high blood pressure. These drugs are useful for lowering blood pressure, but there is some controversy about their effects. Specifically, "potassium-wasting" diuretics deplete your body of potassium and magnesium, two essential minerals for a healthy heart. If your level of these minerals drops too low, you could have cardiac arrest. Except for Lozol, diuretics also can raise your cholesterol. That is why periodic blood tests are crucial.

When taking potassium-wasting diuretics, you will need to eat foods high in potassium to lower your risk.

FOODS HIGH IN POTASSIUM

Apricots, artichokes, asparagus, bananas, beets, bell pepper, blackberries, blackstrap molasses, broccoli, Brussels sprouts, buttermilk, cabbage, cantaloupes, carrots, cauliflower, chicken, fish, kidney beans, lima beans, nectarines, oatmeal, onions, oranges, peaches, plums, potatoes, prunes, raisins, raspberries, spinach (uncooked is best), squash, tomatoes, and yogurt (low-fat is best). It is also a good idea to pursue the self-care things you can do to lower your blood pressure (see below).

The effects of diuretics include increased urination (so take the medication early in the day unless you want to be up all night), muscle cramps, upset stomach, loss of appetite, diarrhea, dizziness, sexual difficulties, increased susceptibility to sunburn, blurred vision, and headache. **Caution:** Report any rash or itching to your doctor; it may be a sign of allergy. If you have kidney or liver disease, lupus, or asthma, some of these diuretics could worsen your condition. They also may increase blood sugar (bad if you have diabetes) or aggravate gout.

Many arthritis/pain relievers do not combine well with diuretics. It would be especially dangerous to take them with Lasix or Bumex. Other drugs that do not combine well with diuretics are Colestid, Questran, Eskalith, Lithobid, DiaBeta, Diabinese, Glucotrol, Orinase, laxatives, and Lanoxin.

If your potassium level is depleted, you will notice specific symptoms, including muscle cramps, confusion, mood changes, weakness, difficulty breathing, dry mouth, thirst, fatigue, lethargy, nausea, vomiting, and irregular heart rhythms.

Potassium-sparing diuretics preserve potassium but still can deplete magnesium. They also can interact with blood pressure medicines called ACE inhibitors (discussed later) and include Accupril, Altace, Capoten, Lotensin, Monopril, Prinivil, Vasotec, and Zestril. Because these ACE inhibitors also *preserve* potassium, dangerous levels of this electrolyte can occur. If you're taking these two drugs in combination, you must watch for a dangerous rise in potassium level. Symptoms of too much potassium are weakness, confusion, slowed heart rate, breathing difficulty, and heart rhythm changes.

ACE inhibitors block an enzyme called ACE (angiotensin-converting enzyme). Some may control congestive heart failure and preserve kidney function in people with diabetes. They can cause severe allergic reactions that are life-threatening. At the first sign of a swollen face, tongue, or lips, and difficulty breathing, emergency treatment is essential. Go immediately to the closest emergency room. If you're pregnant, do not take these drugs because they are extremely toxic to the fetus during the second or third trimester. Blood disorders and kidney problems also have been reported. Avoid extra potassium either as a salt substitute or supplement when on these drugs. Some less dangerous but uncomfortable side effects include drops in blood pressure that can create dizziness; dry, hacking cough; rash; itching; stomach upsets; headache;

weakness; irregular heartbeat, fluid retention; sexual difficulties; sensitivity to sunburn; and loss of taste sensation.

Some potassium-sparing diuretics, including Dyazide, Moduretic, Maxzide, and Aldactazide, can cause a dangerous overload of potassium when taken with ACE inhibitors. Other drugs that can interact in unpleasant or dangerous ways include aspirin, allopurinol (for gout), lithium, oral diabetes drugs, and Indocin (for arthritis). Check with your pharmacist and doctor about problems you experience.

Heart Attack Drugs

Drugs that reduce the risk of heart attack include aspirin, beta-blockers, and calcium-channel-blockers. All have side effects, some more serious than others. If aspirin is prescribed, be sure you take only a baby aspirin, or half of a 325 mg coated aspirin every day. One of aspirin's most serious side effects is bleeding in the stomach. Two studies published in *Stroke* and one in the *Journal of Gender Specific Medicine* show a higher than usual occurrence of brain hemorrhage and strokes in patients taking aspirin.

Beta-blockers have been used for more than thirty years to treat angina (heart pain), high blood pressure, and fast heartbeat due to anger. Some of the more commonly prescribed beta-blockers are metoprolol, propranolol, timolol, atenolol, carteolol, betaxolol, penbutolol, acebutolol, metoprolal, pindolol, bisoprolol, and nadolol. They all have side effects, including decreased sexual interest and orgasm, fatigue, fainting, difficulty breathing due to constricted airways, slowed heart rate, cold hands and feet, stomach upset, difficulty sleeping, skin rash, hair loss, blurred vision, dizziness, joint pain, cholesterol elevation, and reduced effect when taken with arthritis drugs. *If you have asthma or severe lung disease, avoid beta-blockers.* If you have peripheral vascular disease, your leg pain may worsen when they take them. **Caution:** Cutting off these drugs abruptly can cause a dangerous rise in blood pressure and bring on a heart attack. Always talk to your physician and follow a plan for gradually reducing the dosage over several days or a week.

Calcium-channel-blockers help the heart muscle relax. Their side effects include ankle swelling, flushing, nausea, headaches, dizziness, fluid retention (swollen ankles or hands), irregular heartbeat, breathing difficulties, sleep disorders, sexual difficulties, muscle cramps, constipation, hair loss, fatigue, rashes, and swollen gums (especially with Amlodipine). A recent article in the *Mayo Clinic Proceedings* revealed that grapefruit juice increases the potency of calcium-channel-blockers, so if you do take any of these drugs, don't take them with grapefruit juice. (Orange juice is okay.)

There have been few long-term studies on calcium-channel-blockers' safety or effectiveness, and in fact some research shows that these medications may actually cause heart attacks or at least set the stage for them! Calcium-channel-blockers include nifedipine (Adalat or Procardia), verapamil (Calanor, Isoptin, or Verelan), nicardipine (Cardene), dilitiazem (Cardizem and Dilacor XR), isradipine (DynaCirc), amlodipine (Norvasc), felodipine (Plendil), and nisoldipine (Sular).

If you are taking both calcium-channel-blockers and beta-blockers you may be on dangerous ground. The combination can sometimes cause serious slowing of the heart, or even heart block and fainting. *Note:* Calcium-channel-blockers can interact with antidepressants, barbiturates, carbamzepine (Tegretol), cimetidine (Tagamet), cyclosporine (Sandimmune), digoxin (Lanoxin), and theophylline.

Angina-pain-reducing drugs include nitroglycerin (side effects can be furious headaches, giddiness, and weakness), and beta-blockers and calcium-channel-blockers (see above). Stress-induced angina can be controlled with self-care actions (see "Self-Care Measures You Can Take" in this chapter) that have no side effects or dangers and little if any cost.

Blood-Thinning Drugs

Dicumarol has become the primary drug used to prevent blood clots. Sold as Coumadin, the drug can cause serious bleeding in the brain and intestines, so the dosage must be scrupulously monitored or the blood can become too thin and hemorrhage can result. Aspirin or phenobarbital can double Coumadin's blood-thinning effects, so do not take them together. Serious trauma to the head and body also can result in hemorrhage in those patients taking blood thinners. The drug must be discontinued for at least three days prior to dental extraction or any surgery.

Surgical Procedures

If you have blocked arteries, your doctor may suggest balloon angioplasty. During the procedure, a long catheter is inserted into the artery in the upper thigh and snaked up to the coronary artery. Although similar to cardiac catheterization, this procedure takes two to three hours and is a treatment, not a diagnostic procedure. Angioplasty is more successful in men because they have larger and less twisted arteries. It is less successful in women, people with diabetes, and individuals who are obese. Risks include a 30 to 50 percent recurrence rate within six months and a 4 percent rate for reblock of the artery within forty-eight hours after the procedure. To lower the risk of reblockage, you will have to follow a low-fat diet, exercise, and quit smoking. About 5 percent of the time during the procedure, a coronary artery goes into spasm or hemorrhage and becomes 100 percent obstructed. When that happens, emergency bypass surgery is necessary. To avoid bleeding at the catheter site of entry, you will have to lie perfectly still with your leg straight for twelve hours after the procedure.

If your coronary arteries are blocked or if an angioplasty procedure fails and you have a heart attack or go into shock, your doctor will tell you to have coronary artery bypass surgery. Get a second opinion. You will be put on a heart-lung machine. An artery from your chest or a vein from your leg will be removed and reconnected between the aorta and a point on the coronary artery downstream from the obstruction. If the surgeon needs multiple grafts, he might take an artery from your chest and one from your leg.

What are your risks with bypass surgery? Three percent of the people who have bypass surgery have a heart attack during the operation as a result of the procedure. If that happens to you, your heart will be damaged. If the damage is severe enough, heart failure can result. A few patients suffer so much damage to their heart that they need a heart transplant to survive. Hemorrhage and stroke also can occur. In rare cases the heart won't restart after the arteries are bypassed. A heart transplant probably will be necessary then, too.

What are the aftereffects of bypass surgery? Depression is a common reaction to the surgery. If you have sleep disturbance, loss of concentration or memory loss, you could be suffering from depression. Pain in a leg (due to use of the vein in the operation) is a common effect. Chest pain is another, since the breastbone is opened and the area is sewn closed. Chest pain after surgery also can be due to the trauma of surgery or to the coronary artery getting clogged again if you don't change your lifestyle and eat healthier. You won't be able to travel in a vehicle for six weeks or so, because if you are in an accident, you could injure your chest wall before it is properly healed.

Bypass surgery that occurs soon after a heart attack may increase your risk for stroke, according to a study reported in the *Journal of Cardiac Surgery.* Other studies, reported in the *New England Journal of Medicine* and the *Journal of the American College of Cardiology,* found that angioplasty with stenting showed at least as good survival rates as did bypass surgery. As angioplasty with stenting is less invasive than surgery and is associated with a faster recovery, talk to your surgeon about both and remember the pros and cons of each.

What are your alternatives to bypass surgery? Besides angioplasty, there is *Dr. Dean Ornish's Program for Reversing Heart Disease.* Patients in his program are often seriously disabled by chest pain and fatigue. The program includes a very-low-fat diet, exercise, and instruction on how to relax, not be lethargic, manage stress, and how to live fully in the world. The program will teach you how to feel freer and happier. It is based on love, knowledge, and compassion rather than just drugs and surgery. The program has proven effective, and many insurance companies will now reimburse you for taking this program.

Self-Care Measures You Can Take

There are many actions you can take to prevent or treat heart and blood vessel disorders. Select as many as you can from the following descriptions, keeping in mind that the more you change your lifestyle, the more you reduce your risk.

Learn How Your Feelings Are Affecting Your Heart and Blood Vessels

Get in touch with your feelings. Work your way through the following activities in any order that pleases you. Be sure to make a commitment to begin one of these actions today!

Start to pay attention to what your body is doing below your neck. Buy a small notebook, and keep it with you. Write down what your body is doing while you're watching television, working at your desk or in your office, riding in a car, and in other situations. See which ones upset you and if your heart beats faster or your hands get cold and your stomach ties in knots. As you begin to identify your feelings and experience them, you will not need to hold them in your body or let them fester and become part of a disease process. You may wish to take an assertiveness class or find a cognitive-behavioral therapist who can help you find a way to channel your feelings into productive action.

Get Sufficient Touch

Obtain at least ten hugs a day. Research reported in *Research in Nursing and Health* and *Journal of Advanced Nursing* showed that touch can reduce or affect blood pressure and enhance the immune response. Begin by asking your spouse or partner for a hug once every hour. Expand to asking friends for a hug. Touch will not only lower your blood pressure and cholesterol, it will also bring you closer to other people and provide the love and nurturance you may need.

Get in Touch with Nature

Spend time in nature, hiking, watching birds in the trees, and noticing flowers and animals. Take a family member or a friend with you and share the thrill of the outdoors and each other.

Go fishing. Concentrate on the rhythmic motion of casting. Enjoy the fresh air and sunshine. Focus on being, not on doing.

Meditate on the Meaning of Your Life

Contemplate the words that follow and see what meaning they have for your life:

1. "In the greater scheme of things, how much does this current stressful situation matter?"
2. "I have all the time in the world to accomplish what I want to accomplish."
3. "To heal my heart, I must grant forgiveness to the people I feel have hurt me."

Exercise to Strengthen Your Heart and Blood Vessels

Exercise daily. Walking is best, as running or jogging may be too stressful. Walk at your own comfortable rate and not in the heat of the day, slowly building up the distance and quickness with which you walk. Walk only as fast as you can comfortably talk to someone while walking.

Exercise reduces stress and gives your heart and blood vessels the nurturing they need. A study reported in the *American Journal of Cardiology* concluded that the intensity of exercise doesn't matter, but the regularity of it does.

Open Your Heart to Life

Practice opening up your heart by doing any or all of the following activities:

- Lie on your back on a bed, carpet, or pad. Hold one hand over your abdomen. Breathe in through your nose and then breathe out naturally, feeling your abdomen fall beneath your hand.

- When you can do the above activity comfortably, try this. Focus on your breath, and exhale and inhale three times naturally. As you feel the air moving in through your nose and back down your throat, say "one." Feel the air moving back out of your lungs and say "two." As the next breath begins to fill your lungs, say "three." Feel the air moving back out and say "four." Repeat these four actions three more times.

- Lie on the floor or in bed and slowly massage your chest. Start anywhere and gently and tenderly massage. If you find a sore or tight spot, massage that spot a little more until it feels better. Keep breathing evenly and deeply as you massage. When you've massaged your whole chest, see how your heart is feeling. Let your hand rest over your heart, as if you're going to say the Pledge of Allegiance. Feel your heart beating. Tell it to beat calmly and peacefully. Fill it up with peace and love.

- Picture your heart healthy and happy. See the cells in your heart looking healthy and joyful. Fill your heart with a joyful and relaxed color. Feel the positive energy flowing through your heart. Let a healing color expand, filling your heart, chest, and your whole body with soothing light. Give the color a voice. What does it say to you? Make it a joyful sound. Ask the color in your heart to give you a sign, to tell you what you're feeling. Tell your heart it's healing. Tell your heart you'll take care of it and protect it. Repeat as often as you need to until you can see the healing color and hear the voice of your heart.

- Put some stiff pillows on the floor in a pile or fold a blanket and lie down on it, arching your back over the hump. Allow yourself to surrender, letting your shoulders relax and your head relax back into the softness of the pillows or the blanket. Let your breathing slowly and naturally drop lower in your body all the way down to your abdomen. Hum or groan, releasing the tension in your throat and jaw. Take your time. Settle in. Feel any sadness or anger in your throat and shoulders. Let it dissolve or come out as a sound or a color. Replace it with forgiveness and joy.

- Stand up and reach toward the ceiling. Feel your fingertips pulsating with energy. Open your eyes and mouth wide and feel the tension in your face. Then close your eyes and mouth and feel the relaxation. Bend over at the waist, letting gravity pull your head and arms down toward the floor. Feel the energy flowing up through your feet and into your pelvis. Let your head bob like a flower in the breeze. Inhale and let the oxygen flow through your body and into your body tissues. Make soft sounds with your lips, recalling any sadness or loss of a loved one.

- Stand up or sit down on the floor and look at your hands. Picture the face of a loved one in your palm. Let any feelings come. Crying is healing. Let the tears flow.

- Put your hand over your heart and listen for any feelings inside. Feel the comfort that the beating of your heart provides. Feel any sadness or anger, then let it flow away like a quiet river.

- Hold a tennis racket or your fists over your head. Propel your arms forward with a hitting motion. Picture the person you are angry with. Let out any sounds or words you feel as you hit.

- Lie on your back on the floor on a carpet or pad. Do a scissors kick, building up to two hundred times. Shake your head back and forth saying, "No!" or "Why?"

- Rent a movie that makes you sad. Let yourself cry while you watch. It will cleanse your eyes and produce chemicals in your body that will help your cells relax.

- Rent a movie that makes you laugh. Watch it and laugh out loud. Allow yourself to really enjoy the movie. Go ahead; you deserve it.

- Use gentle acupressure to strengthen your heart. Hold the little finger of your left hand with the index, middle, and fourth fingers of your right hand. Hold it gently until you feel a pulse in it, and then in each holding finger of your right hand, that is steady, strong, and comforting. It may take a few minutes. If you're holding the finger too lightly, tighten your grip just a little. Eventually you will feel the pulsations as any blockages begin to open. Persevere. After you feel the pulsations in little finger of your left hand, repeat with your right.

- Recite or write twenty times a day the following affirmations to counteract the negative thoughts and feelings you have. Also, put the words of affirmations you like on 3x5 cards and place them in prominent places around your home and workplace so you will read them frequently. Suggested places include your refrigerator, medicine chest, and any mirror, desk, computer, or television set.
  1. My heart beats to the rhythm of love and understanding.
  2. I bring joy to the center of my being.
  3. I express love to all.
  4. Joy. Joy. Joy.
  5. Joy is circulating through me now and forever.

Learn to Relax

Use the relaxation script on pages 88–89 to relax and heal your heart and reduce your stress. You especially need to do this if you get angry when:

- you get cut off in traffic
- the person in the express checkout lane has too many items
- your spouse, partner, employee, teacher or student is late
- someone doesn't perform to your standards

Mend Your Relationships

Start with your father (or any other loved one from whom you feel distant). If, for example, your father is still alive, practice forgiveness and invite him to lunch. Only talk about neutral topics or things he likes. Get to know him as a person. Ask him questions, and then listen to his answers without judging what he says. Ask, "What are your hobbies? What do you like to do with your spare time? What are the best things in your life? What was it like when you were growing up? How did you get along with your father? What suggestions do you have for getting along better with you?" If you get into an argument, or if being with your father touches off remembrances of old arguments, before you separate, say, "I'm sorry." Those may be the two most healing words you can say to mend your broken heart.

If your father is dead or otherwise unavailable, write letters to him. Pour out your heart. There is no need to actually send them. You just need to get your feelings straightened out. Forgiveness is a major issue for you to deal with. Complete the same process for any other relationship that requires mending. Read and take to heart at least one of the following books: Thom Rutledge, *The Self-Forgiveness Handbook* (Oakland, Calif.: New Harbinger, 1997); Mona Gustafson Affinito, *When to Forgive* (Oakland, Calif.: New Harbinger, 1999); Virginia Sara Fair, *The Art of Forgiveness* (Monongahela, Pa.: Threesie Publications, 1997).

Massage Yourself, or Find Someone to Massage You

Add massage to your daily routine. Either find a massage or Rolfing therapist you like, or start to massage your feet while you're watching television or before you go to bed. Better yet, find a partner. You massage your partner's feet and then let your partner massage yours. Not only is it relaxing, but you will give and get healing touch. For more thoughts on massage, see the third paragraph of "Open Your Heart to Life" earlier in this chapter.

Start Eating Better

Change your eating patterns to cut down on saturated fats and sugar. Eat less or no meat, dairy products (milk, cheese, butter, eggs), fried foods, desserts (except for a piece of fruit), chips, French fries, and sugar. According to a study by Stampfer, these saturated fats and sugar raise triglyceride levels, now linked with an increased risk of heart attack.

Avoid eating salty foods or adding salt to your food if you have high blood pressure. Also, following the *DASH* (Dietary Approaches to Stop Hypertension) Diet has resulted in significant blood pressure reductions. The food plan includes eating many fruits, vegetables, low-fat dairy products, whole grains, poultry, fish, and nuts, and reducing intake of fats, red meat, and refined sugars. Potassium supplements or potassium-rich foods (bananas, cantaloupes, orange juice, baked potatoes, and low-fat yogurt) also can lower blood pressure, according to the *Journal of the American Medical Association*.

Stop drinking coffee. At least one study reported in the *American Journal of Clinical Nutrition* correlated coffee drinking with homocysteine, a blood risk factor for heart and blood vessel disease.

Take vitamins C and E supplements. The Honolulu Heart Program, which has been studying heart disease and stroke since 1965, found that vitamins C and E may boost mental ability and ward off blood vessel dementia, especially if you take them regularly over the years.

Remember that old adage "An apple a day keeps the doctor away"? It's true. Apples are especially good for the heart, according to research reported in the winter 2001 edition of the *Journal of Medicinal Food*. Researchers at the University of California at Davis found that drinking 12 ounces of apple juice or eating 2 apples a day can dramatically reduce the amount of LDL ("bad" cholesterol) in the blood and enhance the lag time for cholesterol to oxidize (which is associated with a reduced risk of heart disease). So if you have heart disease or don't want to get it, eat 2 apples a day or drink 12 ounces of apple juice a day; you should see results in six to eight weeks.

Eat at least one green salad a day. Forget about iceburg lettuce—it doesn't have enough nutrients. Try kale, arugula, escarole, spinach, parsley, romaine, and/or endive. Top it off with a tablespoon of olive oil and some cider or plum vinegar. Olive oil is heart-healthy, so use it for salads and cooking.

Eat at least five fruits or vegetables each day and more fish—the oilier, the better. Mackerel, salmon, and sardines are best. They all contain coenzyme Q10, a vital heart nutrient that will protect you against high cholesterol and irregular heartbeat.

Add soy foods to your food plan. There are many kinds; try them all, for example, soy milk (in strawberry, chocolate, vanilla, carob); tofu (scramble this instead of eggs, adding a little onion and fresh parsley or basil in olive oil, or put 2 to 4 ounces in a smoothie with frozen strawberries and enough cherry juice to make it a good consistency); tempeh (an exotic-tasting form of tofu that you can cube and put in salads or stir-fry with vegetables); and soyburgers (much better than hamburgers and much, much healthier).

Get a juicer. Use fresh and, if possible, organic vegetables. Studies show that organic fruits and vegetables have more vitamins and minerals. Cut the tops and bottoms off carrots and beets. Have several glasses of one or more of the following to help combat your heart or blood vessel disorder. Sip the juices slowly and enjoy their fresh taste: (a) carrot juice with 2 ounces of spinach juice; (b) carrot juice with 2 ounces of spinach juice, 1 ounce of celery juice (or more, according to taste and perceived benefit), and an ounce of parsley juice; or (c) carrot juice with 2 ounces each of cucumber juice and beet juice. *Note:* Because all fiber is removed from the vegetables, they are easy to digest. Make sure you get sufficient fiber from whole grain breads, cereals, and whole fruits and vegetables, because it can help you reduce cholesterol.

B vitamins can enhance the health of your heart. Eat the following foods to increase your intake of B vitamins: lentils, chicken, peanuts, sunflower seeds, tuna, turkey, brown rice, bananas, walnuts, sweet potatoes, cooked cabbage, sesame seeds, cauliflower, mushrooms, lima beans, prunes, green peas, asparagus, raisins, liver, and spinach. Niacin can help lower cholesterol and protect against heart and blood vessel disorders, according to *The Doctor's Vitamin and Mineral Encyclopedia*. Foods rich in niacin include wheat germ, wheat bran, brewer's yeast, salmon, prunes, lentils, chicken, peanuts, sunflower seeds, tuna fish, turkey, and rabbit.

Avoid Hormone Replacement

If you're a post-menopausal woman, avoid taking estrogen and progestin. They can increase your risk for heart disease, stroke, and blood clots, according to the National Institutes of Health (2002).

Learn to Play

Remember what it was to be a five-year-old, chasing a butterfly or picking up shells on the seashore and being delighted at the shapes and colors. Swing on a swing. Finger-paint. Play catch with someone, maybe your father.

Get on the floor with a dog or cat and roll a ball; scratch behind the animal's ears and snuggle up to it. Run in a field of wild flowers. Pick berries. Sit by the ocean or a lake and just watch the water for half an hour. Run in the sand and pretend you're a bird. Play has no outcome, no directions. Just enjoy.

Investigate Herbs

Investigate the use of herbs. If you are taking any medications, make sure they mix well with the herbs you plan to take by checking with your doctor first. Ginger has been shown to significantly reduce plaque and clotting in arteries, according to a study published in *Biomedical Biochemistry Acta*. In China, in one study 90 percent of participants with coronary artery problems were able to stop using nitroglycerin regularly after taking safflower and other herbs, according to *Chinese Herbal Medicine, Materia Medica*.

Ginkgo biloba has been shown to lower blood pressure and improve circulation. Garlic can enhance heart and blood vessel health. These herbs can increase the effect of blood thinners and aspirin, so you may want to talk to your physician about switching to ginkgo and garlic and getting off blood thinners and aspirin, which have side effects. Ginkgo also may affect the performance of Prozac and other antidepressants. Consider using more natural methods of reducing depression, such as enlisting the assistance of a cognitive nurse psychotherapist and taking a B vitamin supplement. If your depression and sleeplessness are due to perimenopause, consider taking black cohosh. Talk to a qualified herbalist who can help you coordinate your care with your physician.

Try Yoga and/or Dancing

Learn yogic breathing technique. Find a local yoga instructor who can help you learn the technique. Research published in the *International Journal of Neuroscience* reported that unilateral forced nostril breathing can positively affect heart function. Also, yoga and/or dance can put you in touch with your body and your feelings. Try taking a class in both to see which one suits you.

Stay Away from Pollution

Avoid going outside during times of high air pollution and/or move to an area that is less polluted. A recent study reported in *Lancet* found that heart attack symptoms correlated with times of high daily air pollution.

Engage in Meditation

Learn to meditate. Twenty minutes a day decreases carotid atherosclerosis, according to a study in *Stroke*, and can reduce blood pressure, in a study published in the *International Journal of Neuroscience*.

Monitor Your Own Blood Pressure

Purchase an easy-to-use home blood pressure monitor, and keep a diary of readings to be shared with your healthcare provider. In this way you can measure your blood pressure under work, stress, and relaxed situations. This can help you find the most appropriate treatment for high blood pressure. When you are in your doctor's office and your pressure is being measured, ask for a large cuff if you have a large arm (putting an average-size cuff on an arm that is bigger than thirteen inches around can lead to a falsely elevated blood pressure reading), keep your arm resting at the same level as your heart, and avoid talking or listening (ask whoever is taking it not to talk, because talking or listening can raise your blood pressure).

Hemorrhoids and/or Varicose Veins: Self-Care Measures

If you have hemorrhoids and/or varicose veins:

- Eat plenty of high-fiber foods every day (nuts, seeds, vegetables, fruits, and whole grains).

- Elevate your feet on a slant board or facsimile twice a day (at least two hours after eating). Start with a few minutes and work up to fifteen to thirty minutes a day. Check with your healthcare practitioner prior to doing this, to ask if there is any reason why you shouldn't. **Warning:** Avoid slant-boarding if you have had retinal detachments, glaucoma, or other conditions where increased pressure in your head is dangerous, or if you have an irritated hiatal hernia.

- Avoid wearing tight clothes, and don't sit or stand in one position too long. Walk around for a minute or two at least every hour, and do some stretches—reach for the ceiling with your right hand and for the floor with your left, keeping your body straight. Separating your fingers and gently stretching them, stretch some more until you feel a tingle in your fingers.

- Squeeze the juice of a quarter of a lemon in a glass of warm water and drink it first thing in the morning or if you are constipated and can't move your bowels.

- Oil your anus with olive or castor oil prior to having a bowel movement to protect it from pain and bleeding. Never strain. Breathe deep in your abdomen while you are sitting on the toilet. Never sit on the toilet to do your reading. Focus on staying calm and breathing. (Also see the immediately preceeding paragraph.) Elevate your feet on two or three bricks when you sit on the toilet to reduce abdominal pressure. After a bowel movement, gently dry with cotton balls soaked in castor oil, and apply vitamin E to your anus (to help heal and reduce pain), alternating with witch hazel (to shrink hemorrhoids and reduce itching).

- Take 2 ounces of aloe vera juice after each meal. **Caution:** Do not use the juice from an aloe vera plant. Purchase aloe vera juice from a health food store.

- Massage your feet, lower legs, and hands daily. Use olive oil or castor oil. Check with your healthcare practitioner to make sure it is okay to massage each area. If it is okay, place your hand on your umbilicus. If you have constipation, massage clockwise out in larger and larger circles, and then massage in until you reach your umbilicus again. Massage counterclockwise if you have diarrhea. If you have neither, first massage clockwise and then counterclockwise to maintain a healthy colon. Massage along your Achilles tendon gently. Massage your feet, especially the middle of the bottom of your feet. Massage on the inside of your palm in a line down from the area between your thumb and index finger.

- Use gentle acupressure. Put three fingers (index, middle, and fourth) on your hemorrhoid and the same three fingers of your other hand on the middle of your calf of the corresponding leg. (*Note:* This will work whether or not you're wearing clothes.) Hold both points until you feel a gentle, open, and strong pulse in all three fingers of both hands; then relax and focus on breathing in your abdomen. (This could take a while if there are energy blockages. At first you may not feel anything, then a pulse may begin, but it may come and go in one or more fingers. You also may feel some bursts of pulsation in one or more fingers until the pulse evens out and balances in a smooth, even flow in all three fingers.

- Between two of your meals, put 1 teaspoon of psyllium husks (available from a health food store) in a glass of water or juice, stir quickly, and drink before it thickens. If this stabilizes your bowel movements and reduces pressure in your hemorrhoids, continue; otherwise, stop.

- Sleep with a small, soft pillow between your knees to take the pressure off your hemorrhoids.

- To improve vein elasticity and strength, take vitamin C (1,000 mg two to three times a day with a full glass of water each time), vitamin E (400 to 800 mg a day), and zinc (up to 30 mg a day). Take bioflavonoids, or vitamin C with added bioflavonoids. Also try horse chestnut capsules (from a health food store).

- Get plenty of exercise, especially walking. Even walking ten thousand steps a day (an amount equivalent to what workers walked daily as measured by a pedometer) can reduce blood pressure that may be causing your hemorrhoids or varicose veins, according to a study in *Hypertension Research*.

- Lie on your back on a soft carpet or your bed. Bring your knees to your abdomen, then stretch them out straight (so you are lying flat), then bring your legs back up to your abdomen. Repeat, working up to twenty times a day. Remember to breathe from your abdomen with each cycle.

- Take milk thistle capsules (follow the directions on the bottle) to cleanse your liver.

Kidney Disease

Your kidneys are small, about the size of your fist, and are in the back, just below the rib cage. These small organs perform many vital functions that help maintain your overall health, including filtering waste and excess fluids from your blood. Every day, your kidneys filter about 200 quarts of fluid. About 2 quarts leave the body in the form of urine; the rest remains in your body. Besides filtering wastes, your kidneys also release hormones that help regulate your blood pressure, control the production of red blood cells, and make vitamins that control growth

When your kidneys no longer can perform these functions, your body may give you early warning signs, including high blood pressure; blood and/or protein in the urine; more frequent urination, especially at night; difficult or painful urination; puffiness around the eyes or swelling of hands or feet, especially in children; and a creatinine blood level greater than 1.2 for women and 1.4 for men.

An infection in the kidney may be proceeded by a *urinary tract infection* lower in the urinary tract. If you have a urinary tract infection, you will probably have some of the following symptoms:

- an urgent need to urinate, often with only a few drops of urine to pass
- a burning feeling when urinating
- an aching feeling, or pressure or pain in your lower abdomen

- cloudy or blood-tinged urine
- a strong odor in your urine

An acute infection of the kidney is usually due to a bacterium. Infections usually occur by ascending up from the bladder. Urine flow usually prevents infectious agents from traveling up from the bladder, but obstructions, tumors, and other conditions can make this journey possible. *Escherichia coli* is the most common bacterium found, and accounts for nearly 75 percent of kidney infections. This bacterium is normally found in the intestine and can be inserted in the urethra in women by wiping from back to front after urinating or after having a bowel movement.

Glomerulonephritis is a disease that damages the kidney's filtering units or glomeruli. The cause of this condition is not always known, but some cases may be inherited, while others may be triggered by an infection.

Other conditions that can affect your kidneys include kidney stones and inherited diseases such as *polycystic kidney disease*. In kidney disease, there is often loss of protein in the urine, called proteinuria.

A *kidney stone* is a crystallization of material (stone) formed in the kidney. Most stones are composed of calcium oxalate, but some are made of calcium phosphate, uric acid, or other chemicals. Stones sometimes stay in the kidney and grow, while others dislodge and try to pass down the narrow ureter, and in this location may be more likely to cause disabling pain. It's hard to predict which stones will cause pain and which won't. Sometimes pain comes and goes. When pain is present, it most commonly occurs in the low back to the side, but it also can occur in your abdomen. If you believe you have kidney stones, drink lots of water until you can get treatment.

Your Risk for Developing Kidney Disease

A kidney infection is more likely if you've had urinary catheterization. Infectious organisms have been found in patients who have indwelling catheters, who become infected while in the hospital, who are on chronic antibiotics, or who are being treated by steroids (such as prednisone) or immunosuppressive drugs (such as methotrexate, azathioprine, prednisone, cyclosporine, or cyclophosphamide) used in severe rheumatoid arthritis or after organ transplantation.

It used to be thought that eating foods high in calcium would cause kidney stones. Now, according to the *New England Journal of Medicine*, a high intake of calcium can reduce the urinary excretion of oxalate, which can lower the risk. A study in the *Annals of Internal Medicine* reported that eating dairy foods can decrease the risk of kidney stones. The same study found that sucrose (sugar) and sodium (salt) intake were associated with stone development.

Another major risk factor for kidney stones is a low intake of fluids, especially water. This produces a low urine volume which can lead to kidney stones, according to a report in *Nephron*.

The two leading risk factors for kidney failure are diabetes and high blood pressure. When these two conditions are controlled, the associated chronic kidney disease can often be prevented or slowed. If they are not controlled, kidney failure can occur, and regular dialysis or transplantation is necessary. A third cause of kidney failure is glomerulonephritis.

A study in the *New England Journal of Medicine* concluded that heavy use of acetaminophen (Tylenol) may cause kidney failure. Ibuprofen (Advil and Nuprin) and Naproxen (Aleve) also may damage the kidneys. For alternatives to pain management see the chapter "Pain" in this book.

According to *Prescription Alternatives*, other drugs that can stress or damage the kidneys include ACE inhibitors, Acyclovir, Allopurinol, aminoglycosides, Amphotericin, azathioprine, beta-blockers, Captopril, Cephalothin, chemotherapy drugs, Chlorothiazide, Chloropropamide, Clofibrate, cyclophosphamide, Cyclosporine, diuretics, Furosemide, Isoproterenol, Lithium, Macanylamine, Methotrexate, Methysergide, Morphine, penicillins, Phenylbutazone, Phenytoin, Piperdine, prednisone, Probenecid, Procaine, Quinidine, Salicylate, sulfonamides, and Tolazoline.

A metaphysical explanation for kidney disease focuses on how thought patterns form physical experience. According to Hay, holding on to old ideas, being "pissed off," and fear of letting go can result in bladder infections. Kidney stones are reflections of undissolved angers from the past. Other kidney conditions could result from feeling criticized, disappointed, shamed, or like a failure.

Six thousand years ago in China, the Yellow Emperor developed the Tao of Realization, a philosophy and method of thinking, breathing, and moving. In the Taoist system, a kidney ailment means excessive fear.

According to this system (see *The Complete System of Self-Healing Internal Exercises*), there are internal exercises that can heal and energize the internal organs, including the kidneys.

How the Doctor Diagnoses Kidney Disease

If you have a kidney infection, you may know it because your face or ankles will become puffed. You may feel an ache in your kidney region in your lower back above your waist on one side or the other, and your tongue may be discolored or "furred." You also may experience chills, fever, flank pain, nausea, vomiting, urinary frequency, and/or trouble passing urine, all of which may have come on quickly.

Upon physical examination of you, your doctor will note that your kidney is enlarged and ask if you're in pain. Diagnosis will be confirmed with laboratory tests, including urinalysis.

An X ray called an intravenous pyelogram or IVP is used to see where a kidney stone is lodged. A substance injected into a vein concentrates in your kidney and shows up on the X ray, detailing whether you have a kidney stone, an obstruction, or some other change from normal renal function.

If you have acute or chronic kidney (renal) failure, a number of other imaging techniques may be ordered to visualize the kidney. Some of these are ultrasonography, computer tomography (CT), angiography, venography, and magnetic resonance imaging (MRI).

What the Doctor Will Probably Prescribe

A kidney infection is usually treated with gentamicin, cephalosporin, or cotrimoxazole. All of these are antibiotics to quell bacteria. If you're not too ill, you may be prescribed tablets or capsules. If you're more ill, you may receive intravenous (IV) therapy. The length of therapy is usually two weeks, but up to six weeks may be required in men to prevent relapse. The doctor may order cultures four to six weeks after treatment to make sure an infection has not recurred. If you have a recurrent infection, you may be put on three-times-a-week therapy or even daily therapy with cotrimoxazole, trimethoprim, or nitrofurantoin.

The majority of kidney stones will pass spontaneously. All small stones should be given time to pass. If a stone doesn't pass, the doctor may suggest Extracorporeal Shock Wave Lithotripsy (ESWL). In this treatment, shock waves are passed through a water medium into your body and to the stone. These fragment the stone without injuring your body, allowing you to pass small pieces of the stone. Another technique involves placing a scope into your urethra, up the bladder, and finally into the narrow ureters. This scope then engages the stone and either fragments it or extracts it. If your stone is large, the doctor may place a scope directly through the skin in your back into the kidney. The stone may then be removed or fragmented through the scope. Fewer than 1 percent of stones end up requiring open surgery.

One treatment for kidney stones is often up to twelve tablets of hypocitraturic calcium or numerous crystal packages or liquid supplements taken through the day. Because this method is cumbersome and expensive, it isn't easy to keep up with the treatment, and this can lead to an increase in kidney stones.

Pain medication also may be prescribed or suggested. If it is, be sure you don't take acetaminophen (Tylenol), ibuprofen (Advil or Nuprin), or naproxen (Aleve). All three have been associated with damage to the kidneys.

Kidney or renal failure can be acute or chronic, and often is treated by dialysis. During this process, elements in the blood are separated in a solution by diffusion across a semipermeable membrane. Toxic products such as urea nitrogen are removed and a balance of appropriate substances is achieved. The dialysis machine achieves what a normally functioning kidney would. Depending on the health of the kidney, water and other fluids may be restricted to maintain specific levels of sodium.

Self-Care Measures You Can Take

There are many measures you can take to prevent or treat a kidney condition when action is necessary. First, when taking antibiotics, it is suggested that you either eat plain yogurt that contains acidophilus or purchase acidophilus at a health food store to replace the friendly bacteria in your gut that the drugs will kill. Without the "good" bacteria in your intestines, you will have difficulty digesting your food and may have cramps, pain, and other feelings of discomfort.

For any kidney condition, try this kidney exercise (from *The Complete System of Self-Healing*); use it every morning and whenever you have pain.

1. Stand up or sit in a chair, leaning a bit forward so you can easily put your fists on your back.

2. Rub your hands together vigorously until you feel the energy flowing in your palms and fingers.

3. Place your palms on the small of your back on each side of your spine, feeling the heat and energy flowing into your back. Keep your upper body tilted slightly forward.

4. Rub up and down and then massage your back in a circular motion.

5. Form two fists and pummel the small of your back for several seconds.

6. Rub and pummel the small of your back two more times.

For Urinary Tract Infections

- Drink plenty of fluids every day, including a large glass of cranberry juice, which has been shown to help prevent bacteria from attaching to urinary cells.

- Urinate immediately when you feel the urge; never wait.

- Empty the bladder completely each time during urination.

- Wipe from front to back after going to the bathroom.

- Clean the area around the rectum, vagina, and in between daily and before sex.

- Say or write at least one of the following affirmations at least twenty times every day:

  1. I am safe and secure.

  2. I release old angers and disappointments.

  3. I welcome the new into my life.

- If you are taking gentamicin, you may have kidney toxicity. A study in *Phytomedicine* found that the herb ginkgo biloba reduces this toxicity. Talk to your doctor about taking this herb.

For Kidney Stones

- Drink more water. Not drinking enough water is a frequent cause of kidney stones. Water helps flush toxins out of your body, so it's a good idea to drink *at least* ten glassfuls a day.

- Eat more foods rich in essential fatty acids. Not eating enough essential fatty acids may be a cause of some kidney conditions, according to a report in the *American Journal of Clinical Nutrition.* The benefits of polyunsaturated fatty acids have been shown in the prevention of some renal diseases. Some foods to eat include fatty fish (tuna, salmon, mackerel, herring, whitefish), green leafy vegetables, flaxseed (add to salads, soups, yogurt, cereals, baked goods, or fresh juices), olive oil, seeds, and nuts.

- Eat foods rich in magnesium. This mineral is an effective inhibitor of the formation and growth of calcium oxalate kidney stones. Eating an ovo-lacto-vegetarian diet (vegetables, fruits, whole grains, milk and milk products, and eggs) is a good way to get and keep the magnesium your body needs to ward off kidney stones, according to a study in the *British Journal of Nutrition.* You also might consider taking a magnesium supplement. According to a study in the *Journal of Urology*, oral supplementation of magnesium in patients with kidney stones resulted in a reduced risk for stone formation.

- Drink reconstituted lemonade. In a study reported in the *Journal of Urology.* the drink increased urinary citrate levels and lowered urinary calcium levels, two things that will reduce kidney stones.

- Reduce your consumption of protein, salt, and foods high in oxalates such as peanuts, cocoa, and chocolate, and the following cooked vegetables: beets, spinach, collards, rhubarb, or chard, because when you cook them, the heat from cooking turns the calcium they contain into calcium oxalate, and stone formation can occur *(Journal of Urology)*.

- Avoid drinking apple juice and grapefruit juice. Both were correlated with stone formation in a study reported in the *American Journal of Epidemiology.*

- Eat more dairy foods to boost your intake of calcium, and if you take calcium supplements, make sure you take them with meals. A study in the *Journal of Urology* found that restriction of dairy products in those prone to kidney stones was not necessary.

- According to findings reported in the *Annals of Internal Medicine*, kidney stones are correlated with sucrose and sodium intake. To reduce your chance of kidney stones, avoid eating sugar and salt.

- Another action you might consider is to lower your intake of animal protein (meat, chicken, eggs, cheese). This is not a settled issue, though. Some research shows that low-protein diets are helpful, but another study, in the *American Journal of Epidemiology*, found that lowering your intake of animal protein, eating a high-fiber diet, and being on a high-fluid diet have no advantage over just increasing your fluid intake.

- Eat more foods high in vitamin B_6, including brewer's yeast, sunflower seeds, toasted wheat germ, brown rice, soybeans, white beans, liver, chicken, mackerel, salmon, tuna, bananas, walnuts, sweet potatoes, and cooked cabbage. A study published in the *Journal of the American Society of Nephrology* found that a high intake of vitamin B_6 through food or supplements protected against kidney stone formation. This study also found that vitamin C need not be restricted, because it is not associated with risk for kidney stones.

- Avoid colas, even sugar-free ones. In one study, individuals who completely banned phosphoric acid-containing colas reduced their risk of recurring kidney stones by 38 percent.

- Eat rice-bran products. A report in *Drugs in Experimental Clinical Research* reviewed the phytonutrients from rice bran that have shown promise in preventing kidney stones. Rice-bran products were one of them, including crackers, cereal, and bread.

- Eat more foods high in potassium (shredded raw cabbage, bananas, turkey, apples, fresh apricots, cooked broccoli, baked potatoes, wheat germ, spinach, dried fruit, and fresh fruit). A study reported in the *Journal of Urology* found that a high-potassium diet may prevent stone growth.

- If you have an active, painful stone and your doctor sends you home to pass a stone, this kidney flush formula may assist you. Take two alfalfa tablets every hour. For the first day, take the juice of six lemons in a gallon of distilled water. Drink all of this the first day. If the stone hasn't passed, on the next days, only use water with the alfalfa tablets. Continue to eat lightly during this time.

- Say or write one of the following affirmations at least twenty times daily:

1. I let go of all anger.
2. I easily dissolve my past problems.

For Progressive Kidney Disease/Chronic Renal Failure

- Eat polyunsaturated fatty acid foods. The benefits of polyunsaturated fatty acids have been shown in the prevention of some renal diseases, including chronic progressive renal disease, according to a report in the *Journal of Nephrology*. Some foods to eat include fatty fish (tuna, salmon, mackerel, herring, whitefish), green leafy vegetables, flaxseed (add to salads, soups, yogurt, cereals, baked goods or fresh juices), olive oil, seeds, and nuts.

- Fish oil may reduce high blood pressure, prevent the development of proteinuria (protein in the urine), and minimize lesions, according to studies published in *Clinical and Experimental Pharmacology & Physiology* and the *American Journal of Kidney Disease*. To ensure these effects, take fish oil capsules and/or eat fish daily.

- Eat a high soy (especially tofu) and vegetarian diet, and include flaxseeds. A report in the *American Journal of Kidney Disease* reviewed recent findings from dietary intervention studies and found that both soy and flaxseed protect against kidney disease.

- Increase your intake of garlic. It can protect the kidney cortex *(Free Radicals in Biological Medicine)* and stop kidney damage in chronic kidney syndrome *(Molecular and Cell Biochemistry)*.

- Vitamin B$_6$ supplementation can improve tingling, numbness, and burning pain in fingers and toes that sometimes accompanies chronic kidney failure, according to a study in *Nephrology Dialysis and Transplants*.

- A Chinese herbal recipe called Yishen Huanshuai can markedly retard the rate of progression of chronic kidney disease when combined with a low-protein diet and controlled blood pressure, according to a study published in *Zhongguo Zhong Xi Yi Jie He Za Zhi*.

- Drink a pint of raw carrot juice mixed with one pint of raw spinach juice daily. It would be best to purchase a juicer, because the juice must be made fresh daily and drunk immediately. To juice spinach, roll several leaves up, then stick them, including the stems, in the juicer end, stems first. You can use a blender to blend the vegetables very finely, adding a small amount of distilled water. After blending, strain and drink immediately.

- Try to eat the following foods; they are considered kidney tonics in Chinese medicine: beef kidney, chestnuts, cinnamon, cloves, dill, fennel, fenugreek, lobster, pistachios, raspberries, and strawberries.
- To balance negative thoughts, say or write one of the following affirmations twenty times every day:

  1. It is safe to grow and be joyful.
  2. The right action is always taking place in my life.
  3. All things good come into my life.

Liver and Gallbladder Diseases

The liver is your body's largest internal organ, weighing 2.5 to 3.3 pounds. Your liver performs more than five thousand vital life-sustaining functions and is an incredibly resilient organ. Almost three-quarters of its cells must be destroyed or removed before it will stop functioning. Here are some of the things your liver does for you: produces bile, which helps remove waste products and aids in the digestion of fats; produces proteins that assist in blood clotting; produces and excretes cholesterol, which distributes fat around your body; and resists infection by producing immune factors.

There are a number of conditions that can disable your liver. *Liver failure* can occur due to an acute overdose of the mild analgesic acetaminophen (Tylenol), among other drugs. *Chronic liver disease* can occur gradually due to the use of prescribed, over-the-counter, or recreational drugs. *Postoperative liver disorders* can occur after surgery and reflect poorly understood effects of anesthetic and operative stress. *Cirrhosis* involves the development of scar tissue on the liver and loss of normal liver tissue. It is caused by chronic liver disease such as hepatitis, but also can be caused by alcoholism.

If you have hepatitis, you may think you have the flu. Symptoms include mild fever, fatigue, muscle or joint aches, nausea and vomiting, vague abdominal pain, loss of appetite, and diarrhea. You also may have dark urine and light-colored feces as well as *jaundice*, or yellowing of the skin and white of your eyes. Many people infected with hepatitis show no symptoms.

The gallbladder is a small sac in the upper right portion of your abdomen, under the liver and near the pancreas. It stores bile, but it also helps digest fat and absorbs some vitamins and minerals. The most significant gallbladder disease is the production of gallstones. Twenty million Americans have gallstones, and five hundred thousand of them undergo operations every year to have them removed. Eighty percent of all gallstones are made of cholesterol; the remaining 20 percent are bile pigment. Most are less than an inch across, but when an acute gallstone attack occurs, the gallbladder contracts and squeezes out one or more stones into the bile duct, along with its bile. The duct is small, and the stone causes a severe colicky pain. If a stone obstructs the duct long enough, bile backs up into the liver and then to the bloodstream, turning the skin and eyes yellow (jaundice). Gallstone pain can be severe, radiating around to the right lower scapular. Nausea and vomiting are usual.

Your Risk for Developing Liver and Gallbladder Diseases

Acute or Chronic Liver Disease

If you take prescription, over-the-counter, or recreational drugs, you are at risk for acute or chronic liver disease. Combined with alcohol, other liver-stressing drugs, or pesticides, your liver is at risk for damage.

All drugs stress the liver to some extent, but those hardest on this body organ are INH (isoniazid, a treatment for tuberculosis), chemotherapy drugs, methyldopa (Aldomet and Aldoril, used to lower blood pressure), monoamine oxide inhibitors (Nardil and Parnate are prescribed to treat mood disorders), all painkillers, anesthetics given during surgery, antibiotics, "blood thinners," antihistamines, cholesterol-lowering drugs, oral diabetes drugs, heart disease drugs, oral contraceptives, and Parkinson's disease drugs. One of the biggest reasons why natural remedies and lifestyle changes are preferable to using prescription drugs is that for the most part, natural remedies tend to be much gentler and safer, even if you take too much.

Hepatitis

Each type of hepatitis has specific risks. You are at risk for hepatitis A if you or your children are from a developing country or have been exposed to contaminated food or water.

You are at risk for hepatitis B if you do not use a condom, are exposed to blood and other bodily fluids at work, have hemophilia, take intravenous drugs, work in a long-term-healthcare facility, are an Alaskan native, had a blood transfusion prior to 1975, or were adopted from Eastern Europe, Africa, South America, Asia, the Middle East, or Pacific islands.

You are at risk for hepatitis C if you are exposed to blood on the job (healthcare, dental, funeral director, emergency worker, etc.), accidental needle sticks (if you're a healthcare worker), household transmission through shared razors or toothbrushes, take drugs intravenously, have your body pierced or tattooed, engage in intranasal cocaine use, or have a history of a sexually transmitted disease or prison stay. You are at risk for hepatitis D if you are an intravenous drug user who is a carrier of hepatitis B.

The major serious consequence of hepatitis C is cirrhosis. Factors that may be predictive of cirrhosis are being older at the time of infection, a longer duration of infection, being a man, using alcohol, coinfection with hepatitis B, and a compromised immune system. Factors that may affect disease progression include smoking and exposure to environmental contaminants.

Gallstones

You are at risk for developing gallstones if you are overweight, don't exercise daily, fast regularly, are female and are between ages twenty and sixty, have been eating fewer than eight hundred calories a day for twelve to sixteen weeks, have had a gastric-bypass operation to lose weight, have been on birth-control pills or hormone replacement therapy, or are a Native American man, a Pima Indian woman of Arizona, or a Mexican American of any age or either sex. A study published in the *European Journal of Gastroenterology & Hepatology* reported two other risk factors: wine consumption and laxative use.

How the Doctor Diagnoses Liver and Gallbladder Diseases

The liver is a complex organ, and no single or simple test assesses overall liver function, so your doctor probably will order several of the most useful screening tests to determine the extent of liver damage, including urine bilirubin (detects bilirubinuria, an early sign of liver disease that develops in acute viral hepatitis even before jaundice appears), urobilinogen (is very difficult to interpret, but may be sensitive for mild liver disease), and 5'-nucleotidase (detects an enzyme that increases in liver diseases). Some of these tests are available at your local pharmacy in commercial urine strip tests. Other tests might be ordered by your doctor.

Symptoms the doctor will ask you about are pain in your abdomen and the upper right quadrant or the upper middle of your abdomen that may radiate to your back below your right shoulder blade, pain that starts after eating fatty or greasy foods, jaundice, fever, nausea and vomiting, heartburn, indigestion, and abdominal fullness. *Cholecystitis* is the diagnosis the doctor will make for an acute inflammation of the gallbladder wall, usually as a response to obstruction in the bile duct by a gallstone. The most widely used test to confirm the presence of a gallstone is an abdominal echo (ultrasound). It is painless, noninvasive, and 98 percent accurate.

If a gallstone has lodged in a bile duct, your doctor may want you to have an ERCP (endoscopic retrograde cholangio-pancreatography) examination. You swallow a long, thin, lighted flexible tube connected to a computer and a TV monitor. A special dye is injected that stains the bile ducts, making them more visible. Any stone can be removed at that time.

What the Doctor Will Probably Prescribe

Abstinence from alcohol can reverse cirrhosis of the liver if it is due to drinking. Acute alcohol withdrawal usually occurs in a hospital. Regardless of the cause of cirrhosis, withdrawal of toxic agents, good nutrition (including supplemental vitamins), and adequate fluids are the most important treatments. Sedatives can lead to further liver damage.

There is no medical treatment for hepatitis A and hepatitis B. Like most viruses, they run their course. Appetite usually returns after the first several days, and confinement to bed is not necessary. Refrain from using any drugs, since they place an undue burden on an already weakened liver. You can safely return to work after the jaundice resolves. The treatment for hepatitis D is to get into a drug rehabilitation program.

The treatment for hepatitis C is interferon, but a new drug, ribavirin, has been approved for use along with interferon. See "Self-Care Measures You Can Take" in this chapter if drugs are prescribed for you. Liver transplantation is the only medical treatment when hepatitis is so severe it damages the liver irreversibly.

Side effects of interferon are flulike and usually occur within the first two weeks of treatment. Serious adverse effects can occur, including severe fatigue, muscle aches, headache, backache, difficulty concentrating, mental clouding, decreased sex drive, hair loss, decrease in white blood cells and platelets, anemia, fever, thyroid disorders, irritability, anxiety, sleep disturbances, severe depression, and suicide. Side effects of ribavirin include anemia and genetic defects in fetuses. Your doctor or nurse probably will caution you to use birth control during therapy.

A typical gallstone episode improves in two to three days and resolves within a week. If your gallstones don't bother you, leave them alone, because there's only a 2 percent chance they will ever act up. If you have chronic pain, you can take a pill (ursodeoxycholic acid) that will dissolve them, but it could take months or longer. There is no guarantee that new ones won't bother you in the future unless you change your lifestyle. *Shock wave lithotripsy* fragments the stone into small pieces that can then be passed, sometimes with a great deal of pain. Your doctor will probably suggest that your gallbladder be removed and tell you that you can live without this organ. You can, but all gallbladder functions, including absorbing vitamins and minerals, will be lost. Get a second opinion before having any surgery.

Self-Care Measures You Can Take

Symptoms of pain and even jaundice are messages from your body to take better care of it and change your lifestyle. Taking too many drugs or drinking too much alcohol or being around pesticides or other toxic materials can lead to liver problems. Eating too many animal fats (butter, bacon, cream, cheese, red meat, and chicken or turkey skin) can lead to gallstones. Vow to change your lifestyle by using one or more of the self-care measures suggested. The more you incorporate these measures into your life, the healthier will be your liver and gallbladder.

For Your Liver

Jaundice or deep-seated pain in your right side near your rib cage are messages from your liver that it needs to be cleansed. Follow the suggestions below to prevent liver disease, or to treat it should your liver become weakened.

- Drink a flush drink for breakfast: juice of 1 to 2 grapefruits or 2 oranges, 1 clove of garlic, 1 tablespoon of olive oil, and the juice of 2 fresh lemons. A sprinkle of cayenne pepper is optional. Drink the mixture for breakfast. Follow with 2 glasses of warm water or herbal tea (dandelion leaf or root, oatstraw, peppermint, yarrow, chickweed, or red clover). Eat nothing solid until lunch.

- Eat the following foods to cleanse your liver: artichokes, watercress, fresh lemon juice, celery, and papaya.

- Take milk thistle to help cleanse your liver. Use it to keep your liver clean and functioning if your doctor prescribes any drugs. *Alternative Medical Review* published information on its effectiveness and use in the treatment for hepatitis, fatty liver, cirrhosis, and viral hepatitis.

- Take SAMe for pain. This popular supplement works as well as ibuprofen and other painkillers but fewer adverse effects, according to *Clinician Reviews*. It also may help relieve liver symptoms.

- Avoid all red meats. Eat only fish and chicken. Do not have any sugar, alcohol, coffee, or tea (except herbal), fried foods, processed foods or flours, salt, strong spices, preservatives, additives, or synthetic vitamins. Eat pickles, sauerkraut, and other fermented vegetables to stimulate the healthy functioning of your liver. Other cleansing foods include pineapple, celery, parsley, watercress, and fresh grapes. Eat a lot of steamed vegetable and tofu meals, concentrating on green vegetables. With lunch and dinner have 2 tablespoons of grated beets with 1 tablespoon of olive oil and 1 teaspoon of fresh lemon juice. Eat bland, avoiding onion, garlic (except in the liver flush drink), radishes, and spices. Avocados also are good to eat.

- For infectious hepatitis take 1,000 mg of vitamin C every two to four hours with a full glass of water; a calcium citrate-magnesium capsule; and a B complex capsule, vitamin E, and lecithin *(Vegetarian Times/Well-Being)*.

- If you have cirrhosis, try taking zinc as a supplement. In a study reported in the *Romanian Journal of Internal Medicine*, patients who were given zinc improved considerably after thirty days.

- Use licorice abstract (not the candy). In Chinese medicine this herb has been used for thousands of years as a treatment for liver dysfunction *(Designer Foods III, Proceedings)*. A study in *Hepatology* found that licorice (glycyrrhiza root) prevents progressive disease in hepatitis C. Another study, in *Cancer*, found that licorice extract was effective in preventing liver cancer in individuals with chronic hepatitis C.

- Consider using black pepper. In a study reported in *Cancer Letters*, black pepper was shown to be a potent liver detoxifier.

- Complete the following exercises morning and night, working up to three to four times a day:

  1. Stand with your arms hanging freely. Twist vigorously from side to side, inhaling deeply while twisting to the left and exhaling when you twist to the right. Repeat up to twenty times.

  2. Inhale and reach up with your arms, clasping your hands above your head. Bend to the left while you exhale, and hold for five slow counts. Inhale slowly, bringing your arms back above your head. Bend to the right while you exhale, and hold for five slow counts. Inhale slowly, bringing your arms back above your head. Repeat up to five times.

  3. Kneel on the floor, extending your left leg to the side and stretching your right arm up and over your head while sliding your left arm down your leg toward your foot. Keep your elbows and unbent knee straight. Hold while inhaling and exhaling slowly for ten breaths. Picture your liver releasing toxins on each exhalation and cleansing itself as you inhale *(The Foot Book)*. Repeat, using the right leg and right arm.

  4. Sit or lie down in a quiet, comfortable place. Place the palm of your right hand on the side of your body next to the bottom of your rib cage. Rub your hand across the bottom of your rib cage

up to your sternum (center of your rib cage). Rub up and back thirty-six times *(The Complete System of Self-Healing Exercises)*.

- Avoid taking acetaminophen (Tylenol). A study published in the *Journal of the American Medical Association* found that Tylenol was associated with liver toxicity. Use SAMe instead (see the fourth item above in this list).

- Use affirmations to heal your liver. Say or write at least one of the following statements 20 times each day to counter your negative emotions:

  1. I feel only peace.

  2. I feel only love.

  3. I feel only joy.

For Your Gallbladder

- Change your lifestyle patterns and switch to eating a healthy, low-fat diet. Stay away from greasy, high-fat foods, and stick with lean sources of protein (turkey, fish, chicken, tofu and other soy products), fresh fruits and vegetables, and whole grains. A vegetarian diet has shown promise for people with gallbladder problems, according to a study published in *Digestive Diseases*. A large Harvard study found that women who ate lots of fruits and vegetables were least likely to have gallstone symptoms. The foods especially effective at promoting bile flow and strengthening your gallbladder are apple juice, radishes, Brussels sprouts, artichokes, and bitter greens (radicchio, dandelions, escarole, arugula, and endives) Try to eat 75 percent raw fruits and vegetables. Avoid sugar and products containing sugar in any form, commercial salad oils (stick to olive oil for salads and cooking), coffee, chocolate, and refined flour products (any pasta, cereal, bread, or dessert that isn't made with whole grains).

- Avoid diets. A study reported in the *Annals of Internal Medicine* linked rapid weight change and temporary weight loss with increased risk of gallstones. Dieting boosts the need for gallbladder surgery by up to 70 percent; women with severe weight cycling (more than one diet a year) had a 68 percent greater risk.

- For five days consume as much pure apple juice as possible. Add pear juice occasionally. Beet juice also will cleanse your liver. Use a juicer, and put 2 to 3 ounces of beet juice in a glass of carrot juice.

- If you have gallstones; combine 3 tablespoons of olive oil with the juice of 1 lemon or ½ grapefruit. Take it before retiring and upon awakening. Many stones pass in the stool with this technique.

- If you are having gallstone pain, heat a piece of flannel or cotton with ½ cup of castor oil. Place the castor oil pack on the gallbladder area for at least an hour. For a more powerful pack, lay a plastic bag on top of a heating pad and then the soaked flannel pieces. Keep the heating pad setting on the highest tolerable temperature.

- Investigate the use of the herbs wild yam, dandelion root, and peppermint. Be sure to consult with a healthcare practitioner with expertise in herbology, although all three are relatively safe. You also can eat dandelion greens if you're worried about taking herbs. You can obtain essential peppermint oil in a health food store. (Don't use the cooking variety, which is not pure oil.) Peppermint can be taken in tea, tincture, capsule, and oral peppermint. It is effective for the aggravating chronic burping that often accompanies gallbladder disease.

- Take up to 3,000 mg of vitamin C (ascorbic acid) daily. In a study published in *Archives of Internal Medicine*, men and women who had a high level of ascorbic acid in their blood had 13 percent fewer incidents of gallbladder disease. Other studies have shown that vitamin C helps to turn cholesterol into bile acids.

- Keep physically active. Exercise (the more vigorous the better) has been linked with reduced risk for gallstone disease in a study reported in *Annals of Internal Medicine*.

Multiple Sclerosis

Multiple sclerosis (MS) is a progressive, degenerative disorder affecting the white (and occasionally the gray) matter of the central nervous system. The result is abnormal nerve conduction. The cause is not clear, but some research suggests an immune-mediated response to a viral trigger *(American Journal of Nursing)*. Heredity, a virus, and poisons in the environment, especially heavy metals, also are at the top of the list of possible causes. Chemical poisoning by pesticides, industrial chemicals, or heavy metals also may play a part in the development of MS. Many experts suspect that mercury poisoning is behind many cases of MS, especially due to amalgam dental fillings. (The levels of mercury in people with MS have been found to be an average of seven times higher than those in healthy people.) There is also a theory that MS is caused by food intolerances or allergies, especially to dairy products and gluten. Diet may play a key role in the development of MS. The condition is common in the United States but is almost unheard of in Japan, Korea, and China. Asian fare is typically low-fat, and the diet is rich in marine foods, seeds, and fruit oil, which are high in essential fatty acids, which have an inhibitory effect on inflammation. Consumption of saturated fats, cholesterol, and alcohol in the United States leads to the production of a hormonelike substance called prostaglandin 2, which worsens symptoms of MS and promotes the inflammatory response.

MS is widely believed to be an autoimmune disease in which the body is attacked by its own immune system, instead of protecting the body against harmful invaders. In MS, the target of the attack is the myelin sheath that protects nerves in the brain and spinal cord. When this protection is destroyed, signals are no longer reliably transmitted to the muscles.

Another explanation for multiple sclerosis is metaphysical. This philosophy states that both the good things in life and the diseases result from negative thought patterns. *Heal Yourself* lists mental hardness, hard-heartedness, iron will, inflexibility, and fear as the negative thought patterns correlated with multiple sclerosis.

Your Risk for Developing Multiple Sclerosis

If you have MS in your family, are exposed to heavy metals, eat a lot of fatty foods, drink alcohol, or are between ages twenty and forty, your risk for developing MS may be increased.

How the Doctor Diagnoses Multiple Sclerosis

There is no single test for MS, and all its symptoms could be caused by some other condition. Symptoms also tend to appear and then disappear for long periods of time, so it could take years to get a clear diagnosis. Symptoms that may lead your doctor to diagnose you with MS include pain, tremors, speech impairment, blurred or double vision, and dizziness. The disease can progress to a stage of needing a wheelchair and indwelling urinary catheter.

What the Doctor Will Probably Prescribe

One of the most recently approved medications for MS is Novantrone (mitoxantrone), which works by suppressing the T cells, B cells and macrophages believed to lead the attack on the myelin sheath. Other commonly prescribed drugs are Betaseron, Avonex, and Copaxone, but they are very expensive (up to ten thousand dollars a year), even if you have a medigap policy. Also, all treatments are administered by injections, sometimes daily, and you will have to be taught to give yourself the shots.

Other problems with the drugs include their side effects. For example, Betaseron has the following adverse reactions: injection site reactions and harm to the tissues, flulike symptoms, menstrual disorders, mental disorders, depression, sleepiness, palpitations, high blood pressure, blood vessel problems in the arms and legs, stomach and intestinal upset, destruction of blood cells, trouble breathing, laryngitis, bladder infections, pain, and more (*Nurse Practitioners' Prescribing Reference*).

A significant number of individuals with MS suffer from fatigue. (See "Chronic Fatigue Syndrome.") One drug frequently prescribed for this symptom is Amantadine, but no reliable studies on its use have been published to date. Pemoline is another drug used for fatigue, but a meta-analysis published in *Health Technology Assessment* found it was no better than a placebo (sugar pill) in reducing fatigue. A study reported in *Health Expectations* found that of the 318 individuals diagnosed with MS they surveyed, 47 percent reported using evening primrose oil and 8 percent used cannabis for help in treatment.

Self-Care Measures You Can Take

The prevalence of MS has been increasing, and traditional medical therapies and treatments are only temporarily effective (*Cleveland Clinic Journal of Medicine*). A report in the *Journal of Holistic Nursing* found that 56 percent of patients diagnosed with multiple sclerosis had their mercury dental fillings removed; 50 percent tried homeopathy; 50 percent tried massage; 44 percent changed their eating patterns; 32 percent tried physical therapy; 32 percent tried psychological counseling; 19 percent participated in aquatic therapy; 13 percent used shiatsu, biofeedback, or chelation; and 6 percent tried therapeutic touch or yoga to stop progression of the disease. All respondents reported that the severity of their symptoms decreased as a result of the therapies they tried. There was a statistically significant improvement in symptom severity following use of complementary therapies. Some complementary therapies you might want to try are discussed below.

- Say or write one of the following affirmations twenty times a day to counteract the negative mental patterns that may have a hold on you:

  1. I choose loving, joyous thoughts.

  2. I am safe.

3. I am free.

4. I create love and joy.

- Rub any sore, cold, or inflexible body parts with gentle compassion, bringing fresh blood and energy to those spots.

- Lie prone on your side with one hand over your head and the other resting on a soft mat, rug, or mattress beneath you. Bend the knee of your top leg, but keep the bottom leg straight. Breathe in and out very slowly while tightening the muscles of your anus. Hold the muscles tight for as long as you can, then relax. Repeat until you feel weary or strained, then stop and relax (*The Complete System of Self-Healing*).

- Change your eating patterns. According to the *Journal of Neurovirology*, a good diet to treat or prevent MS includes fresh prepared fruits and vegetables to aid in remyelination of your spinal cord and nerves. Replace all animal fat (meat, milk, eggs, cheese) with plenty of monosaturated fat (olive oil to cook with and put on your salads), and move to a vegetarian diet, suggests a report in *Medical Hypotheses*. Eat plenty of omega-3 fatty acids (found in salmon and other cold-water fish and in flaxseeds). Also take in capsule form 500 mg of evening primrose oil or black currant oil to reduce inflammation (*Integrative Medicine*). If this doesn't help, eliminate bread, pasta, rice, cereals, and all grains.

- To prevent urinary infections, take vitamin C every day (*Journal of Neurovirology*).

- Enroll in a tai chi or exercise class. A study reported in *Alternative Therapies in Health and Medicine* found that walking speed, hamstring flexibility, and psychosocial well-being improved. In another study, published in *Annals of Neurology*, fifty individuals diagnosed with MS were randomly assigned to a three-times-a-week exercise class or to nonexercise groups. Participants in the exercise class had improved bowel and bladder function and significant increases in upper and lower extremity strength, aerobic capacity, and triglycerides, and in combating depression, anger, and fatigue.

- Investigate bodywork/massage and psychological counseling to combat depression anxiety and to improve self-esteem (*Complementary Therapies in Medicine*).

- Look into aquatic exercise. A study reported in *Physical Therapy* found that aquatic therapy with a pool temperature of 94°F improved mobility.

- Join a music therapy group. A study reported in *Rehabilitative Nursing* found that patients who received music therapy showed more expiratory muscle strength than patients who attended music appreciation class.

- If you have constipation, fecal incontinence, or a combination, sign up with a biofeedback specialist. A study reported in the *Journal of Neurology and Neurosurgical Psychiatry* found a beneficial effect after biofeedback sessions for patients whose bowel symptoms were having a major impact on their life.

- Try yoga. Its gentle stretches can help you maintain strength, flexibility, and balance. This focused breathing exercise can reduce stress and symptoms. Look for an instructor in your yellow pages or watch for flyers about yoga classes.

- Take extra B vitamins to help form and maintain the myelin around your nerves. Foods that contain vitamin B_{12} are especially important, including sardines, herring, nutritional yeast, mackerel, trout, sea vegetables (kombu, dulse, kelp, and wakame), and fermented soyfoods (tempeh, natto, and miso).

- Try the Ayurvedic tonic herb ashwagandha. You probably will have to visit an Ayurvedic practitioner to obtain the herb. It could protect your body against stress and counter fatigue *(Integrative Medicine)*.

- Investigate hypnosis. A study in the *American Journal of Hypnosis* reported use of hypnosis with individuals with multiple sclerosis. Hypnosis helped patients get out of wheelchairs, walk with better balance, and experience reduced pain. A secondary effect of hypnosis was an increased sense of hopefulness.

- Drink fresh juices every day. Start with a pint (2 glasses) of carrot juice, or 9 ounces of carrot juice with 5 ounces of celery juice and 2 ounces of parsley juice, or 12 ounces of carrot juice mixed with 4 ounces of parsley juice. Work up to several quarts of fresh juice a day.

Osteoporosis

Osteoporosis is a progressive condition with deterioration of bone tissue that results in loss of bone mass. When bone mass diminishes, bones become fragile, and the risk of fractures from minimal trauma rises.

Your Risk for Developing Osteoporosis

Age and gender are risk factors. Ninety percent of women over age seventy-five have osteoporosis. Being postmenopausal, engaging in excessive exercise, having had a hysterectomy, early menopause, and anorexia nervosa all lower estrogen levels and accelerate loss of bone.

Stress increases the release of adrenal hormones that stimulate the cells that break down bone tissue. Caucasian and Asian women are more likely to develop the condition than African American women. Anyone who's had a previous fracture is more likely to develop osteoporosis. If you're chronically thin, smoke, drink alcohol, lack aerobic and weight-bearing exercise, have a calcium deficiency, are a high-performance athlete, indulge in extreme diets, or carry the genes for osteoporosis, you're more likely to get the condition.

High blood pressure in elderly women has been linked with abnormalities in calcium metabolism leading to calcium losses, according to a study reported in the *Lancet*. A number of studies have linked excessive meat consumption to greater bone loss. Because meat is acidic, it causes the body to use calcium to buffer acids, thereby depleting the available calcium from healthy bone. Red meat also contains phosphorus, which can facilitate the loss of calcium.

Drinking cola beverages also is a risk factor for osteoporosis. A survey reported in the *Journal of Adolescent Health* found that girls who drank cola drinks, which are high in phosphoric acid that can cause calcium to leave the bones, were more apt to have bone fractures.

Other medical conditions and medications can increase your risk. If you have diabetes; kidney or liver disease; thyroid or parathyroid disease; Cushing's syndrome; stomach or intestinal disorders; or use thyroid medication, steroids, diuretics, or phenytoin, you are at greater risk for osteoporosis.

While fiber has a positive effect on your digestion and cholesterol, eating too many fiber-rich foods when you eat calcium-containing foods can interfere with your body's ability to absorb calcium. Too much salt also can lead to your body excreting calcium; so can drinking carbonated beverages, because the phosphate in the drinks binds with calcium, reducing its absorbability. Lack of essential fatty acids also can lead to osteoporosis *(Progress in Lipid Research)*. Avoid taking benzodiazepines (Dalmane, Doral, and Halcion), which increase your risk for osteoporosis *(Nurse Practitioners' Prescribing Reference, New England Journal of Medicine)*.

A metaphysical approach to osteoporosis examines the connection between the mind and the body. Mental thought patterns are believed to inform physical life experiences. Disease is created by negative thoughts. In this framework, osteoporosis is interpreted as feeling there is no support left in life *(Heal Your Body)*.

How the Doctor Diagnoses Osteoporosis

Osteoporosis is rarely diagnosed before major bone loss has occurred. Often the condition is only found by mistake, when your doctor looks at your X rays for some other reason and sees that you have the condition.

There are some conditions that mimic osteoporosis, including disk disease, osteomalacia, degenerative arthritis, and vitamin D deficiency, which makes diagnosis even more difficult. The primary ways your doctor can tell if you have osteoporosis are by bone density measurement tests (BDM), which measure bone strength, and skeletal imaging studies. Blood and urine tests also can show bone disease.

What the Doctor Will Probably Prescribe

Hormone replacement therapy (HRT) is one of the most used treatments for osteoporosis. It can prevent fractures associated with the condition. It also relieves hot flashes, protects against atrophy of the bladder and vagina, and may reduce risk of heart blood vessel disease. According to the National Heart, Lung and Blood Institute, it also can increase the risk of endometrial cancer, heart attack, stroke, breast cancer, blood clots in the lungs, make your breasts tender, and cause vaginal bleeding. You can't take HRT if you have active liver or gallbladder disease, are pregnant, use oral contraceptives, or have breast or endometrial cancer. Many women start taking HRT and then drop the treatment due to the inconvenience of vaginal bleeding and the fear of breast cancer.

Biphosphonates were approved by the FDA in 1997 for the prevention of osteoporosis. Alendronate can decrease the possibility of fractures, but should be taken upon waking on an empty stomach with a full glass of water. You shouldn't sit or lie down for thirty minutes, to prevent acid regurgitation, and refrain from eating and taking calcium supplements and antacids for at least thirty minutes, either. Adverse effects you might experience include abdominal pain, upset stomach, nausea, constipation, diarrhea, gas, ulcers in your esophagus, pain in your muscles or bones, and headache. Stomach and intestinal ulcers also could result (*Nurse Practitioners' Prescribing Reference*).

Calcitonin is a hormone secreted by the thyroid in response to increased calcium in the blood. With aging, the level of this hormone decreases, and the hormone is less effective. You may get a prescription for calcitonin if you are postmenopausal and unable to use HRT. It can't be taken by mouth, so you'll either have to receive an injection or use a nasal spray (Micalcin). Calcitonin has been shown to reduce new spinal fractures by 36 percent. Adverse reactions to expect if you take this drug include back pain, stomach and intestinal upset, dizziness, tingling of the hands, rash, antibody formation, and facial flushing. You won't get flushing or stomach or intestinal symptoms, but you may get ulcers in your nasal passages, and nasal and lung congestion.

Selected estrogen receptor modulators (SERMs) are another category of drugs used to prevent osteoporosis. Raloxifene (Evista) is an alternative to hormone therapy. The drug can boost bone density and reduce serum cholesterol. It can cause blood clots, leg cramps, hot flashes, may antagonize blood thinners, and shouldn't be used if you take diazepam (Valium).

Fluoride has been used in clinical trials, but it hasn't been approved by the FDA. It may decrease fracture, but it can produce nausea, diarrhea, vomiting, hemorrhage, pain in the joints and stomach and intestinal symptoms, and/or rashes and may be more prone to bone fractures and osteosarcoma (a form of bone cancer). With fluoride now being added to water, toothpaste, mouthwashes and other products, there is a danger of overfluoridation (*Review of Fluoride*).

Self-Care Measures You Can Take

- Eat more foods high in calcium. If you don't eat these foods already, add them to your menus: tofu, broccoli, kale, raw spinach, perch, turnip greens, okra, beet greens, collards, sardines, salmon, dried beans (pinto, black), chickpeas, sesame seeds, almonds, brazil and hazel nuts, some mineral waters (check the label), and nonfat yogurt. Avoid eating them with bran or other high-fiber foods when eating calcium-rich to enhance their absorption. Eliminate animal proteins (meat, cheese, eggs, milk) that increase the elimination of calcium. When your diet consists of more than 15 percent of protein, your kidneys require much more water than usual to excrete it. As a result, calcium is flushed out. At the very least, reduce your intake of animal protein to 3 to 6 ounces a day (*Z Arztl Fortbild*). A great way to protect your bones is to drink 3 glasses of carrot juice mixed with 2 ounces of parsley or spinach juice. You will exceed the U.S. RDA for calcium if you do, but you will also build bone strength, strengthen your eyes, and aid your digestion. Also eat lots of fruits, vegetables, and dried beans. They contain boron, which has a positive effect on calcium absorption; reduces excretion of calcium; and lowers blood phosphorus levels, another factor associated with osteoporosis (*American Journal of Natural Medicine*).

- Take 1,500 mg of calcium citrate daily to maintain bone strength (*Journal of Clinical Pharmacology*). Take it in divided doses every other day to increase bone resorption and to protect against osteoporosis (*Calcification Tissues*). If you aren't in sunlight daily, take a vitamin D supplement to further prevent postmenopausal bone loss (*Journal of Bone Mineral Research*).

- Eat more soy products. A report in *Menopause* found that eating whole soy foods resulted in significant reductions in clinical risk factors for osteoporosis, while a study in the *American Journal of*

Clinical Nutrition found that soy protein stops bone loss in the lumbar spine in women who are at about menopausal age. Consider using soy as your main source of protein. Most people eat too much protein, and it increases calcium excretion according to a report in *International Journal of Sport Nutrition*.

- Exercise. Men who used vigorous to moderate levels of physical activity were protected from future hip fractures, according to a study in *Archives of Internal Medicine*. Women who folk-danced or participated in gymnastics showed improved muscular performance and body balance in addition to increased bone mass, according to a study in the *Journal of Bone and Mineral Research*. The Rehabilitation Institute of Chicago recommends weight-bearing exercise to help develop bone mass and strength; do this for twenty to thirty minutes three to four times a week, or for three minutes ten times a day. Even walking, as long as it is performed briskly, can enhance the minerals in your bones (*International Journal of Sport Nutrition*). Back-strengthening exercises also are beneficial. If you spend fewer than four hours a day on your feet, you are at increased risk for hip fracture (*New England Journal of Medicine*). Weight lifting can maintain bone mineral density and ward off osteoporosis, according to a study conducted at the University of Florida in Gainesville. But you don't have to do something that energetic. Gardening once a week can prevent osteoporosis, according to a study presented at the annual meeting of the American Alliance for Health, Physical Education, Recreation, and Dance. Women over age fifty who did yard work at least once a week had stronger bones than women who jogged and did aerobics. Weight training was the only other activity that significantly strengthened bones.

- Avoid antacids as a regular source of calcium. They can interrupt the effect of other drugs and are damaging to you if you have kidney disease (*Drugs*).

- Don't smoke. Smoking reduces bone mass and increases your risk of fractures.

- Avoid heavy alcohol use. Heavy drinking results in decreased bone mass and increased risk for falls and fractures. A maximum of two drinks a day is a good rule.

- Eliminate caffeine (coffee, caffeinated tea, colas, chocolate, and cocoa) from your meal plan. High caffeine intake is associated with increased risk for hip fracture, according to a study in the *New England Journal of Medicine.* Avoid carbonated drinks, even noncolas, because they make calcium less absorbable.

• Eat lettuce and green leafy vegetables at least once a day. A study in the *American Journal of Clinical Nutrition* found that women who ate lettuce once a day had half the risk of hip fractures of women who didn't. Vitamin K was thought to play a key role in allowing certain proteins to be taken up by the bones. Other foods to eat that are rich in this vitamin are broccoli, Brussels sprouts, cabbage, kale, and spinach.

• Eat more prunes. They are a source of boron, which is believed to play a role in the prevention of osteoporosis *(Critical Review of Food Science Nutrition).*

• Move toward a plant-based diet. It is beneficial to bone health *(American Journal of Clinical Nutrition).*

• Maintain your weight. Women who weighed less than they had at age 25 had two times the risk of hip fracture, according to a study in the *New England Journal of Medicine.*

• Take a multivitamin along with your calcium and vitamin D. It can help you increase spinal bone mineral density, according to a study in *Osteoporosis International.*

• Encourage your children and grandchildren to take part in sports. A study in *Bone* reported that those who participated in sports during adolescence had less osteoporosis later in life.

• Avoid taking steroids (prescribed for asthma, rheumatoid arthritis, glaucoma, and other conditions). Corticosteroids are linked to bone loss, according to the American College of Rheumatology.

• Make sure you get enough vitamin C. It is a cofactor in collagen formation, the glue that holds your bones in place *(Yale Journal of Biological Medicine, Physiological Review).* Eat plenty of foods high in vitamin C, including green peppers, honeydew melons, cooked broccoli or Brussels sprouts, cooked kale, cantaloupes, strawberries, papaya, cooked cauliflower, oranges, watercress, raspberries, parsley, raw cabbage, grapefruit, blackberries, lemons, onions, sprouts, raw spinach, and tomatoes.

• Vitamin B_6 can function as a cofactor to build up cross-links, which stabilize the collagen chains of the bone. A study reported in *Acta Orthop Scandinavia* found that participants in one study who had low vitamin B_6 blood levels were more likely to sustain hip fracture. Make sure you eat foods rich in this vitamin, including brewer's yeast, sunflower seeds, toasted wheat germ, brown rice, soybeans, white beans, liver, chicken, mackerel, salmon, tuna, bananas, walnuts, peanuts, sweet potatoes, and cooked cabbage.

- Eat foods and take supplements rich in essential fatty acids. Some of the best sources are fish and fish oils, flax oil, olive oil, borage oil, and evening primrose oil.

- Eat plenty of onions, and use onion powder in cooking. A study reported in *Nature* found that a dried onion daily prevented the bone loss that would normally occur due to the decrease in estrogen levels. It also reversed the bone loss seen in osteoporosis, and the effect was greater than that available using the osteoporosis prescription drug Calcitonin.

- Say or write one of the following affirmations twenty times a day:
  1. I stand strong and healthy.
  2. Life itself supports me.
  3. I walk forward in love.

- Complete a bone breathing exercise: Lie on your back in a comfortable place or sit in a chair once you've mastered the process. Keep your arms next to your body and your feet slightly apart. Keep your eyes closed and take a few easy breaths, letting your breathing move toward your center. When you exhale, let go of everything it's time to let go of, letting it flow down your body and out your toes. When you inhale, let energy come in your toes and flow up through the bones of your legs, up through your spine and neck. and out the top of your head. Exhale again. On the next inhale, let energy flow through the bones of your chest, down your arm bones, and out your fingertips. Repeat the whole sequence three to four times.

Overweight/Obesity

Carrying around extra weight is hard on your heart, but dieting is harmful, too, and it isn't effective. Research published in *Obesity Research* found that frequent dieters showed significantly more weight regain than less frequent dieters.

Taking appetite suppressants and using laxatives don't work either. Research published in the *Journal of Consulting Clinical Psychology* found that even among young girls, those who dieted were more likely to weigh more, and obesity was strongly associated with trying to control weight. The researchers concluded that weight-reducing efforts lead to dysregulation of the normal appetite system, resulting in weight gain from erratic eating behaviors and decreased efficiency in metabolism.

According to Louise Hay, our thoughts shape our life and experiences. Metaphysical models are based on the idea that awakening the ability to actively contribute to your healing positive thought patterns can lead to a positive outcome. A belief in fear, a need for protection, running away from feelings, insecurity, self-rejection, and eating to seek fulfillment are some of the beliefs you may hold if you are overweight.

Your Risk for Developing Overweight/Obesity

Being overweight is correlated with diabetes, heart disease, breast cancer, backache, gallstones, high blood pressure, and joint and muscle conditions, among other conditions. According to a report in *Preventive Medicine*, these conditions may be compounded if you eat meat.

Stress can affect your eating patterns and could be a significant risk factor. When you are under continual stress, you do not pay attention to the signals inside you that tell you when you're hungry and when you're full, according to studies in the *Journal of Clinical Psychology*, *Physiological Behavior*, and *Obesity*. When you aren't in touch with your inner signals, you will eat beyond being full and eat to reduce stress.

How the Doctor Diagnoses Overweight/Obesity

The *Body Mass Index* (BMI) is used to determine overweight and obesity. It is determined by multiplying your weight in pounds by 703 and dividing that result by your height in inches squared. The following BMIs are used by your doctor: normal weight between 18.5 and 24.9, overweight between 25 and 29.9, obese between 30 and 34.9, and very obese over 35.

What the Doctor Will Probably Prescribe

Your doctor may give you a diet to follow or may just suggest you lose weight. He probably won't have the time to make sure you follow up, although the nurse or nurse practitioner may help you. If not, you may decide to look into diet drugs or just follow the latest fad diet you see advertised.

WHY DIETING ISN'T THE ANSWER

Dieting may sound like an easy way to lose weight. The latest fad diet brings hope that "this will be the one," but it never is, at least not for long. Once you return to old eating habits, the weight piles back on.

The real problem with all of these diets is that eating so much protein is very unhealthy. It leaches minerals from your bones and accumulates ketones that are bad for your kidneys and that can give you headaches, bad breath, and dizziness.

Because they lack sufficient fiber, these diets don't protect you from toxins and can leave you constipated. What is more dangerous about these diets is the intake of saturated fat that is encouraged is one of the major risk factors for strokes, certain cancers, and heart attacks. Your risk for these conditions increases even more because you are restricting intake of the very foods that could protect you—fruits, vegetables, and grains

Yo-yo dieting or weight cycling is even worse because you lose weight quickly and regain it, increasing your risk for gallstones and the need for gallbladder surgery (*Annals of Internal Medicine.*)

Dieting regularly is also bad for your heart. Losing weight may help, but when you gain it back, rebound effects are unhealthy. Your blood pressure may soar, you may have disturbances in heart rhythm, and defects in heart function can occur. Yo-yo dieting and its resultant weight fluctuation yielded death rates that were higher by 50 percent (*Journal of the American Medical Association*).

When you diet, by definition you restrict intake of some foods. High-protein, high-fat diets restrict the very natural antioxidants in vegetables, fruits, and grains that can protect you. These are the very substances that fight the cellular damage that can be done by free radicals found in pesticides, acid rain, artificial preservatives, additives, and environmental pollutants.

Taking a vitamin pill will not correct the problem, according to reports in *Haemostasis* and *ASCD Journal of Dentistry and the Child*. Other substances may be contained in vegetables, fruits, and grains that could protect you that we haven't even identified yet. Eating a small amount of foods rich in antioxidants confers more protection than thousands of units of vitamins.

Dieting also is harmful because it leads to false hope, making you think the weight will stay off, according to a report in the *International Journal of Eating Disorders*. When weight is regained, as it is for 90 percent of dieters, depression and feelings of failure arrive. These bring more stress.

Dieting is stressful and leads to binge eating, which is correlated with bulimia. As tension builds from feeling deprived of certain foods, binge eating occurs. According to a study in the *Journal of Eating Disorders*, women most likely to binge had dieted one or more times in the past year. The more that participants in the study tried to restrict what they ate (dieted), the more they binged and exercised excessively and were apt to be bulimic.

Dieting also can affect your reactions and mental performance, according to a study in the *Journal of Clinical Psychology*. When participants were tested on reaction and mental performance tests, dieting was comparable to having had two alcoholic drinks. The ones who did the worst on the tests were the ones who were dieting but weren't losing any weight.

DIET DRUGS DON'T WORK EITHER

If dieting isn't the answer, neither are diet pills. Many drugs, such as Benzedrine and Dexedrine, have been banned due to their addictive qualities. Dexatrim and Acutrim have been banned because of their stroke risk. Fenfluramine was first reported to be safe, then pulled off the market when people started dying. Herbal weight loss products haven't been tested for long-term weight loss effectiveness.

Self-Care Measures You Can Take

- Develop a contract with yourself or a trusted significant other to get yourself going. The idea is to identify a specific goal you want to work on and then take active steps to meet that goal. This works even better if you do it with a supportive friend—someone who will help you along, not discourage you.

- Chart your food and mood. Keep a food/stress diary for at least a week. Write down each time you eat something, what it was, and what you thought and did while eating it. After several days you will begin to see patterns of how stress leads to eating too much or too little; then you can begin to plan ways to prevent stress eating. Finding patterns is the first step on the path to controlling your weight.

- Eliminate sugary foods, which can aggravate tension, increase stress, and add unwanted pounds. They taste good, but studies in *Nutrition Report, International Journal of Eating Disorders,* and *Behavioral Neuroscience* found that the mood enhancement that sugar brings lasts briefly. After one or two hours, fatigue and decreased energy resume. With this dip in mood, the urge to eat more sugar recurs, and you'll probably reach for a sweet. A cycle is reinforced, and weight gain is not far behind.

  A study in *Behavior Therapy* found that eliminating sugar from the diet reduced symptoms of depression, and returning it to the diet brought the depression back. This showed that the effect of sugar on mood was a real one.

  Eating low-fat sweet foods will not help in weight loss because sugar is usually used to replace the fat that is removed. Sugars that may be the worst for weight loss are refined sugars. These are sugars added to foods to make them taste better, instead of unrefined sugars that occur naturally in fruits and some vegetables. The sugar in cookies is refined, while the sugar in a banana is unrefined. A study in the *Journal of the American Dietetic Association* concluded that in a group of men and women who ate the same number of calories, the ones who ate refined sugars gained more weight.

  Eating sugary foods that are also high in fat puts on even more weight because the foods taste good, yet are not satisfying for long because they're not nutritious. This leads to eating more and more cookies, candy bars, doughnuts, cakes, pies, ice cream, Danish or sweet rolls, and other baked goods.

- Eliminate artificially sweetened foods. Some are linked to cancer. Aspartame is methanol or wood alcohol and contributes to the formation of formaldehyde in the body. Reported reactions to aspartame (NutraSweet and Equal) include mood swings, headaches, changes in vision, sleep disorders, memory loss and confusion, nausea and diarrhea, and even convulsions, according to studies in *Neurology, Biological Psychiatry, Journal of Neuropathology and Experimental Neurology,* and *Life Science.*

- Avoid processed foods; they don't have enough fiber in them to keep blood glucose levels low. Consuming too many processed foods can produce insulin resistance and send blood glucose to fat depositories on your body.

- Eliminate the stress of caffeine (coffee, tea, colas, chocolate, cocoa, some prescription and over-the-counter drugs), which can raise your blood pressure, contribute to adrenal exhaustion, create hormonal imbalances, and has even been linked to cancer (*American Journal of Cardiology*). *The Merck Manual of Diagnosis and Therapy*, a medical text that has been relied on by physicians for a hundred years, lists caffeine as a poison. And homocysteine, a risk factor for heart disease, is correlated with coffee drinking, according to a study in the *American Journal of Clinical Nutrition*. Caffeine creates more stress by leaching calming B vitamins, bone-strengthening calcium, and relaxing magnesium (*American Journal of Clinical Nutrition, Journal of the American College of Nutrition*).

- Avoid gluten if you find that after you eat bread, cake, pie, cereal, or canned goods, you find you have abdominal cramping, gas, bloating, chronic diarrhea or constipation, fatigue, depression, or bone or joint pain. These are signs of gluten intolerance. Every time you eat this substance, a portion of the lining of your small intestine is damaged, creating stress in the intestine and making it nearly impossible to absorb vital stress-reducing nutrients.

- Eliminate oxidized transfats from your diet. These products were developed by a food process called hydrogenation, which transforms vegetable oils into solid substances that can alter the composition, size, and number of your fat cells, promoting weight gain. Transfats are found in almost all commercially made doughnuts, crackers, cookies, pastries, fried foods, potato and corn chips, baked goods, frosting, candy products, and most margarines. A study of eighty-five thousand nurses confirmed that those who consumed more transfats, and especially margarine, had higher rates of both heart disease and cancer (*Health and Stress*). Use olive oil instead.

- Stay away from meat and animal products that can stress your kidneys and liver and leave less room for the fruits, vegetables, and grains you need to stay healthy and lose weight. A vegetarian eating plan is associated with less heart disease, diabetes and other chronic illness, and lower weight, according to studies in *Public Health Nutrition, American Journal of Clinical Nutrition*, and *Preventive Medicine*.

- Eat a variety of foods. When you eat, always sit down to do it. Don't eat while driving, and never do anything else while you're eating. Concentrate on chewing, tasting, enjoying. Don't think or talk about upsetting topics while you eat. Listen to your "fullness" signals and stop eating. Even if you think you're still hungry, wait at least five minutes before you eat more. Let your digestive processes catch up with your brain.

- Don't drink alcohol while you're eating if it makes you eat more. Sometimes it works to drink half a glass of wine right before you sit down to eat. It relaxes you and slows you down. Experiment and find out whether you eat more or less. Use the method that works for you. Be careful, though—drinking more than half a glass will short-circuit your fullness signals and may lead you to eat way beyond your nutritional needs.

- Always drink a glass of water before you eat. Sometimes that will fill you up enough so you won't eat as much. Drink at least ten glasses of water a day. When you feel hungry between meals, drink a glass of water. You need water to digest your food and move toxins and wastes through you. Your brain is about 75 percent water and is the first part of you affected when you don't drink enough. Although you might not notice, dehydration can lead to headaches, fatigue, poor physical performance, and bad food choices.

- Always eat breakfast, even if you're not hungry. Examine your eating patterns if you don't want breakfast. Chances are you're eating after 7:00 P.M., which is a no-no if you want to lose weight. Better to go to bed hungry. Drink a glass of water and go to sleep. Get up and eat a big breakfast. Your metabolism will work the best and work off the calories the best the earlier in the day you eat your biggest meal. If you skip breakfast, eat a salad for lunch, and pick at food all night, there is no way you can lose weight. Reverse your eating patterns and you will lose weight. A study in *Medicine and Science in Sports and Exercise* backs this up. The researchers found that eating light all day but having a large evening meal made participants store more fat. Even when they reduced their daily calories and exercised vigorously, they could not lose weight. Some even gained weight.

- If you get hungry, eat five or six meals a day. This is an especially good tactic if you suffer from low blood sugar. You can tell if you have low blood sugar because you will experience sugar craving, headache, palpitations, jitteriness, weakness, or fatigue. In this case, eat five or six small meals that are high in protein (tofu, fish, and skinless chicken are good bets) and low in carbohydrates (especially fruits, cereal, pasta, bread, and rice) at spaced intervals. Don't cut out vegetables, though, because they provide so many vitamins and minerals and protect you in other ways.

- Eat high-satisfaction foods. Some foods fill you up better than other foods. Focus on eating them instead of reaching for a sugary sweet or a nonnutritious snack. One study ranked the following foods in order from most satisfying to least satisfying: potatoes, fish, oatmeal, oranges, apples, whole-wheat pasta, baked beans, grapes, whole-grain bread, popcorn, bran cereal, eggs, cheese, white rice, lentils, brown rice, and rice crackers. You can lose more weight and make it stay off if you eat foods high in starchy carbohydrates such as potatoes and rice because they weigh more than high-fat foods but contain fewer calories (*Journal of the American College of Nutrition*).

- Eat foods high in fiber to reduce stress to your digestive system and lose weight. Eating a moderate amount of high-fiber foods helps you lose weight because they fill you up and take longer to eat. (It takes longer to eat an apple than drink a glass of apple juice, and crunching is more satisfying than drinking.) If you eat more digestible fibers (cereals, fruits, vegetables, beans, whole-grain breads, nuts, and seeds), you'll not only regulate your blood sugar and feel more satisfied, you'll also reduce your risk of heart disease and high cholesterol.

- If you have any elimination problems or suffer from abdominal discomfort or heartburn, purchase psyllium husk powder, an indigestible fiber available at health food stores. Put a teaspoonful in a glass of water, stir quickly, and drink.

- Use tryptophan (an amino acid found in all protein-rich foods) to reduce cravings and enhance sleep. If you're a woman and premenopausal, you may experience carbohydrate craving and depression before your menstrual period. If you live in the northern part of the United States, you may experience depression with a lack of exposure to sunlight. These conditions are stress-related and are associated with tiny chemical messengers in your brain (neurotransmitters) that affect your mood, appetite, cravings, sleep, and basic drives. If you are stressed and can't sleep, have a piece of tuna or chicken on half a slice of bread, or eat fish for dinner and have a piece of fruit an hour before bedtime. If you're vegetarian, have cooked dried beans or peas for dinner and half a piece of bread or half a cup of rice about an hour before you go to bed.

- Use monounsaturated oil to reduce afternoon cravings. If you eat a salad for lunch, make sure you drizzle olive oil on it. According to a study presented at the Experimental Biology 2000 Conference in San Diego, men who were served lunch prepared with monounsaturated oil were significantly less hungry than the group who were served a lunch prepared with polyunsaturated oil.

- Eat high-zinc foods to lose weight. A study reported in the *Journal of the American College of Nutrition* found that zinc may influence leptin, a hormone that plays a key role in maintaining energy balance. Leptin can make you feel full even when you're not. If you're overweight, you're probably not producing enough leptin to curb your food cravings. Men who were fed zinc-deficient diets produced less leptin. The researchers concluded that when fat is lost, leptin production decreases, which may explain why dieters regain weight. If you maintain high leptin levels by eating foods high in zinc, it may help you keep weight off once you've lost it. Zinc-rich foods include oysters, herring, eggs, nuts, wheat germ, liver, and red meat. Dietary fiber, calcium, and foods that contain phytate (dried beans, whole grains, and peanut butter) can interfere with your body's ability to absorb zinc, so have them at times other than when you're eating zinc-rich foods.

- If you crave chocolate and find that eating it prevents you from losing weight, you may wish to eat more foods high in magnesium. Research published in the *Journal of the American Dietetic Association* found that chocolate can be used as a self-medication for dietary deficiency, especially magnesium. Foods high in magnesium include whole-grain breads and cereals, brown rice, fresh peas, wheat germ, nuts, soy products, Swiss chard, figs, green leafy vegetables, and citrus fruits.

- Increase your intake of B vitamins to help metabolize fatty foods (and lose weight) and raise your mood. Since stress is linked to overeating, calming your mood also can help. Foods to concentrate on include sunflower seeds, rolled oats, lima beans, soybeans, raisins, wheat germ, peas, whole-wheat-flour foods, asparagus, brown rice, chicken, peanuts, raw spinach, kale, eggs, tuna, turkey, salmon, mackerel, sweet potatoes, cooked cabbage, bananas, sardines, trout, sea vegetables (dulse, kombu, kelp, and wakame), fermented soy foods (tempeh, natto, and miso), fresh green uncooked vegetables, lobster, broccoli, cauliflower, sesame seeds, mushrooms, yogurt (plain, low-fat), oranges, grapefruit, peaches, lettuce, and molasses.

- Train yourself to stop binge eating. One thing that may drive binges is a lack of serotonin, a feel-good brain chemical that can help calm you. Eating carbohydrates increases serotonin levels, while eating protein reduces them. This could be why being on a high-protein, high-fat diet will lead to stressful feelings and binge eating, while chocolate, pasta, and bread may make you feel relaxed. If you feel stressed, take a bite of bread or a mouthful of pasta or rice. (Chocolate is not recommended because of its high fat and sugar content.)

  Another action you can take to reduce binge eating is to start a binge journal. Write down when you binge; the trigger experiences that precede your binge eating; and your thoughts and feelings before, during, and after your binge. After recording several episodes, you will begin to see patterns and situations that set you up to binge.

  You also can use distraction when the urge to binge strikes. Count to ten, read a favorite book, exercise, get a hug or massage, or get involved in some activity you enjoy. Make sure you don't get overly hungry, fatigued, hung over, lonely, or stressed, as any of these situations can lead to binge eating. Carry a handful of unsalted and nonoiled nuts with you to snack on so you won't be overly hungry. While you're chewing on them, ask yourself, "Am I really hungry, or am I angry or hurt?" If you're angry or hurt, listen to a relaxation tape (buy one in advance for moments such as these). Take a relaxation break instead of a coffee break every day as a preventive action. If you don't have a tape, find a quiet, comfortable spot, kick off your shoes, sit, place one hand over your abdomen, close your eyes, and gently suggest that you will breathe in your center, about navel level. As your breathing relaxes and moves lower in your body, it will gradually push out your hand. Sit there quietly, breathing. You can combine this with a meditation to stop bingeing. Breathe in and say to yourself, "I am in control of what I eat." Then breathe out and say to yourself, "I eat only what I need to stay healthy." Alternative statements are to inhale and say, "I breathe in calm and control," and to exhale and say, "I breathe out all fear (worry, anger, hurt)."

  Eat at least one portion of a "forbidden food" every day. Restricting yourself from eating the foods you adore and then bingeing on them, then feeling guilty and restricting yourself again is a common cycle that you can choose to stop by eating one portion of a food you've restricted yourself from eating.

Make sure you eat enough protein to help eliminate cravings. Some good snacks to carry are a couple of crackers with cheese or peanut butter on them, a hard-boiled egg, or a couple of slices of chicken or turkey.

Drink half a glass of unsweetened fruit juice when you start to crave food. If you crave fatty foods (e.g., French fries, burgers, or chips), take a tablespoon of flaxseed oil or several flaxseed capsules when you get an urge to binge. Or eat only a handful of walnuts, a good source of fatty acids.

If chocolate is your downfall, eat foods high in magnesium (discussed earlier in this section). Moderate exercise, such as brisk walking, can help your body use insulin more effectively so you'll be less apt to binge.

Avoid bringing binge foods into the house and don't plan for a time to eat them. If you live with someone else, ask that person to help you and not bring binge foods home. On days when you have spare time and could binge because you're bored, plan an activity with someone else, and keep your promise. Eat your forbidden foods somewhere other than your home, or only bring home one portion.

- Use imagery to picture yourself fitting into the clothes you want to wear, meeting your eating goals, and letting go of any failures or angers. This will help control your eating.

- Do at least one active thing after you eat dinner: walk, dance, clean your house. Choose something that engages your mind so you're not thinking about food.

- Use affirmations to put positive thoughts in your mind to counter any negative ideas you have. Choose one of the following statements, and say or write it twenty times a day:

  1. I am safe.

  2. I love myself and approve of my actions.

  3. I create my own peace and security.

For a complete weight loss plan see *De-Stress, Weigh Less: A Six-Step No-Diet Plan for Relaxing Your Way to Permanent Weight Loss* by Paul J. Rosch and Carolyn Chambers Clark (New York: St. Martin's Press, 2001).

Pain

Pain is an unpleasant sensory and emotional experience associated with actual or potential tissue damage. Since there are no biological markers for pain, you are the best source of what kind of and how much pain you have. How much pain you feel is subject to your memories, expectations, and emotions.

Chronic pain is a persistent pain that does not respond to routine pain control methods. Despite the fact that chronic pain doesn't respond to medication, a recent Louis Harris telephone survey found that one in five older Americans is taking pain medication several times a week or more, and 63 percent had taken prescription pain medications for more than six months *(The Study of Pain and Older Americans)*.

The results of chronic pain include depression, decreased socialization with others, sleep disturbance, difficulty walking, and increased visits to the doctor or other healthcare provider. You also may be more irritable and even confused when the pain takes over. You may find yourself calling out, crying, or moaning in pain.

Chronic pain can occur just about anywhere, from the feet and the legs to the head, where recurrent tension headaches, migraines, and mixed headaches are found. Pain can have its source in nerves or muscles or bones. Pain that seems to be located in one spot but actually is due to tissue damage somewhere else in the body is called *referred pain*.

One explanation for chronic pain is that it is caused by damaged and inflamed nerves, muscles, or blood vessels. This damage makes the pain very real. Your body can become locked into a vicious cycle when you limit movement in the painful area and as a result lose strength and flexibility. If you try to guard against the pain, muscle tension and spasms can result. This can lead to frustration, anger, and depression. Friends and family may not understand how much of your life pain has taken control of and may underestimate its hold over you. This can lead to more frustration and depression and even more pain. Others may coddle you. This can make you feel dependent and out of control. All these negative emotions can perpetuate more pain. The more negativity you feel, the more pain you experience. The more pain you experience, the more negativity you feel *(Emotional Wellness Matters)*.

Your Risk for Developing Pain

If you're older, you're more apt to suffer from arthritis, bone and joint disorders, back problems, and many other chronic conditions. Besides age, cultural group can influence pain and how it is perceived. Contrary to popular belief, pain is not a necessary part of aging *(Nursing Home Medicine)*.

How much pain you complain about and even how much pain you feel can be affected by your cultural and family groups. Some families focus on and complain about pain openly. Other families and cultural groups are more stoic and prefer to suffer in private. If you were raised in an environment that didn't focus on pain and even taught you to deny it, chances are you won't be very verbal about your pain, may think it's not worth mentioning, and may suffer needlessly. If you've come from the opposite kind of environment, you may be very verbal about your pain and very in touch with every aspect of it.

Unmet psychological, social, economic, or sexual needs may be at the root of much chronic pain. High emotion or increased stress can bring on headaches or chest pain. Anxiety and fear also can have a strong effect on how much pain is experienced. Sometimes chronic pain is related to old, unhealed emotional wounds due to incest, rape, or other traumatic experiences that have not been resolved.

How the Doctor Diagnoses Pain

Effective January 1, 2001, all nursing homes, hospitals, and clinics certified by the Joint Commission on Accreditation of Healthcare Organizations (JCAHO) must institute new standards of pain assessment and relief. This means you have the right to have your pain assessed and managed appropriately, that you should be asked to rate your level of pain on a scale from 0 to 10 (children may be shown pictures), results of this assessment must be documented, and appropriate pain relief should be initiated (*American Journal for Nurse Practitioners*).

Because the majority of people with chronic pain have few if any abnormal physical findings, the doctor will probably ask you a number of questions to determine the type and effects of your pain. Some questions you may be asked include: "When did the pain start?" "How long have you had the pain?" and "What kind of pain is it?" Some descriptive terms you can use to tell your doctor about your pain are "burning," "discomfort," "aching," "soreness," "heaviness," "tightness," "shooting," "radiating," "ripping," "stabbing," and "stinging." You may be asked to describe the pain's intensity, character, frequency, patterns, location, duration, what helps and what makes the pain worse. You may want to write this all down to give to the doctor, or bring along a family member who knows about your pain if you anticipate experiencing a lot of pain during the visit.

Because chronic pain can influence your daily activities, the doctor also may ask if you've had any changes in daily activities, have suddenly stopped common routines, or have decreased your interaction with friends or family due to your pain. The doctor may observe your facial expressions for signs of pain and see if you rock or change position because of the pain.

Be prepared to either show or tell the doctor what kind of pain medications you are taking, both prescribed and over-the-counter and any complementary remedies you are using, especially herbs. The doctor or nurse practitioner will probably give you a physical examination to determine if there may be some unidentified sources of your pain. You may be asked to fill in a scale that evaluates your mood, especially depression.

The doctor also may want to see you walk and see what effect if any your pain has on your gait. You may be asked how your pain has affected your ability to function or the quality of your life. Pain should be assessed by a pain intensity scale, which starts at 0, or no pain, and goes to 10, or the worst possible pain. The doctor may give you a pain scale and ask you to fill it in daily (or more frequently) to help judge whether the medications or treatments that have been ordered are effective.

What the Doctor Will Probably Prescribe

Pain medications, especially nonsteroidal anti-inflammatory drugs (NSAIDS), are usually prescribed, but if you're over age sixty, you are more likely to experience side effects. Old adults who take NSAIDs are four times as likely to develop peptic ulcer disease and five times as likely to die from gastrointestinal bleeding as those who do not take NSAIDs (*American Journal of Nursing*).

The NSAID most likely to irritate your stomach and intestines is aspirin. If you have a history of stomach or intestinal irritation, are taking steroids, smoke, have abnormal kidney function, drink alcohol, or take high doses of NSAIDs, you are at greater risk for developing adverse effects. According to *The Management of Chronic Pain in Older Persons*, other side effects to watch out for are liver damage (Tylenol), abnormal kidney function, constipation, confusion, and headaches (Motrin, Advil, Nuprin, Naprosyn, Trilisate, and related drugs).

If you take NSAIDs, it is better to take them as needed, not daily or around the clock. Never use more than one NSAID at a time (*The Management of Chronic Pain in Older Persons*). Even one or two ibuprofen (Motrin) capsules taken two or three days a week can cause kidney damage (*Health and Stress*). They may also depress healing. So although they reduce pain in the short run, the longer-term healing process is hampered.

Sometimes opiates are prescribed. One opiate that has many problems is Norpropoxyphene. It can bring about fluid in the lungs, heart toxicity, difficulty breathing, cardiac arrest, and even death. If this drug is prescribed with diazepam (Valium), the occurrence of adverse effects is increased, including falls, an already serious problem among older adults (*American Journal of Nursing*).

Steroids may be prescribed or injected into your back or joints. They have the most serious side effects and should not be accepted unless you've tried everything else. Their side effects can cause serious demineralization on your bones and fluid retention.

You may not want to take drugs because you fear the side effects or are worried you might get addicted to medicines. All drugs do have side effects, so it is wise to make sure you don't start or continue taking any medications that create new symptoms for you. Some chronic pain responds to anti-inflammatory medications or antidepressants, but many people find they don't help at all, and they all have side effects. Look up any drugs you are prescribed in *Physicians' Desk Reference*, at the reference desk of your local library, or check them out online.

Your doctor also might suggest local anesthetics or surgical procedures. A surgeon will be more apt to recommend surgery. If you have back pain, always get a second opinion from a neurologist prior to having back surgery. Studies reported in *Spin, Medical Clinics of North America*, and *Mayo Clinic Proceedings* found that most patients with low back pain recovered with conservative treatment and did not need surgery unless they were having difficulty urinating or wet the bed.

Other treatment and referral possibilities include physical therapy (which can include range-of-motion exercises and the use of ice packs for up to fifteen minutes at a time), chiropractics, electrotherapy (passing a mild electric current from an electrode pad placed on the surface of the skin), and ultrasound (using a high frequency radio crystal to transmit sound waves through your skin into the painful area or areas of your body). Also, ask your doctor for a referral to a mental health nurse practitioner or a holistic practitioner who is skilled in working with pain.

Self-Care Measures You Can Take

Pain is a message you give yourself that something is wrong. Do not ignore that message. You may not know exactly what is wrong, but your body does. Try to listen to it, and tune into what is wrong under the pain. Finding that out can break the negative spiral of chronic pain that has gained a hold over you. The realization that nothing else medically can be done can help you to focus on what *you* can do. This realization can be a blessing if you take action to reduce your own pain. What steps are suggested?

For All Kinds of Pain

- Find a massage therapist who can work at separating the fibrotic muscle fibers, relaxing any muscles in spasm and increasing circulation in painful muscles. Look in the yellow pages and ask around. If there is a massage school near you, call up and see what services they offer. Also, interview the massage therapist on the phone and or in person, and obtain a minimassage to see if that person works well with your body and you.

- Try a psychotherapeutic approach. If you've tried drugs and massage to no avail, consider working with a mental health nurse practitioner who has pain management skills. Ask friends, attend free community workshops on the topic (or related ones), or check your yellow pages.

  With good therapeutic support and hard work on important life issues, your chronic pain can be managed. It can help you from falling into the role of victim, or help you out if you've already slipped into that role.

  You will need to examine in depth the cost of pain in your life. How does it decrease your ability to enjoy beloved activities, your family, your friends, your peace of mind? It can help to explore what hidden benefits pain has brought you. This is called "secondary gain." It could be that the only time anyone pays any attention to you is when you are in pain. Studies have shown that people who get support from their pain usually have high levels of pain and are more disabled than others who don't. Pain also can be used as an excuse for not dealing with other problems in life such as a bad marriage or fear about discussing important issues. It is not easy to talk about some of these topics, but a good therapist can help you do it and keep you feeling safe. A major goal of this kind of approach is to find a way for you to meet your goals in a healthy way rather than relying on being in pain to achieve them.

  Mind/body strategies have been known to work even when all else failed. People who have been through a therapeutic experience that addressed their pain report significant reductions in pain severity, depression, anxiety, and feeling out of control. They even report that pain interferes less in their activities of daily life. Even if the pain continues, the negative emotions, which make the pain worse, are reduced, and participants can take an active role in life again.

- Start a pain diary. It can help you become more aware of what is adding to your pain. Record your level of pain every hour and see how it is related to the time of day, your mood, fatigue, stress, what you are doing, and with whom.

- Embrace your pain. Avoid thinking of it as the enemy. You must take ownership of the pain to try to understand how pain fits into the whole of your life experience. Listen to the message of pain deep within you. It is a valuable gift that can be understood. Once you hear and understand the basis of your pain, you can regain control of the pain and of your life.

- Express your feelings. Keeping pain to yourself will only increase your pain. This does not mean complaining more; it means saying, "I feel angry when . . ." or "I'm afraid of . . ." and then being very specific about what is angering you or making you fearful. This kind of assertive communication isn't easy, because you may end up blaming another person. If you find it difficult, take an assertiveness course or seek out a mental health nurse practitioner with assertiveness skills who can teach you.

- Learn to relax your body. According to the *Journal of the American Medical Association*, the evidence is strong for the effectiveness of relaxation as a class of techniques to reduce chronic pain. Many people think they are relaxed when they watch TV or read a book, but they're not. Their muscles may be taut and their heart may be racing. True relaxation includes deep breathing techniques and methods of relaxing all the muscles in your body. Find a relaxation tape you like and listen to it in the morning and before you go to bed, at the minimum. For quicker results, leave it playing at low volume all day long, except when you're driving or using heavy machinery.

- Learn massage techniques. Purchase a book on self- or couple massage, and practice the techniques with a friend. Even rubbing someone else's feet and having that person rub yours can bring many benefits. A study in *Journal of Burn Care and Rehabilitation* found that a twenty-minute massage once daily just before the morning debridement of skin in burn patients provided a measurable decrease of anxiety after the massage session and significant lower pain ratings after a week of treatment. Another study reported by the University of Florida in Gainesville found that both massage and relaxation therapy reduced pain. The researcher believed it is because both treatments cause blood vessel to dilate, improving blood flow.

- Exercise. Movement distracts you from pain and helps your body to release endorphins, natural body painkillers. Exercise also strengthens muscles, improves joint mobility, promotes comfort, restores coordination and balance, and improves sleep. There is no evidence that one type of exercise is better than another, but slow movement such as walking or tai chi is less stressful. A study reported in *Aging* found that fitness walking reduced pain more than a pain education program (instruction in and demonstration of the use of heat, cold, massage, relaxation, and distraction) or usual medical care.

To get started exercising, purchase a book on exercising, join a health club, or get a personal trainer to work with you so you exercise in the most effective and safe manner. Your schedule should be gentle, regular, and gradual to avoid introducing additional pain.

- Meditate. If you are constantly thinking about your pain meditation can help you. One technique, called "mindfulness," encourages you to stay passively focused on your pain and just observe it. This can help you distinguish between pain and its experience. Once you get to that point, you will realize you can control your pain. You may purchase a meditation tape or work with a professional who is skilled in meditation.

- Use guided imagery. Work with a trained professional, or purchase a pain reduction tape. Bookstores often carry an assortment of tapes to help you relax, meditate and use guided imagery.

- Nurture yourself. Stop feeling guilty about comfort and pleasure. at least half an hour a day doing some activity that gives you pleasure *(Emotional Wellness Matters)*. Put that activity on your calendar and then take a walk, listen to music, soak in a bubble bath, read a book, see a play, or do whatever you enjoy. Rediscover how joyful you can feel!

- Use affirmations. Write or say one of the following statements at least twenty times a day, and stop yourself when you hear words that are in opposition to it:

  1. I release the past and let it go.
  2. I am free and everyone is free.
  3. I forgive myself and everyone else.
  4. I deserve to be free and pain-free.

- Try Feldenkrais for headaches or musculoskeletal problems. Feldenkrais is the use of small body movements to reduce muscular tonicity and spasticity to change self-image. A study reported in the *American Journal of Pain Management* found that patients with chronic headaches and/or musculoskeletal problems reported more mobility and decreased pain up to a year after treatment compared to comparison groups.

- Reiki could work. Reiki uses ritual meditations and the laying on of hands in a series of positions on the body to unblock energy centers so healing can occur. A study reported in *Cancer Prevention Control* found that Reiki treatments reduced pain.

- Herbs reduce pain. A study in the *American Journal of Medicine* reported a reduction in pain after taking ginkgo biloba for leg pain. The herb also increased walking distance. Other herbs that have shown promise for pain treatment include garlic and feverfew (especially for headaches because it either prevents blood vessel spasm or blocks prostaglandins that increase inflammation). Cayenne has been shown to reduce arthritis pain *(British Journal of Rheumatology)*. A useful topical agent, cajeput oil, which is usually combined with peppermint, clove, menthol, eucalyptus, cayenne, or arnica oil, can relieve musculoskeletal pain, headache, hemorrhoid pain, neuralgia, rheumatic pain, and pain resulting from sports injuries.

- Learn self-hypnosis. The evidence supporting the effectiveness of hypnosis in alleviating chronic pain, especially with cancer, is strong. It is also effective for reducing pain in irritable bowel syndrome, TMJ, and tension headaches.

- Massage the ileocecal valve points to relieve low back pain, chest pain, or headaches. See the chapter "Digestive Problems" in this book.

- Drink six to eight glasses of water every day. Much pain is due to dehydration.

For Back Pain

Examine your beliefs. A study published in the *Clinical Journal of Pain* found that participants with low back pain had more catastrophizing thoughts ("It only feels bad. I cannot think or do anything.") and higher levels of psychological distress.

For Stomach Pain

Investigate cognitive-behavioral family intervention. A study in the *Journal of Consulting and Clinical Psychology* found that children with recurrent abdominal pain reported complete elimination of pain and lower levels of relapse after completing a round of cognitive-behavioral family therapy.

For Headache

- A study reported in *Advances in Migraine Research and Therapy* found that sufferers of migraine headaches who took more than thirty pain tablets a month had twice as many headaches as those who took fewer than thirty pain tablets a month.

  In another study patients with daily headaches were told to stop taking pain medication. A month later, 66 percent were improved, and by the end of the second month 81 percent were improved *(Cephalgia)*. If you take a large number of analgesics (e.g., Advil, Aleve, or Motrin) and have migraine headaches, the medicines you are taking may be causing them. Many headache medicines also contain caffeine or a sedative. Eliminating these drugs can lead to withdrawal symptoms (nausea, abdominal cramps, diarrhea, restlessness, sleeplessness, or anxiety), but they won't last for more than twenty-four to forty-eight hours.

  Withdrawal of ergotamine also can produce rebound headaches. Since most migraine headaches do not occur more frequently than every few days, you can be pretty sure that you are having an ergotamine rebound effect if you have daily headaches.

- Try herbs. Feverfew is a herb that also shows promise. A study published in *Lancet* found that feverfew was associated with a reduction in the number and severity of migraines and in the degree of vomiting. There were no serious side effects.

  Apply a topical ointment with cayenne in and around the nostril several times a day. Use a little and it may burn a little at first.

  Try a couple of sprinkles of ginger or a ginger extract. Repeat every two hours as needed. Ginkgo, 50 mg, three times a day with water or as a tincture might help because it increases circulation to the brain, but check with your pharmacist first to make sure it won't interact with any other medications you're taking.

  Take 750 mg willowbark up to three times daily. It also can be taken as a tincture or a tea. It contains the same active ingredients as aspirin but has none of its adverse effects.

  Try massaging the affected area with a 10 percent solution of peppermint oil.

- Take complete breaths. If you're like a lot of people under pressure, you're breathing in the upper part of your chest. Give your brain the oxygen it needs by learning how to breathe from your abdomen. Place your hand at navel level and gently try to push that hand out every time you exhale. Put reminders around you to "breathe in your abdomen." If that doesn't help, take a yoga or meditation class to help you slow down and breathe right.

- Set reasonable limits on your activities and responsibilities. Feeling overstressed can make you tighten up your muscles, cut off your blood supply to neck and shoulders, and bring on a headache. Consider professional time management or counseling help with this.

- Get adequate rest. Fatigue can bring on headaches and so can too much sleep.

- Rotate your neck every hour. Headaches can result from neck and shoulder tension. Prevent them by gently rotating your neck from side to side and shrugging your shoulder to break the tension you are holding in your muscles. Do this at least every hour, and more frequently if you are sitting at a monitor or holding your head still.

- Several times a day or at the first hint of pain, take a B complex supplement that contains all the B vitamins. It will improve your mood, too.

- Take more essential fatty acids. EFAs, including salmon and evening primose oil (EPO), are anti-inflammatory substances that can relieve headache. Find EPO at your health food store. Eat fish for your protein source every day, especially the oily varieties such as salmon, tuna, sardines, and mackerel.

Parkinson's Disease

The classic symptom of Parkinson's Disease (PD) is tremor. These tremors are often intensified when you are stressed or fatigued, but disappear during sleep or concentrated effort. Fatigue and muscle cramps in the legs, neck, or trunk are also common.

Muscle stiffness or rigidity slowly begins to impede your movement, and your body movements slow. As the disease progresses, you may start to shuffle and have less control over your posture and body movement. You may develop a stooped position and lose your balance easily, and you may notice skin oiliness (especially on your forehead and scalp), perspiration, difficulty sleeping, mood changes, speech changes, loss of facial expression and finger dexterity, loss of control of automatic movement (blinking, swallowing saliva), and difficulty adjusting your posture when you are seated. Usually the condition does not require hospitalization unless you fall and injure yourself.

Your Risk for Developing Parkinson's Disease

The cause is unknown in about 90 percent of PD cases. The following situations are correlated with an increased risk for PD: exposure to neurotoxic drugs (compazine, trilafon, mellaril, Prolixin, Stelazine, Thorazine, Trilafon, Haldol, reglan, Clozaril, Risperdal, Zyprexa, and other tranquilizers, tetrabenazine, cinnarizine, flunarizine, amiodarone, bethanechol, pyridostigmine, lithium, Valium, Prozac, Nardil, Demerol, amphotericin B, caphaloridine, 5-fluorouracil, vincristine-doxorubicin, and the synthetic heroin compound MPTP), poisoning by chemicals (manganese dust, carbon disulfide, copper, or carbon monoxide), arteriosclerosis associated with a cerebral vascular accident (stroke), secondary to other conditions (tumor, repeated head injury, genetic malformation, or infections such as tuberculosis or syphilis), or due to encephalitis.

Three recent studies concluded that diets high in animal fat or cholesterol are associated with substantial increase of risk for PD. In contrast, fat of plant origin does not appear to increase risk. There is a possibility that vegetarian diets are beneficial in PD because they slow the loss of surviving dopaminergic neurons, retarding the progress of the syndrome *(Medical Hypotheses)*.

Some research shows that there is a greater prevalence of PD in rural areas and among farming communities. This suggests a link to agricultural chemicals, especially the herbicide Parquat, which has a structure similar to that of MPTP *(Nursing Spectrum)*. Another study, in the *Scandinavian Journal of Work Environment and Health*, concluded that statistically significantly high risks for PD were found for farmers and for all men in agriculture and horticulture.

Damage in some form precedes the condition and blocks dopamine production. This interrupts the ability of your muscles to receive messages from your brain. A sudden injury or exposure to a chemical agent can bring on the condition, but the disease usually develops slowly.

How the Doctor Diagnoses Parkinson's Disease

Because it is difficult to trace back to the onset of the condition, symptoms may be dismissed as part of the normal aging process. This makes diagnosis difficult. CAT scans, EEGs, and MRIs can only rule out other underlying disorders, and laboratory tests provide little evidence. Only SPECT scans can show the degeneration of neurons *(Journal of Neurological Transmission)*.

Your doctor will probably do a thorough neurological examination or refer you to a neurologist. Your history of what toxic situations you've been exposed to will be key to your doctor's diagnosis.

What the Doctor Will Probably Prescribe

There is no cure for Parkinson's disease. Treatment is used to reduce symptoms and to keep your body functions for as long as possible. Medication, some dietary changes, and occupational and physical therapy may be ordered.

Levodopa (L-dopa) is the standard treatment. It replaces and mimics dopamine in the brain. It takes several weeks for L-dopa to take effect, and its effect diminishes over time. The drug has many adverse effects, including nausea, vomiting, lack of appetite, low blood pressure, heart irregularities, confusion, delirium, depression, uncontrollable movement of the face (grimacing, yawning, tightening of the muscles of the neck and face, abnormal movement of the eyes), and repetitive foot tapping.

To counteract these annoying effects, L-dopa is usually given with Sinemet (carbidopa). This combination may bring earlier results, and can reduce nausea and vomiting. Unfortunately, Sinemet has its own set of adverse reactions, including stomach and intestinal upset, hallucinations, confusion, psychological disturbances, depression, dizziness, headache, dream abnormalities, low blood pressure, back pain, eyelid spasms (especially if the dose is too high), kidney and liver disorders, seizures, heart arrhythmias, neuroleptic malignant syndrome (drooling, decreased consciousness, restlessness, fever, high blood pressure, racing heartbeat, and sweating), and blood clots in the lungs. Other drugs may be prescribed to reduce these effects, but they also will have adverse effects.

L-dopa interacts with many other drugs, so you will need to consult with your doctor before taking any over-the-counter medicines. Sometimes selegiline (Eldepryl) is used in combination with levodopa or carbidopa, but its adverse effects are similar to those of L-dopa. Foods and beverages containing caffeine (colas, chocolate, tea, cocoa) and certain cheeses and meats should be avoided because of the risk of high blood pressure.

Swimming, stationary cycling, and stretching exercises can help for a while, but only for a few years. Surgery can relieve some symptoms, but it is only used for young, otherwise healthy patients. Brain surgery for Parkinson's disease carries many risks, is very expensive, and is usually not covered by HMOs, Medicare, or private insurance because of its experimental status. There haven't been any clinical trials to prove the worth of surgery, from which 5 to 10 percent of patients have suffered vision loss from inadvertent damage to the optic nerve, and from which 10 percent have had unsatisfactory or adverse reactions, including hemorrhage.

Self-Care Measures You Can Take

- Avoid using herbicides and pesticides. Use natural substances such as garlic, soap and water, and oil to spray outdoor plants and protect them from insects. Learn to live with the balance of nature (i.e., there will be insects). Besides, insects perform a useful function. Consider digging up your lawn and using the Xeriscape method in your yard, with native plants and flowers that are insect-resistant. If you live in an apartment or condo complex that sprays for insects, get a note from your doctor stating that you are allergic to the substance and do not wish to participate in the program.

- Cleanse your liver. If you've been exposed to damaging toxics, as most people have been, take silymarin (milk thistle) to cleanse your liver, and take large doses of vitamin C to counter toxins.

- Learn relaxation procedures. A study in *Biofeedback and Self-Regulation* found that tremors were reduced significantly after biofeedback training.

- Work with an Alexander Technique therapist. This technique focuses on creating the right amount of tension necessary for activities to sustain a proper relationship of the head and neck to the back, and attaining a calmer and clearer state of mind. A study in *Clinical Rehabilitation* found that patients with Parkinson's disease who used the Alexander Technique showed reduced depression and improved ability to manage their disability.

- Find an Ayurvedic practitioner. A study in the *Journal of Alternative and Complementary Medicine* reported that an Ayurvedic approach showed statistically significant reductions in symptoms of sixty patients with Parkinson's disease. Call a holistic or wellness center, or look in the yellow pages for a practitioner.

- Start an exercise program. A study reported in the *Journal of the American Geriatric Society* found that a ten-week exercise program improved spinal flexibility and function in people with Parkinson's disease who were in the early or midstages of PD. Swimming, stationary biking, or walking (if balance is good), might be appropriate choices, but consult with a personal trainer, or find a special exercise program for people with PD.

- Get osteopathic manipulation. An osteopath is a medical doctor who also uses physical manipulation skills. A study reported in the *Journal of the American Osteopathic Association* found that standard osteopathic manipulative treatment improved the gait in patients diagnosed with PD.

- Eat more foods high in zinc, and consider taking supplements. A study in the *Journal of Alternative and Complementary Medicine* found that patients with PD showed a significantly decreased zinc status as compared to a control group. Foods high in zinc include wheat germ, eggs, nuts, herring, and oysters. Zinc supplementation has been shown to significantly increase superoxide dismutase, which aids in the protection of neurons from free radicals. Invest in a good multimineral that includes at least the minimum daily requirement for zinc.

- Find a music therapist. A study reported in *Psychosomatic Medicine* found that music therapy (including choral singing, voice exercise, rhythmic and free body movements, and collective invention) had a significant overall effect, increasing happiness and ability to control walking patterns.

- Investigate Chinese herbs. A study reported in *Phytomedicine* found that a Chinese traditional medicine, banxia heupo tang (BHT), significantly improved the swallowing reflex in PD.

- Consider butcher's broom for low blood pressure. A study in the *Journal of Alternative and Complementary Medicine* found that butcher's broom *(Ruscus aculeatus)*, a herb, may be of benefit in treating chronic low blood pressure (orthostatic hypotension), which can accompany this condition.

- Acupuncture may help. A study in the *Journal of Traditional Chinese Medicine* found that acupuncture reduces PD symptoms, delays the disease's progression, and decreases the dosage needed for anti-Parkinsonian drugs.

- Take coenzyme Q-10 and sesame oil. A study reported in *Neurotoxicology* found that coenzyme Q-10 and N-acetylcysteine provided protection against toxicity. Coenzyme Q-10 is found in mackerel, salmon, sardines, peanuts, and spinach. You also can purchase the enzyme as a capsule in a health food store. Look for a liquid or an oil form that contains a small amount of vitamin E to preserve the coenzyme. N-acetylcysteine helps detoxify harmful toxins and protect the body. (**Caution:** Do not use if you have diabetes because it can inactivate insulin.)

- Start eating vegetarian. Animal fat and cholesterol are associated with PD, while fat of plant origin (olive oil, sesame oil) isn't. Fruits and vegetables also will help clear toxins and rebuild tissue.

- Drink green tea. Green tea has neuroprotective properties and has been shown to guard against neurotoxins.

- Take vitamins C and E. These vitamins are antioxidants that offer protection against the free radicals produced by L-dopa. Taking these vitamins before symptoms appear may protect against the condition developing *(Archives of Neurology)*. Take 1,000 to 3,000 mg a day of vitamin C and 800 mg a day of vitamin E.

- Eat foods high in lycopene. A study reported in *Movement Disorders* found an association between lycopene, found in tomatoes and tomato products, and protection against PD risks.

- Maintain bone strength. People with PD tend to have lower bone mineral density, more severe osteoporosis, and more falls and fractures. Take calcium citrate, the most absorbable form. Make sure you get at least 1,200 mg a day, and eat calcium-rich foods that are easy to absorb, including broccoli, kale, green leafy vegetables, tomatoes, whole wheat bread, yogurt, canned sardines, molasses, almonds, soy milk, buttermilk, and tofu.

- Eat foods rich in B vitamins. Foods rich in B vitamins can elevate mood and reduce tingling or burning sensations in the feet or legs. Eat more sunflower seeds, rolled oats, lima beans, soybeans, raisins, wheat germ, peas, whole-wheat-flour foods, asparagus, brown rice, chicken, peanuts, raw spinach, kale, eggs, tuna, turkey, salmon, mackerel, sweet potatoes, cooked cabbage, bananas, sardines, trout, sea vegetables (dulse, kombu, kelp, and wakame), fermented soy foods (tempeh, natto, and miso), fresh green uncooked vegetables, lobster, broccoli, cauliflower, sesame seeds, mushrooms, yogurt (plain, low-fat), oranges, grapefruit, peaches, lettuce, and molasses.

Sleep Disorders

You're not alone. About 35 percent of the American population complains of insomnia (difficulty falling asleep or staying asleep). Although the ability to maintain sleep decreases with age, the need for sleep does not change over time. If you awake feeling refreshed, no matter how long you've slept or how often you've been awakened during the night, your sleep is within normal bounds *(Insomnia)*.

Not getting enough quality sleep can leave you feeling listless, fatigued, and irritable during the day. It also can affect your ability to fight off infection and contribute to depression. Without proper sleep, your body is not rested and ready to carry out its daily functions, and that can affect your ability to heal from other conditions *(American Psychological Association Monitor)*.

Even one night of disturbed sleep can affect your daytime sleepiness, mood, attention span, and mental flexibility, so sleeping well is important. *Sleep apnea* is characterized by long, frequent pauses during sleep.

Your Risk for Developing Sleep Disorders

Medical problems and treatments can cause sleep disorders. Medicines your doctor orders that can interfere with sleep include Norpramine, Prozac, sarafem, efflexor, Wellbutrin, Tofranil, Nardil, and Zoloft. Mood disorders such as depression can result in disturbed sleep. Acute pain can make sleep difficult. If you take a narcotic to help you sleep, you may find yourself waking up more often. Sleep disturbances are common with chronic pain conditions such as Huntington's disease, fibromyalgia, cancer, and Parkinson's disease *(Clinician Reviews)*.

Many unsuspected items that you eat or drink can block sleep. You probably know that caffeine in coffee can keep you awake. Many over-the-counter painkillers, cold and allergy remedies, diet pills, and other drugs contain caffeine, one of the greatest sleep robbers that make you feel fatigued and depressed.

Some drugs to avoid are Anacin, Aqua-Ban Plus, Caffedrine, NoDoz, Quick Pep, Tirend, Midol, Vanquish, Vivarin, Extra Strength Excedrin, and Bayer Select Maximum. Herbal products that contain ephedra, caffeine, or guarana also can keep you awake. Allergy and cold medicines that can rob you of sleep include Sudafed, Bronkaid, Primatene, and Tedral. Cortisones such as prednisone, heart drugs such as propranolol, furosemide, and lovastatin, thyroid medication such as synthroid, and even antidepressants can interfere with sleep.

Sleeping pills cause either dependence or addiction, lose their effectiveness quickly, suppress the dream and REM sleep you need to stay mentally healthy, and also have a rebound effect, so if you stop taking them your insomnia worsens. Alcohol also is a sleep robber. In addition, drinking a lot of fluids before going to sleep can keep you up at night.

If you drink alcohol, you are probably at risk. More than one or two drinks will prolong the first two stages of sleep and stop you from entering deep sleep. This results in fragmented sleep patterns and reduced sleep quality. Whether due to prescribed drugs, over-the-counter drugs, or alcohol, if you don't experience deep sleep, the REM stage will not occur and you will awake fatigued. Daytime sleepiness will follow *(Clinician Reviews)*.

Watching stimulating or violent shows before going to bed can keep you up. If you have an important or tense day coming up, spend time before you go to bed making sure you are fully prepared.

Noise is a major sleep robber. If you travel a lot, live in a noisy neighborhood, or have a family member who stays up late, making noise, part of you will remain on alert until the noise stops or you fall asleep due to exhaustion.

Phase changes from shift work, jet lag, or just changing the time you retire can result in poor-quality sleep. Even sleeping later than usual can disturb sleep patterns *(Clinician Reviews)*.

Another risk for sleeplessness is a nighttime breathing disorder called sleep apnea. The upper airways close for more than ten seconds. Each time this happens, the oxygen levels in your blood decrease, making your heart pump harder, so your blood pressure rises while the muscles that control breathing struggle to restore airflow. When this happens many times a night, you increase your risk for a heart attack *(The National Center for Sleep Disorders Research)*.

You're at a higher risk for sleep apnea if you're obese, male, and have high blood pressure. Sleep apnea can produce feelings of fatigue, sleepiness, memory and judgment problems, irritability, difficulty concentrating, and personality changes. Your heart and blood vessel systems also are adversely affected by sleep apnea. High blood pressure and heart arrhythmias are associated with sleep apnea.

You're at high risk for sleep apnea if you exhibit loud, chronic snoring; choke or gasp during sleep; are obese; have a large neck girth (seventeen inches for a man and sixteen inches for a woman); have excessive daytime sleepiness (especially drowsy driving); have automobile- or work-related accidents due to fatigue; or have personality changes or thinking difficulties due to fatigue.

How the Doctor Diagnoses Sleep Disorders

Your doctor will probably ask you to keep a one- to two-week sleep diary. This tool usually records bedtime, total sleep time, time to sleep onset, number of awakenings, use of sleep medications, time out of bed in the morning, and a rating of subjective quality of sleep and daytime symptoms. This diary can serve as a baseline for assessing what works to help you sleep and what doesn't.

Your doctor will probably try to rule out drinking alcohol or coffee and any other stresses or physical disorders that may be keeping you awake. It could be that your insomnia is due to a transient event such as loss or promotion, some world event, or a great deal of air travel. It also could be that you are suffering from sleep apnea, a more complex condition.

If you complain of sleepiness but don't have the other symptoms and signs of sleep apnea, a review of sleep habits may be helpful. Your doctor may also ask you how many hours of sleep you average per night, recent changes in your schedule, and recent lifestyle changes. If you wake up with a headache and dry mouth, have to get up to urinate during the night often, have enuresis (bed-wetting), excessive daytime dozing (especially while driving or during sedentary activities), or sexual dysfunction, your doctor may conclude that you have obstructive sleep apnea syndrome.

If your child has sleep apnea, your doctor can make the diagnosis by finding out from you about the child's snoring, labored breathing, weight loss or failure to reach a normal weight, poor school performance, bed-wetting, or behavioral problems.

Your doctor will probably refer you to a sleep specialist, who will conduct a sleep study. Polysomnography is the optimum test for a diagnosis of sleep apnea. The test includes an overnight stay, an evaluation of sleep staging, airflow and ventilatory effort, oxygen saturation, electrocardiogram, body position, and periodic limb movements. If polysomnography is not available, portable (home) monitoring of your heart and lungs may be used *(Sleep Apnea)*.

The severity of your symptoms will determine how quickly a sleep study should be obtained. If you fell asleep while driving or have heart failure or angina, you need to have a sleep study and rapid treatment immediately.

What the Doctor Will Probably Prescribe

You doctor may recommend that you stop drinking coffee or alcohol prior to sleep or try to help you to sleep with a medication prescription. Sleeping pills may work for a short time (after that they become less effective), and they make it more difficult for you to wake up feeling rested and alert. Currently there are no safe and effective medications in the routine treatment of sleep apnea, either (NIH publication 95-3802, 1995). If you are grieving from a major loss or have other signs of psychiatric disturbance, you may be referred to a psychiatrist, psychologist, or mental health nurse practitioner.

If you have signs of sleep apnea, your doctor may send you to a sleep disorders specialist. A common treatment for sleep apnea is nasal continuous positive airway pressure, or CPAP. This is delivered by a device consisting of a small blower attached with a flexible tube on a snug-fitting mask placed over your nose. Air pressure delivered through the device keeps the airways open during the night, restoring uninterrupted sleep. According to the American Lung Association, the treatment can rapidly reverse daytime sleepiness caused by breathing disorders during sleep.

CPAP may be difficult to tolerate because you must wear a mask, and it can be inconvenient to be connected to a machine, which is why only 50 to 80 percent of those with the condition use the machine and then less than 70 percent of the time and never all night *(Consultant)*. Common side effects include nasal stuffiness, inflammation in the nose, facial skin discomfort, and discomfort with the pressure. Humidifiers, variations in pressure application, or different masks may relieve side effects. Nasal sprays are sometimes used, but your body will build up a tolerance, and you may get rebound rhinitis (nasal inflammation or irritation) if you use it regularly *(Consultant)*.

Oral or dental appliances may help with mild to moderate sleep apnea. These devices displace the tongue forward or move the jaw forward to improve the airway. Side effects of these devices include excessive salivation and TMJ discomfort. A dentist or orthodontist will fit you, and be sure to have a sleep study to make sure the device is properly fitted. None of these treatments is a cure. At best, they only treat the symptoms.

Surgery also is a possibility, but none of the procedures is 100 percent effective, they are invasive, and they carry a risk. Uvulopalatopharyngoplasty, or UPPP, is a procedure that resects the uvula and portions of the soft palate to widen your airway. It's hard to predict who will respond well to this surgery, and the overall success rate is only about 40 percent. Nasal surgery may be used alone or with other procedures. By itself, it will not cure the problem.

In children and adolescents, adenotonsillectomy *(Lancet)* may be useful. Tonsillectomy alone in adults is usually not helpful but is often done in conjunction with UPPP *(Archives of Internal Medicine)*. Laser-assisted uvulopalatoplasty (LAUP) has received attention, as has electrical stimulation and oxygen, but none has been shown to be effective *(American Sleep Disorders Association; Chest)*.

Carefully weigh your options before choosing surgery. CPAP is highly effective when used properly and is safer and reversible *(Chest; Sleep)*.

The goals of treatment for sleep apnea include eliminating sleep fragmentation, apnea, and lack of oxygen. Other goals include eliminating snoring and sleepiness and improving quality of life. Behavioral interventions include losing weight, eliminating evening alcohol and sedatives, and proper positioning. Although difficult to achieve, losing weight may cure the condition. See the chapter "Overweight/Obesity" in this book for suggestions.

Self-Care Measures You Can Take

Keep in mind that natural remedies usually take longer than pharmaceuticals but have fewer side effects, and once you have established a healthy sleeping pattern, you can slowly phase them out.

- Bring your bed partner with you to the doctor. You may not know when you snore or how loudly, if you sleepwalk, or if you kick or thrash during the night, but your bed partner will *(Don't Take Sleep Problems Lying Down)*. If you live alone, turn on your tape recorder, make a permanent record, and bring that along.

- Exercise. Make sure you exercise during the day every day. Do some gentle stretches, but nothing too strenuous before bedtime; it will keep you awake.

- Avoid alcohol. It is a known sleep robber *(Don't Take Sleep Problems Lying Down)*.

- Lose weight if you're overweight. A study reported in the *International Journal of Obesity and Related Metabolic Disorders* found that hypnosis helped clients with sleep apnea lose weight. (See the chapter "Overweight/Obesity" in this book for specific ideas).

- Take a B complex capsule every day. The B vitamins are known to calm you down and can reduce nightmares and restless sleep. Pantothenic acid is particularily good for drying the sinuses and easing breathing.

- Spray your throat with a natural lubricant. While medicated sprays can create a rebound effect and irritate you, natural sprays won't. Try an antisnoring spray formula from your health food store that contains almond oil, olive oil, and/or eucalyptus oil. (Make sure there are no herbs in the spray.)

- Maintain a consistent bedtime routine. Changes in your usual pattern can disturb sleep.

- Eat a light meal no fewer than three hours before retiring. If your body is still digesting food, you will have a difficult time sleeping well.

- Keep your bedroom quiet and dark. Avoid any situation that distracts from sleeping.

- Participate in a relaxing activity prior to sleeping. Read a boring book, take a short walk, or enjoy a warm bath. If these activities are insufficient, purchase a relaxation tape and listen to it while you're in bed.

- Write down your concerns. To keep from worrying instead of sleeping, write down your concerns about upcoming events or the day's events. If necessary, write down your plans for dealing with tomorrow so you won't think about them while trying to go to sleep.

- Have a small evening snack of foods containing trytophan. This substance is known to bring on drowsiness and induce sleep. It is found in milk, turkey, and potatoes.

- Look into taking melatonin. This supplement lessens jet lag and can induce sleep in some people, although there have been no long-term trials *(Annals of Pharmacotherapy; Annals of Medicine; Sleep)*. A method of increasing the production of your own melatonin is to shine a light on the back of the knee. Researchers at Cornell University released a study showing that body temperature and melatonin levels were altered when light was shined on the back of the knee *(Science)*. This may reset the body's (circadian) clock and should work to reduce jet lag, the effects of shift work, and changes in usual sleep behavior.

- Take valerian. This herb has been validated in Europe for its effectiveness in relieving insomnia. Germany's Commission E has approved it for sleep disorders and as a minor tranquilizer. No side effects have been reported. A study reported in *Wien Med Wochenschr* found that valerian was just as good as an antianxiety insomnia (benzodiazepine) preparation, providing evidence that valerian is as effective, but has no withdrawal symptoms. A study in *Schweiz Rundsch Med Prax* found that while medications for insomnia had a "morning hangover" effect, valerian did not. Follow the directions on the bottle.

- Try kava root. Since 1869, European herbal medicine has recommended kava root in many forms as a treatment for anxiety. Several studies comparing kava to tranquilizers have shown that it's very effective for insomnia when 150 to 210 mg are taken in a single dose one hour before going to bed. **Caution:** Do not take kava with alcohol or prescription antianxiety medicines such as Valium. Discuss all herbs with your physician before taking them.

- Use better sleep posture. When you snore, your tongue falls back toward the throat and partially blocks off your airway. If you sleep on your back, you're more apt to snore, but elevating your head with a pillow while sleeping may prevent it. Sleep experts recommend using a cervical support pillow.

- If you aren't asleep after twenty minutes, get out of bed. Avoid letting your bed become perceived by you as a location to be aware. Avoid eating, studying, watching TV, or reading in bed. Any of these behaviors can create negative cues and condition you for insomnia.

- Avoid nicotine. Take a smoking cessation course or hire a hypnotist to help you quit smoking. Until you are smoke-free, at least avoid nicotine near bedtime and upon night awakenings. It is a stimulant.

- Take folate for restless leg syndrome. A study reported in the *Journal of Women's Health and Gender-Based Medicine* found that women who had unpleasant sensations in their legs when falling asleep had lower blood levels of folate. Foods to eat to increase your intake of folic acid include asparagus, fresh liver, fresh dark green uncooked vegetables, turnips, potatoes, orange juice, black-eyed peas, lima beans, watermelons, oysters, and cantaloupes.

  Other remedies that might work are taking additional calcium or vitamin E. Talk with your doctor before trying these supplements if you're taking medications.

- Investigate acupressure. A study reported in the *Journal of Gerontology and Biological Science and Medical Science* found that acupressure produced a significant effect in reducing nighttime awakening and in improving the quality of sleep.

- Avoid salt. Using salt for dinner can aggravate sleep disorders. It can act as a mild stimulant to your adrenal glands *(Alternatives)*.

- Rebalance your blood sugar. If you fall asleep easily but wake in the middle of the night, it could be due to a low blood sugar level. Until you can change your meal plan to include more nutritious foods, a quick fix is to consume a teaspoonful of unsweetened juice, cottage cheese, or peanut butter *(Alternatives)*.

- Change beds. If you can't fall asleep in one bed, try another.

- Try sex. Graedon recommends sex as a wonderful way to help fall asleep.

- Investigate the sleep-robbing effects of every drug you take. Call your pharmacist, or look up every over-the-counter, prescription, or recreational drug you are taking in *Physicians' Desk Reference* (online or in your local library reference department) and avoid them and/or talk to your doctor about the effect or effects they may be having on your sleep patterns, and avoid them if possible.

- Choose one of the following affirmations to replace negative thoughts you may be holding. Say or write at least one of the following statements twenty times every day to balance negative thinking patterns:

  1. I release the day.

  2. I slip into peaceful sleep.

  3. Tomorrow will take care of itself.

References

I have separated the references by condition so you can find the articles and books that may be most appropriate for you should you want to do more reading. You will notice that most of the references are from research studies. Ninety-nine percent of the self-care measures I recommend are research-based. That means they have been tried and found effective for the condition you're interested in. These were the most valuable and up-to-date references on the twenty conditions in this book that I could find when I wrote this book. Since then, more research may have been conducted. You can find both the references I've listed and new research by going to the Internet and typing in "PubMed" in the address section. Once you arrive at the National Library of Medicine, just type in your condition and you will see all the articles about that topic displayed.

AIDS

Allard, J. P., E. Aghdassi, J. Chau, et al. 1998. Effects of vitamin E and C supplementation on oxidative stress and viral load in HIV-infected subjects. *AIDS* 12 (13):1652–1659.

Baum, M. K., and G. Shor-Posner. 1998. Micronutrient status in relationship to mortality in HIV-1 disease. *Nutrition Review* 56 (1 pt. 2):S135–S139.

Berkow, R., and A. J. Fletcher. 1992. *The Merck Manual of Diagnosis and Therapy.* Rahway, N.J.: Merck & Company, pp. 58, 85.

Cloyd, M. W., J. J. Chen, and I. Wang. 2000. How does HIV cause AIDS? The homing theory. *Molecular Medicine Today* 6 (3):108–111.

Collins, R. A., T. B. Ng, W. P. Fong, et al. 1997. A comparison of human immunodeficiency virus type 1 inhibition by partially purified aqueous extracts of Chinese medicinal herbs. *Life Science* 60 (23):PL345–PL351.

Coutsoudis, A., R. A. Bobat, H. M. Coovadia, et al. 1995. The effects of vitamin A supplementation on the morbidity of children born to HIV-infected women. *American Journal of Public Health* 85 (8 pt. 1):1076–1081.

Diego, M. A., T. Field, M. Hernandez-Reif, et al. 2001. HIV adolescents show improved immune function following massage therapy. *International Journal of Neuroscience* 106 (1–2):35–45.

Field, T. 1997. Massage effects on development-immune function of HIV-exposed infants. http://altmed.od.nih.gov/oam/cgi-bin/research. Accessed 7/21/97.

Filteau, S. M., N. C. Rollins, A. Coutsoudis, et al. 2001. The effect of antenatal vitamin A and beta-carotene supplementation on gut integrity of infants of HIV-infected South African women. *Journal of Pediatric Gastroenterology and Nutrition* 32 (4):464–470.

Friedman, H. S. 1991. *The Self-Healing Personality.* New York: Henry Holt & Company.

Gruzelier, J., F. Smith, A. Nagy, et al. 2001. Cellular and humoral immunity, mood and exam stress: The influences of self-hypnosis and personality predictors. *International Journal of Psychophysiology* 42 (1):55–71

Hori, K., D. Hatfield, F. Maldarelli, et al. (1997). Selenium supplementation suppresses tumor necrosis factor alpha-induced human immunodeficiency virus type 1 replication in vitro. *AIDS Research in Human Retroviruses* 13 (15):1325–1332.

Lutgendorf, S. K., M. H. Antoni, G. Ironson, et al. (1997). *Journal of Consulting and Clinical Psychology* 65 (1):31–43.

Methylcobalamin. (1998). *Alternative Medicine Review* 3 (6):461–463. No author.

Newschaffer, C. J., et al. 2000. Can antiretroviral drug cause congenital abnormalities? *Journal of Acquired Immune Deficiency Syndrome* 24 (3):249–256.

Patrick, L. 1999. Nutrients and HIV: part one—beta-carotene and selenium. *Alternative Medicine Review* 4 (6):403–413.

———. 2000. Nutrients and HIV: part two—vitamins A and E, zinc, B vitamins, and magnesium. *Alternative Medicine Review* 5 (1):39–51.

Ross, M. F. 1997. UF researchers: stress can hasten progression of HIV. Gainesville: University of Florida.

Roubenoff, R. 1999. Exercise: a major component in treating HIV. *Tufts Nutrition* (Spring):3.

See, D. M., N. Broumand, L. Sahl, et al. 1997. In vitro effects of echinacea and ginseng on natural killer and antibody-dependent cell cytotoxicity in healthy subjects and chronic fatigue syndrome or acquired immunodeficiency syndrome patients. *Immunopharmacology* 35 (3):229–235.

Sicher, F., E. Targ, D. Moore, et al. 1998. A randomized double-blind study of the effect of distant healing population with advanced AIDS. *Western Journal of Medicine* 169 (6):356–363.

Yao, X. J., M. A. Wainberg, and M. A. Parniak. 1992. Mechanism of inhibition of HIV-1 infection in vitro by purified extract of *Prunella vulgaris. Virology* 187 (1):56–62.

Allergies

Berkow, R., and A. J. Fletcher, eds. 1992. *The Merck manual of diagnosis and therapy.* Rahway, N.J.: Merck Research Laboratories.

Camus, P. 2001. Medicines linked to lung diseases. www.drkoop.com/dyncom/article. Accessed September 6, 2001.

Carey, O. J., J. B. Cookson, J. Britton, et al. 1996. The effect of lifestyle on wheeze atrophy and bronchial hyperreactivity in Asian and white children. *American Journal of Respiratory and Critical Care Medicine*, 154 (2), part 1, 537–540.

Carey, O. J., C. Locke , and J.B. Cookson. 1993. Effect of alterations of dietary sodium on the severity of asthma in men. *Thorax* 48 (7):107–110.

Castes, M., I. Hagel, M. Palenque, et al. 1999. Immunological changes associated with clinical improvement of asthmatic children subjected to psychosocial intervention. *Brain and Behavioral Immunity* 13 (1):1–13.

Clark, C. C. 1999. *Encyclopedia of complementary health practice*. New York: Springer Publishing Company.

———. 2002. Nutrition and weight management. In *Health promotion in communities: holistic and wellness approaches*. New York: Springer Publishing Company, 133–181.

Cohen, H. A., I. Neuman, and H. Nahum. 1997. *Archives of Pediatrics & Adolescent Medicine* 151:367–370.

Ellwood, P., M. I. Asher, B. Bjorkstein, et al. 2001. Diet and asthma, allergic rhinoconjunctivities and atopic eczema symptom prevalence: An ecological analysis of the International Study of Asthma and Allergies in Childhood (ISAAC) data. *European Respiratory Journal* 17 (3):436–443.

Fogarty, A., S. Lewis, S. Weiss, et al. 2000. Dietary vitamin E, IgE concentrations, and atopy. *The Lancet* 356 (9241):1573–1574.

Halper, J. Guided imagery in the treatment of asthma. http://altmed.od.nih.gov/oam/cgi-bin/research/search_simple.cgi. Accessed July 21, 1997.

Hasselmark, L., R. Malmgren, and O. Zetterstrom. 1993. Selenium supplementation in intrinsic asthma. *Allergy* 48:30–36.

Hodge, L., C. M. Salome, J. K. Peat, et al. 1996. Consumption of oily fish and childhood asthma risk. *The Medical Journal of Australia* 164:137–140.

Jick, S. S., C. Vasilakis-Scaramozza, and W. C. Maier. 2001. The risk of cataract among users of inhaled steroids. *Epidemiology* 12 (2):229–234.

Klykov, N. V. 1969. Use of calcium pantothenate in the treatment of cardiac insufficiency. *Kardiologiia* 9 (2):130–135.

———. 1972. Results of complex treatment of patients with chronic circulatory insufficiency using strophanthin, ATP, vitamin B_{12}, folic acid, calcium pantothenate, and unithiol. *Kardiologiia* 12 (1):126–131.

Kohen, D. P., and E. Wynne. 1997. Applying hypnosis in a preschool family asthma education program: Uses of storytelling, imagery, and relaxation. *American Journal of Clinical Hypnosis* 39 (3):169–181.

Kumerova, A. O., L. I. Utno, Z. E. Lipsberga, et al. 1992. Study of pantothenic acid derivatives as cardiac protectors in a model of experimental ischemia and reperfusion of the isolated heart. *Bull Eksp Biol Med* 113 (4):373–375.

Landis, R., and K. P. Khalsa. 1997. *Herbal defense*. New York: Warner.

Maribini, S., P. G. Ciabatta, G. Polli, et al. 1991. Beneficial effects of intranasal applications of capsaicin in patients with vasomotor rhinitis. *European Archives of Otorhinolaryngology* 248 (4), 191–194.

Marini, A., M. Agosti, G. Motta, et al. 1996. Effects of a dietary and environmental prevention programme on the incidence of allergic symptoms in high atopic risk infants: three years' follow-up. *Acta Paediatrica* (Supplement 414):1–21.

Meyer, H. 2001. Antibacterial agent in some asthma medications linked to airway constriction, UF scientists find. Gainesville, University of Florida.

Mindell, E., and V. Hopkins. 1998. *Prescription Alternatives.* New Canaan, Conn.: Keats Publishing.

Mundy, W. L. 1993. *Curing Allergy with Visual Imagery.* Shawnee Mission, Kan.: Mundy & Associates.

Murray, M. 1994. Dietary and life-style factors in treating asthma, hay fever, and allergies. In *Natural Alternatives to Over-the-Counter and Prescription Drugs.* New York: William Morrow & Company.

Oddy, W. H., P. G. Holt, P. D. Sly, et al. 1999. Association between breast feeding and asthma in six-year-old children: Findings of a prospective birth cohort study. *British Medical Journal* 319 (7213):815–819.

Reilly, D.T., M. A. Taylor, C. McSharry, et al. 1986. Is homeopathy a placebo response? Controlled trial of homeopathic potency, with pollen in hay fever as model. *Lancet* 344:1601–1606.

Ritz, T., and A. Steptoe. 2000. Emotion and pulmonary function in asthma: reactivity in the field and relationship with laboratory induction of emotion. *Psychosomatic Medicine* 62 (6):808–815.

Rockhill, B., W. C. Willett, J. E. Manson, et al. 2001. Physical activity and mortality: A prospective study among women. *American Journal of Public Health* 91 (4):578–583.

Shimizu, S. 1999. Pantothenic acid. *Nippon Rinsho* 57 (10):2218–2222.

Smith, C. M., C. M. Narrow, Z. V. Kendrick, et al. 1987. The effect of pantothenate deficiency in mice on their metabolic response to fast and exercise. *Metabolism* 36 (2):115–121.

Smith, J. M., A. A. Stone, A. Hurewitz, et al. 1999. Effects of writing about stressful experiences on symptom reduction in patients with asthma or rheumatoid arthritis. *Journal of the American Medical Association* 281 (14):304–309.

Somerville, R. 1997. *The Alternative Advisor.* Alexandria, Va.: Time-Life.

Tanner, J. O. 2001. Asthma vs. anti-inflammatory drugs. *The Clinical Advisor* (October):45.

Troisi, R. J., F. E. Speizer, W. C. Willett, et al. 1995. Menopause, postmenopausal estrogen preparations, and the risk of adult-onset asthma: A prospective cohort study. *American Journal of Respiratory & Critical Care Medicine* 152 (4, pt. 1):1183–1188.

Troisi, R. J., W. C. Willett , and S. T. Weiss. 1995. A prospective study of diet and adult-onset asthma. *American Journal of Respiratory and Critical Care Medicine* 151 (5): 1401–1408.

Alzheimer's Disease

Arkin, S. M. 1999. Elder rehab: a student-supervised exercise program for Alzheimer's patients. *Gerontology* 39:729–735.

Behl, C. 2000. Vitamin E protects neurons against oxidative cell death in vitro more effectively than 17-beta estradio and induces the activity of the transcription factor NF-kappaB. *Journal of Neural Transmission* 107 (4):393–407.

Clark, M. E., A. W. Lipe, and M. Bilbrey. 1997. Use of music to decrease aggressive behaviors in people with dementia. *Journal of Gerontological Nursing* 24 (7):10–17.

Commenges, D., V. Scotet, S. Renaud, et al. 2000. Intake of flavonoids and risk of dementia. *European Journal of Epidemiology* 15 (4):357–363.

Denney, A. 1997. Quiet music: An intervention for mealtime agitation. *Journal of Gerontologic Nursing* 23 (7):16–23.

Francese, T., J. Sorrell, and F. R. Butler. 1997. Effects of regular exercise on muscle strength and functional ability of late stage Alzheimer's residents. *American Journal of Alzheimer's Disease* 12 (3):122–127.

Gerdner, L. 1997. An individualized music intervention for agitation. *Journal of the American Psychiatric Nurses' Association* 3 (6):177–184.

———. 2000. Effects of individualized versus classical "relaxation" music on the frequency of agitation in elderly persons with Alzheimer's disease and related disorders. *International Journal of Psychogeriatrics* 12 (1):49–65.

Gerdner, L. A., and K. C. Buckwalter. 1994. Assessment and management of agitation in Alzheimer's disease and related disorders. *Journal of Gerontological Nursing* 20 (4):11–19.

Helmer, C., D. Damon, and L. Letenneur, et al. 1999. Marital status and risk of Alzheimer's disease: A French population-based cohort study. *Neurology* 53:1953–1958.

Hong, J. T., S. R. Ryu, H. J. Kim, et al. 2000. Neuroprotective effect of green tea extract in experimental ischemia-reperfusion brain injury. *Brain Research Bulletin* 53 (6):743–749.

Ironson, G., T. Field, F. Scafidi, et al. 1996. Massage therapy is associated with enhancement of the immune system's cytotoxic capacity. *International Journal of Neuroscience* 84 (1–4):205–217.

Itil, T., and D. Martorano. 1995. Natural substances in psychiatry (ginkgo biloba in dementia). *Psychoparmacology Bulletin* 31 (1):147–158.

Kilstoff, K. 1998. New approaches to health and well-being for dementia day-care clients, family caregivers, and day-care staff. *International Journal of Nursing Practice* 4 (2):70–83.

Kontush, A., U. Mann, S. Arlt, et al. 2001. Influence of vitamin E and C supplementation on lipoprotein oxidation in patients with Alzheimer's disease. *Free Radicals in Biological Medicine* 31 (3):345–354.

Lazowski, D. A. 1999. A randomized outcome evaluation of group exercise programs in long-term-care institutions. *Journal of Gerontology* 54 (12):M621–M628.

LeBars, P. L., M. M. Katz, N. Berman, et al. 1997. A placebo-controlled, double-blind randomized trial of an extract of gingko biloba for dementia. *Journal of the American Medical Association* 278:1327–1332.

Liu, F., B. H. Lau, Q. Peng, et al. 2000. Pcynogenol protects vascular endothelial cells from beta-amyloid-induced injury. *Biology Pharmacy Bulletin* 23 (6):735–737.

Masaki, K. H., K. G. Losonczy, G. Izmirlian, et al. 2000. Association of vitamin E and C supplement use with cognitive function and dementia in elderly men. *Neurology* 54:1265–1272.

McKenna, D. J., K. Jones, and K. Hughes. 2001. Efficacy, safety, and use of ginkgo biloba in clinical and preclinical applications. *Alternative Therapies in Health and Medicine* 7 (5):70–86, 88–90.

Pettegrew, J. W., J. Levine, and R. J. McClure. 2000. Acetyl-L-carnitine physical-chemical, metabolic, and therapeutic properties: Relevance for its mode of action in Alzheimer's disease and geriatric depression. *Molecular Psychiatry* 5 (6):616–632.

Rondeau, V., D. Commenges, H. Jacquin-Gadda, and J. F. Dartigues. 2000. Relation between aluminum concentrations in drinking water and Alzheimer's disease: An 8-year follow-up study. *American Journal of Epidemiology* 152 (1):59–66.

Ruether, E., R. Husmann, E. Kinzler, et al. 2001. A 28-week, double-blind, placebo-controlled study with Cerebrolysin in patients with mild to moderate Alzheimer's disease. *International Clinical Psychoparmacology* 16 (5):253–263.

Russell, R. M. 2000. The aging process as a modifier of metabolism. *American Journal of Clinical Nutrition* 72 (2):529S–532S.

Ryden, M. B., M. Snyder, C. R. Gross, et al. 2000. Value-added outcomes: The use of advanced practice nurses in long-term care facilities. *Gerontologist* 40 (6):654–662.

Sano, M., C. Ernesto, R. G. Thomas, et al. 1997. A controlled trial of Selegiline, Alpha-Tocopherol, or both as treatment for Alzheimer's disease. *New England Journal of Medicine* 336:1216–1222.

Sobel, B. P. 2001. Bingo vs. physical intervention in stimulating short-term cognition in Alzheimer's disease patients. *American Journal of Alzheimers Disease and Other Dementias* 16 (2):115–120.

Stough, C., J. Clarke, J. Lloyd, et al. 2001. Neuropsychological changes after 30-day Ginkgo biloba administration in healthy participants. *International Journal of Neuropsychopharmacology* 4 (2):131–134.

Sutherland, J. 1999. Foot acupressure and massage for patients with Alzheimer's disease and related dementias. *Image: Journal of Nursing Scholarship* 31:347–348.

Tabak, N., R. Bergman, and R. Alpert. 1996. The mirror as a therapeutic tool for patients with dementia. *International Journal of Nursing Practice* 2 (3):155–159.

Van der Voet, G. B., E. Schiijns, and F. A. de Wolff. 1999. *Archives of Physiology and Biochemistry* 107 (1):15–21.

Varner, J.A., K. F. Jensen, W. Horvath, et al. 1998. Chronic administration of aluminum fluoride or sodium fluoride to rats in drinking water: Alterations in neuronal and cerebrovascular integrity. *Brain Research* 784 (1–2):284–298.

Wang, H. X., A. Wahlin, H. Basun, et al. 2001. Vitamin B_{12} and folate in relation to the development of Alzheimer's disease. *Neurology* 56 (9):1188–1194.

Wettstein, A. 2000. Cholinesterase inhibitors and Ginkgo extracts–are they comparable in the treatment of dementia? Comparison of published placebo-controlled efficacy studies of at least six months' duration. *Phytomedicine* 6 (6):393–401.

World Alzheimer Congress. 2000. Impaired memory may not indicate Alzheimer's disease. *Clinician Reviews* 10 (11):127.

World Alzheimer Congress. 2000. Does education reduce the risk of Alzheimer's disease? *Clinician Reviews* 20 (11):127–128.

World Alzheimer Congress. 2000. AD risk increases with high-fat diet. *Clinician Reviews* 10 (11):132.

Arthritis

Affleck, G., H. Tennen, S. Urrows, et al. 1994. *Journal of Personality and Social Psychology* 66 (2):329–340.

Anthony, D. D., S. Gupta, N. Ahmad, et al. 1999. Prevention of collagen-induced arthritis in mice by a polyphenolic fraction from green tea. *Proceedings of the National Academy of Sciences* 96 (8):4524–4529.

Bassleer, C., P. Gysent, R. Bassleer, et al. 1987. Proteoglycans synthesized by human chondrocytes cultivated in clusters. *American Journal of Medicine* 83 (5A):25–28.

Bell, K. M., L. Plon, W. E. Bunney Jr., et al. 1988. S-adenosylmethionine treatment of depression: A controlled clinical trial. *American Journal of Psychiatry* 145:1110–1114.

Caruso, I., and V. Pietrogande. 1987. Italian double-blind multicenter study comparing S-adenosylmethionine, naproxen, and placebo in the treatment of degenerative joint disease. *American Journal of Medicine* 83 (5A):66–71.

Creamer, P., M. Lethbriedge-Ceju, and M. C. Hochberg. 2000. Factors associated with functional impairment in symptomatic knee osteoarthritis. *Rheumatology* 39 (5):490–496.

Darlington, L.G., and T. W. Stone. 2001. Antioxidants and fatty acids in the amelioration of rheumatoid arthritis and related disorders. *British Journal of Nutrition* 85 (3):251–269.

Day, J. P., A. Lanas, P. Rustagi, et al. 1996. Reversible prolonged skin bleeding time in acute gastrointestinal bleeding presumed due to NSAIDs. *Journal of Clinical Gastroenterology* 22 (2):96–103.

Dingle, J. T. 1991. Cartilage maintenance in osteoarthritis: interaction of cytokines, NSAID, and prostaglandins in articular cartilage damage and repair. *Journal of Rheumatology Supplement* 28:30–37.

Domijan, Z., B. Vrhovac, T. Dumgi, et al. 1989. A double-blind trial of ademetionine vs. Naproxen in activated gonarthrosis. *International Journal of Clinical Pharmacology and Toxicology* 27:329–333.

Flynn, M. A., W. Irvin, and G. Krause. 1994. The effect of folate and cobalamin on osteoarthritic hands. *Journal of the American College of Nutrition* 13 (4):351–356.

Garfinkle, M. S., H. R. Schumacher Jr., A. Husain, et al. 1994. Evaluation of a yoga-based regimen for treatment of osteoarthritis of the hands. *Journal of Rheumatology* 21 (12):2341–2343.

Gordon, A., J. H. Merenstein, F. D'Amico, et al. 1998. The effects of therapeutic touch on patients with osteoarthritis of the knee. *The Journal of Family Practice* 47 (4):271–277.

Grant, W. B. 2000. The role of meat in the expression of rheumatoid arthritis. *British Journal of Nutrition* 84 (5):589–595.

Hanninen, K. K., A. L. Rauma, M. Nenonen, et al. 2000. Antioxidants in vegan diet and rheumatic disorders. *Toxicology* 155 (1–3):45–53.

Hansen, G. V., L. Nielsen, E. Kluger, et al. 1996. Nutritional status of Danish rheumatoid arthritis patients and effects of a diet adjusted in energy intake, fish meal, and antioxidants. *Scandinavian Journal of Rheumatology* 25 (5):325–330.

Hay, L. 1984. *Heal your body: The mental causes for physical illness and the metaphysical way to overcome them.* Carlsbad, Calif.: Hay House.

Helgeland, M., E. Svendsen, O. Forre, et al. 2000. Dietary intake and serum concentrations of antioxidants in children with juvenile arthritis. *Clinical Experimental and Rheumatology* 18 (5):637–641.

Helmy, M., M. Shohayeb, M. H. Helmy, et al. 2001. Antioxidants as adjuvant therapy in rheumatoid disease. *Arzneimittelforschung* 5 (4):293–298.

Kagan, B. L., D. L. Sultzer, N. Rosenlicht, et al. 1990. Oral S-adenosylmethionine in depression: a randomized, double-blind, placebo-controlled trial. *American Journal of Psychiatry* 147 (5):591–595.

Knekt, P., M. Heliovaara, K. Aho, et al. 2000. Serum selenium, serum alpha-tocopherol, and the risk of rheumatoid arthritis. *Epidemiology* 11 (4):402–405.

Konig, B. 1987. A long-term (two years) clinical trial with S-adenosylmethionine for the treatment of osteoarthritis. *American Journal of Medicine* 83 (5A):89–94.

Kremer, J. M., and J. Bigaouette. 1996. Nutrient intake of patients with rheumatoid arthritis is deficient in pyridoxine, zinc, copper, and magnesium. *Journal of Rheumatology* 23 (6):990–994.

Lapane, K. L., J. J. Spooner, L. Mucha, et al. 2001. Effect of steroidal anti-inflammatory drug use on the rate of gastrointestinal hospitalizations among people living in long-term care. *Journal of the American Geriatric Society* 49 (5):577–584.

Leventhal, L. J., E. G. Boyce, and R. B. Zurier. 1994. Treatment of rheumatoid arthritis with black currant seed oil. *British Journal of Rheumatology* 33 (9):847–852.

———. 1994. Treatment of rheumatoid arthritis with gammalinolenic acid. *Annals of Internal Medicine* 119 (9):867–873.

Lystbaek, B. B., L. B. Svendsen, and L. Heslet. 1995. Paracetamol poisoning. *Nordic Medicine* 110 (5):156–159.

Manicourt, D. H., A. Druetz-Van Egeren, L. Haazen, et al. 1994. Effects of tenoxicam and aspirin on the metabolism of proteoglycans and hyaluronan in normal and osteoarthritic human and articular cartilage. *British Journal of Pharmacology* 113: 1113–1120.

McAlindon, T. E., D. T. Felson, Y. Zhang, et al. 1996. Relation of dietary intake and serum levels of vitamin D to progression of osteoarthritis of the knee among participants in the Framingham Study. *Annals of Internal Medicine* 125 (1):353–359.

Muller, H., F. W. de Toledo, and K. L. Resch. 2001. Fasting followed by vegetarian diet in patients with rheumatoid arthritis: A systematic review. *Scandinavian Journal of Rheumatology* 30 (1):1–10.

Muller-Fassbender, H. 1987. Double-blind clinical trial of S-adenosylmethionine verus ibuprofen in the treatment of osteoarthritis. *American Journal of Medicine* 83 (5A):81–83.

Muller-Fassbender, H., G. L. Bach, W. Haase, et al. 1994. Glucosamine sulfate compared to ibuprofen in osteoarthritis of the knee. *Osteoarthritis Cartilage* 2 (1):61–69.

Murray, M. T. 1996. *Encyclopedia of Nutritional Supplements.* Roseville, Calif.: Primar Publishing.

Muscara, M. N., W. McKnight, S. Asfaha, et al. 2000. Wound collagen deposition in rats: Effects of an NO-NSAID and a selective COX-2 inhibitor. *British Journal of Pharmacology* 129 (4):681–686.

Noreau, L., H. Martineau, L. Roy, et al. 1995. Effects of a modified dance-based exercise on cardiorespiratory fitness, psychological state, and health status of persons with rheumatoid arthritis. *American Journal of Physical Medicine and Rehabilitation* 74 (1):19–27.

O'Leary, A., S. Shoor, K. Lorig, et al. 1990. A cognitive-behavioral treatment for rheumatoid arthritis. *Health Psychology* 7 (6):527–544.

Parker, J. C., K. L. Smarr, S. E. Walker, et al. 1991. Biopsychosocial parameters of disease activity in rheumatoid arthritis. *Arthritis Care Research* 4 (2):73–80.

Perlman, S. G., K. J. Connell, A. Clark, et al. 1990. Dance-based aerobic exercise for rheumatoid arthritis. *Arthritis Care Research* 3 (1):29–35.

Schanberg, L.E., M. J. Sandstrom, K. Starr, et al. 2000. The relationship of daily mood and stressful events to symptoms in juvenile rheumatic disease. *Arthritis Care Research* 13 (1):33–41.

Shapiro, J. A., T. D. Koepsell, L. F. Voigt, et al. 1996. Diet and rheumatoid arthritis in women: A possible protective effect of fish consumption. *Epidemiology* 7 (3):256–263.

Smith, J. M., A. A. Stone, A. Huurewitrz, et al. 1999. Effects of writing down about stressful experiences on symptom reduction in patients with asthma or rheumatoid arthritis. *Journal of the American Medical Association* 281 (14):1328–1330.

Stein, M. B., and E. Barrett-Connor. 2000. Sexual assault and physical health: Findings from a population-based study of older adults. *Psychosomatic Medicine* 62 (6):838–843.

Vahora, S. A., and P. Malek-Ahmadi. 1988. S-adenosylmethione in the treatment of depression. *Neuroscience and Biobehavioral Review* 12 (2):139–141.

Van Deusen, J., and D. Harlowe. 1987. The efficacy of the ROM Dance Program for adults with rheumatoid arthritis. *American Journal of Occupational Therapy* 41 (2):90–95.

Vetter, G. 1987. Double-blind comparative clinical trial with S-adenosylmethionine and Indomethacin in the treatment of osteoarthritis. *American Journal of Medicine* 83 (5A):78–80.

Walco, G. A., J. W. Varni, and N. T. Ilowite. 1992. Cognitive-behavioral pain management in children with juvenile rheumatoid arthritis. *Pediatrics* 89 (6, pt. 1):1075–1079.

Zautra, A. J., J. Hoffman, P. Potter, et al. 1997. Examination of changes in interpersonal stress as a factor in disease exacerbations among women with rheumatoid arthritis. *Annals of Behavioral Medicine* 19 (3):279–286.

Zautra, A. J., and B. W. Smith. 2001. Depression and reactivity to stress in older women with rheumatoid arthritis and osteoarthritis. *Psychosomatic Medicine* 63 (4):687–696.

Cancer

Abrams, M. B., K. T. Bednarek, S. Bogoch, et al. 1994. Early detection and monitoring of cancer with the antimalignin antibody test. *Cancer Detection and Prevention* 18 (1):65–78.

Adebamowow, C. A., and O. O. Adekunie. 1999. Case-controlled study of the epidemiological risk factors for breast cancer in Nigeria. *British Journal of Surgery* 86 (5):665–668.

Adenis, A., N. Leriche, J. M. Pion, et al. 1996. Ineffectiveness of sequential high-dose methotrexate and 5-fluorouracil combined with epirubicin (FEMTX regimen) as a salvage therapy in advanced colorectal cancers and other gastrointestinal tumors. *Anticancer Research* 16 (4A):2063–2067.

Ain, K. B., M. J. Egorin, and P. A. DeSimone. 2000. Treatment of anaplastic thyroid carcinoma with paclitaxel: phase 2 trial using ninety-six-hour infusion. Collaborative Anaplastic Thyroid Cancer Health Intervention Trials (CATCHIT) Group. *Thyroid* 10 (7):587–594.

Alabaster, O., Z. Tang, and N. Shivapurkar. 1996. Dietary fiber and the chemopreventive modulation of colon carcinogenesis. *Mutation Research* 350 (1):185–197.

Amano, G., N. Ohuchi, T. Ishibashi, et al. 2000. Correlation of three-dimensional magnetic resonance imaging with precise histopathological map concerning carcinoma extension in the breast. *Breast Cancer Research and Treatment* 60 (1):43–55.

Aro, A. R., S. Pilvikki Absetz, T. M. van Elderen, et al. 2000. False-positive findings in mammography screening induces short-term distress—breast cancer specific concern prevails longer. *European Journal of Cancer* 36 (9):1089–1097.

Aronson, W. J., J. A. Glaspy, S. T. Reddy, et al. 2001. Modulation of omega-3/omega-6 polyunsaturated ratios with dietary fish oils in men with prostate cancer. *Urology* 58 (2):283–288.

Bagga, D., S. Capone, and H. Wang. 1997. Dietary modulation of omega-3/omega-6 polyunsaturated fatty acid ratios in patients with breast cancer. *Journal of the National Cancer Institute* 89 (15):1123–1131.

Barnes, S., J. Sfakianos, L. Coward, et al. 1996. Soy isoflavonoids and cancer prevention: Underlying biochemical and pharmacological issues. *Advanced Experimental and Medical Biology* 401:87–100.

Batkin, S., S. J. Taussig, and J. Szekerezes. 1998. Antimetastatic effect of bromelain with or without its proteolytic and anticoagulant activity. *Journal of Cancer Research and Clinical Oncology* 114:507–508.

Batty, D, and I. Thune. 2000. Does physical activity prevent cancer? Evidence suggests protection against colon cancer and probably breast cancer. *British Medical Journal* 321:1424.

Bernstein, L., B. E. Henderson, R. Hanisch, et al. 1994. Physical exercise and reduced risk of breast cancer in young women. *Journal of the National Cancer Institute* 86:1403–1408.

Bogoch, S., and E. S. Bogoch. 1994. A checklist for suitability of biomarkers as surrogate endpoints in chemoprevention of breast cancer. *Journal of Cell Biochemistry Supplement* 19:173–185.

Bogoch, S., E. S. Bogoch, and V. M. Illiescu. 1988. *In vitro* production of the general transformation antibody related to survival in human cancer patients: antimalignin antibody. *Cancer Detection and Prevention* 12 (1–6):313–320.

Boik, J. 1997. *Cancer and natural medicine: A textbook of basic science and clinical research.* Princeton, MN: Oregon Medical Press.

Bostick, R. M., J. D. Potter, D. R. McKenzie, et al. 1993. Reduced risk of colon cancer with high intake of vitamin E: The Iowa Women's Health Study. *Cancer Research* 53:4230–4237.

Botti, C., A. Martinetti, S. Nerini-Molteni, et al. 1997. Antimalignin antibody evaluation: A possible challenge for cancer management. *International Journal of Biological Markers.* 12 (4):141–147.

Brahmi, Z., J. E. Thomas, M. Park, et al. 1985. The effect of acute exercise on natural killer-cell activity of trained and sedentary human subjects. *Journal of Clinical Immunology* 5:321–328.

Bretherton-Watt, D., R. Given-Wilson, J. L. Mansi, et al. 2001. Vitamin D receptor gene polymorphisms are associated with breast cancer risk in a U.K. Caucasian population. *British Journal of Cancer* 85 (2):171–175.

Bromelain. 1998. Monograph published in *Alternative Medicine Review* 3 (4):302–305. No author.

Burger, A. M., X. Zhang, and A. Seth. 1998. Detection of novel genes that are up-regulated (De12) or down-regulated (TIA12) with disease progression in breast cancer. *European Journal of Cancer Prevention Supp.* 1:S29–S35.

Calderon-Garciduenas, A. L , F. U. Paras-Barrientos, L. Cardenas-Ibarra, et al. 2000. Risk factors of breast cancer in Mexican women. *Salud Publica Mex* 42 (1): 26–33.

Cardis, E., E. S. Gilbert, L. Carpenter, et al. 1995. Effects of low doses and low dose rates of external ionizing radiation: cancer mortality among nuclear industry workers in three countries. *Radiation Research* 142 (2):117–132.

Chang, S. T. 1986. *The complete system of self-healing.* San Francisco: Tao Publishing.

Chie, W. C., C. Y. Li, C. S. Huang, et al. 1998. Oral contraceptives and breast cancer risk in Taiwan, a country of low incidence of breast cancer and low use of oral contraceptives. *International Journal of Cancer* 77 (2):219–223.

Chiu, B. C.-H., J. R. Cerhan, A. R. Folsom, et al. 1996. Diet and risk of non-Hodgkin's lymphoma in older women. *Journal of the American Medical Association* 275 (17): 1315–1321.

Clawson, G. A. 1996. Protease inhibitors and carcinogenesis: A review. *Cancer Investigation* 14 (6):597–608.

Cos, S., and E. J. Sanchez-Barcelo. 2000. Melatonin, experimental basis for a possible application in breast cancer prevention and treatment. *Histology and Histopathology* 15 (2):637–647.

————. 2000. Melatonin and mammary pathological growth. *Frontiers in Neuroendocrinology* 21 (2):133–170.

Cramer, D.W., R. Liberman, L. Titus-Ernstoff, et al. 1999. Genital talc exposure and risk of ovarian cancer. *International Journal of Cancer* 81 (3):351–356.

Deneo-Pellegrini, H., E. DeStafani, P. Boffetta, et al. 1999. Dietary iron and cancer of the rectum: A case-control study in Uruguay. *European Journal of Cancer Prevention*, 8 (6):501–508.

Doyle, T. J., W. Zheng, J. R. Cerhan, et al. 1997. The association of drinking water source and chlorination by-products with cancer incidence among postmenopausal women in Iowa: A prospective cohort study. *American Journal of Public Health* 87 (7): 1168–1176.

Elmore, J. G., M. B. Barton, V. M. Moceri, et al. 1998. Ten-year risk of false positive screening mammograms and clinical breast examinations. *New England Journal of Medicine* 338:1089–1096.

Ernster, V. L., J. Barclay, K. Kerlikowske, et al. 2000. Mortality among women with ductal carcinoma *in situ* of the breast in the population-based surveillance, epidemiology, and end results program. *Archives of Internal Medicine* 160 (7):953–958.

Epstein, S. S. 1997. *The breast cancer prevention program.* New York: Macmillan.

Fackelmann, K. A., and J. Raloff. 1993. Psychological stress linked to cancer. *Science News* 144:23–29.

Flatin, T. P. 1992. Chlorination of drinking water and cancer incidence in Norway. *International Journal of Epidemiology* 21:6–15.

Franceschi, S., A. Favero, C. La Vecchia, et al. 1995. Influence of food groups and food diversity on breast cancer risk in Italy. *International Journal of Cancer* 63 (6):785–789.

Freudenheim, J. L., J. R. Marshall, and J. E. Vena. 1996. Premenopausal breast cancer risk and intake of vegetables, fruits, and related nutrients. *Journal of the National Cancer Institute* 88 (6):340–348.

Friedenreich, C. M., H. E. Bryant, and K. S. Courneya. 2001. Case-control study of life-time physical activity and breast cancer risk. *American Journal of Epidemiology* 154:336–347.

Frisch, R. E., G. Wyshak, N. L. Albright, et al. 1985. Lower prevalence of breast cancer and cancers of the reproductive system among former college athletes compared to non-athletes. *British Journal of Cancer* 52:885–891.

Frisell, J., and E. Lidbrink. 1997. The Stockholm Mammographic Screening Trial: Risks and benefits in age group 40–49 years. *Journal of the National Cancer Institute Monograph* 22:49–51.

Furberg, H., B. Newman, P. Moorman, et al. 1999. Lactation and breast cancer risk. *International Journal of Epidemiology* 28 (3):396–402.

Gago-Dominguez, M., J. E. Castelao, J. M. Yuan, et al. 2001. Use of permanent hair dyes and bladder cancer risk. *International Journal of Cancer* 91 (4):575–579.

Garland, C. F., F. C. Garland, and E. D. Gorham. 1999. Calcium and vitamin D: Their potential roles in colon and breast cancer prevention. *Annals of the New York Academy of Science* 889:107–119.

Giovannuci, E., E. G. Rimme, and G. A. Colditz. 1993. A prospective study of dietary fat and risk of prostate cancer. *Journal of the National Cancer Institute* 85:1571–1579.

Giovannuci, E., M. J. Stampfer, and G. A. Colditz. 1998. Multivitamin use, folate, and colon cancer in women in the Nurses' Health Study. *Annals of Internal Medicine* 129:S517–S524.

Glasziou, P., and L. Irwig. 1997. The quality and interpretation of mammographic screening trials for women ages 40–49. *Journal of the National Cancer Institute Monogram* 22:73–77.

Goldberg, J. G. 1991. *Deceits of the mind and their effects on the body.* New Brunswick, N.J.: Transaction.

Goldstein, N.S., F. A. Vicini, L L. Kestin, et al. 2000. Differences in the pathologic features of ductal carcinoma *in situ* of the breast based on patient age. *Cancer* 88 (11): 2553–2560.

Goodman, M. T., L. R. Wilkens, J. H. Hankin, et al. 1997. Association of soy and fiber consumption with the risk of endometrial cancer. *American Journal of Epidemiology* 146 (4):294–306.

Gyenes, G., L. E. Rutqvist, A. Liedberg, et al. 1998. Long-term cardiac morbidity and mortality in a randomized trial of pre- and postoperative radiation therapy versus surgery alone in primary breat cancer. *Radiotherapy Oncology* 48 (2):185–190.

Harras, A., B. K. Edward, W. J. Blot, et al. 1996. *Cancer rates and risks.* Washington, D.C.: National Cancer Institute, U.S. Department of Health and Human Services, Public Health Service. National Institutes of Health. NIH Publication No. 96–691.

Hartmann, A. M , L. E. Burleson, A. K. Holmes, et al. 2000. Effects of chronic kombucha ingestion on open-field behaviors, longevity, appetitive behaviors, and organs in c57–bl/6 mice: A pilot study. *Nutrition* 16 (9):755–761.

Hay, L. 1984. *Heal your body: The mental causes for physical illness and the metaphysical way to overcome them.* Carlsbad, Calif.: Hay House.

Hayashi, I., M. Ohotsuki, I. Suzuki, et al. 2001. Effects of oral administration of *Echinacea purpurea* (American herb) on incidence of spontaneous leukemia caused by recombinant leukemia viruses in AKR/J mice. *Nihon Rinsho Meneki Gakkai Kaishi* 24 (1):10–20

Hayes, R. B., R. G. Ziegler, G. Gridley, et al. 1999. Dietary factors and risks for prostate cancer among blacks and whites in the United States. *Cancer Epidemiology Biomarkers for Prevention* 8 (1):25–34.

Heber, D., Q. Y. Lu, and V. L. Go. 2001. Role of tomatoes, tomato products, and lycopenes in cancer prevention. *Advanced Experimental Medical Biology* 492:29–37.

Helzlsouer, K. J., A. J. Alberg, H. Y. Huang, et al. 1999. Serum concentrations of organochlorine compounds and the subsequent development of breast cancer. *Cancer Epidemiological Biomarkers and Prevention* 8 (6):525–532.

Hepp, R., and M. R. Baeza. 1999. Conservative treatments of ductal carcinoma *in situ* of the breast. *Review of Medicine Chile* 127 (11):1345–1350

Hoar, A. S., D. D. Weisenburger, P. A. Babbitt, et al. 1990. A case-control study of non-Hodgkin's lymphoma and the herbicide 2,4-dichloro phenoxyacetic acid (2,4-D) in East Nebraska. *Epidemiology* 1:349–356.

Hoar, S. K., A. Blair, F. F. Holmes, et al. 1986. Agricultural herbicide use and risk of lymphoma and soft-tissue sarcoma. *Journal of the American Medical Association* 256: 1141–1147.

Hogberg, T., B. Glimelius, P. Nygren, et al. 2001. A systematic overview of chemotherapy effects in ovarian cancer. *Acta Oncology* 40 (2–3):340–360.

Holly, E. A., C. Lele, and P. M. Bracci. 1998. Hair-color products and risk for non-Hodgkin's lymphoma population-based study in the San Francisco Bay Area. *American Journal of Public Health* 88 (12):1767–1773.

Inano, H., K. Suzuki, M. Onoda, et al. 1999. Comparative effect of chlormadinone acetate and diethylstilbestrol as promoters in mammary tumorigenesis of rats irradiated with gamma-rays lactation. *Breast Cancer Research and Treatment* 53 (2):153–160.

Ingham, D., K. Sanders, M. Kolybaba, et al. 1997. Case-control study of phytoestrogens and breast cancer. *Lancet* 350 (9083):990–994.

Jatoi, I. 1999. Breast cancer screening. *American Journal of Surgery* 177 (6):518–524.

Julien, J. P., N. Bijker, I. S. Fentiman, et al. 2000. Radiotherapy in breast-conserving treatment for ductal carcinoma *in situ:* First results of the EORTC randomised phase III trial 10853. EORTC Breast Cancer Cooperative Group and EORTC Radiotherapy Group. *Lancet* 355 (9203):528–533.

Kennedy, A. R. 1995. The evidence for soybean products as cancer preventive agents. *Journal of Nutrition* 125 (Supplement 3): 733S–743S.

Kirxhwan, P. E., J. N. Cawson, C. M. Kirshnan, et al. 2000. Axillary dissection and ductal carcinoma *in situ* of the breast: A change in practice. *Australian and New Zealand Journal of Surgery* 70 (6):419–422.

Knight, D. C., and J. A. Eden. 1996. A review of the clinical effects of phytoestrogens. *Obstetrics and Gynecology* 87 (5, pt. 2):897–904.

Kolonel, L. N., J. H. Hankin, A. S. Whittemore, et al. 2000. Vegetables, fruits, legumes, and prostate cancer: A multiethnic case-control study. *Cancer Epidemiological Biomarkers and Prevention* 9 (8):795–804.

LeBlanc, E. S., C. M. Viscoli, and J. B. Henrich. 1999. Postmenopausal estrogen replacement therapy is associated with adverse breast cancer prognostic indices. *Journal of Women's Health and Gender-Based Medicine* 8 (6):815–823.

Lee, I. M., J. E. Manson, U. Ajani, et al. 1997. Physical activity and risk of colon cancer: The Physicians' Health Study. *Cancer Causes Control* 8 (4):568–574.

Lefevre, M. L. 1999. Prostate cancer screening: More harm than good? *American Family Physician* 59 (6):1405–1406.

Le Marchand, L., J. H. Hankin, L. R. Wilkens, et al. 1997. Dietary fiber and colorectal cancer risk. *Epidemiology* 8 (6):658–665.

Levitt, B. B. 1995. *Electromagnetic fields: A consumer's guide to the issues, and how to protect ourselves.* San Diego: Harcourt, Brace.

Li, C. I., K. E. Malone, N. S. Weiss, et al. 2001. Tamoxifen therapy for primary breast cancer and risk of contralateral breast cancer. *Journal of National Cancer Institute* 93 (13):963–965.

Lipworth, L., L. R. Bailey, and D. Trichopoulos. 2000. History of breast-feeding in relation to breast cancer risk: A review of the epidemiologic literature. *Journal of the National Cancer Institute* 92 (4):302–312.

Lu, L. J., K. E. Anderson, J. J. Grady, et al. 2001. Effects of an isoflavone-free soy diet on ovarian hormones in premenopausal women. *Journal of Clinical Endocrinology and Metabolism* 86 (7):3045–3052.

Luettig, B., C. Steinmuller, G. E. Gifford, et al. 1989. Macrophage activation by the polysaccharide Arabinogalactan isolated from plant cell cultures of *Echinacea purpurea. Journal of the National Cancer Institute* 81 (9):669–675.

MacKenzie, R. G., E. Franssen, R. Wong, et al. 2000. Risk-adapted therapy for clinical stage I-II Hodgkin's disease: 7-year results of radiotherapy alone for low-risk disease, and ABVD and radiotherapy for high-risk disease. *Clinical Oncology* 12 (5):278–288.

Martinez, M.E., E. Giovannucci, D. Spiegelman, et al. 1997. Leisure-time physical activity, body size, and colon cancer in women. Nurses' Health Study Research Group. *Journal of the National Cancer Institute* 89 (13):948–955.

Martin-Moreno, J. M., W. C. Willett, L. Gorgojo, et al. 1994. Dietary fat, olive oil intake, and breast cancer risk. *International Journal of Cancer* 58 (6):774–780.

Matthews, J. P., J. F. Bishop, G. A. Young, et al. 2001. Patterns of failure with increasing intensification of induction chemotherapy for acute myeloid leukaemia. *British Journal of Haematology* 113 (3):727–736.

Michaud, D. S., D. Feskanich, E. B. Rimm, et al. 2000. Intake of specific carotenoids and risk of lung cancer in prospective U.S. cohorts. *American Journal of Clinical Nutrition* 72 (4):990–997.

Moerman, C. J. 1993. Dietary sugar intake in the etiology of biliary tract cancer. *International Journal of Epidemiology* 145 (2):117–123.

Morrison, H. I., K. Wilkins, R. Semenciw, et al. 1992. Herbicides and cancer. *Journal of the National Cancer Institute* 84:1866–1874.

Moysich, K. B., C. B. Ambrosone, J. E. Vena, et al. 1998. Environmental organochlorine exposure and postmenopausal breast cancer risk. *Cancer Epidemiological Biomarkers and Prevention* 7 (3):181–188.

Nagata, C. 2000. Ecological study of the association between soy product intake and mortality from cancer and heart disease in Japan. *International Journal of Epidemiology* 29 (5):832–836.

Newcomb, P. A., K. M. Egan, L. Titus-Ernstoff, et al. 1999. Lactation in relation to postmenopausal breast cancer. *American Journal of Epidemiology* 150 (2):174–182.

Pennebaker, J. W. 1989. Confession, inhibition, and disease. In *Advances in experimental social psychology*, vol. 22, edited by L. Berkowitz. New York: Academic Press.

Pennebaker, J. W., J. K. Kiecolt-Glaser, and R. Glaser. 1988. Disclosure of traumas and immune function: Health implications for psychotherapy. *Journal of Clinical and Consulting Psychology* 63:787–792.

Pienta, K. J., H. Naik, and A. Alchtar. 1995. Inhibition of spontaneous metastasis in rat prostate cancer model by oral administration of modified citrus pectin. *Journal of National Cancer Institute* 87 (5):348–353.

Portakal, O., O. Ozkaya, I. M. Erden, et al. 2000. Coenzyme Q10 concentrations and antioxidant status in tissues of breast cancer patients. *Clinical Biochemistry* 33 (4):279–284.

Potter, J. D. 1996. Nutrition and colorectal cancer. *Cancer Causes and Control* 7 (1): 127–146.

Purdie, D. M., and A. C. Green. 2001. Epidemiology of endometrial cancer. *Baillieres Best Practice Research in Clinical Obstetrics and Gynaecology* 15 (3):341–354.

Rafnsson, V., H. Tulinius, J. G. Jonasson, et al. 2001. Risk of breast cancer in female flight attendants: a population-based study. *Cancer Causes and Control* 12 (2):95–101.

Rangavajhyala, N., K. M. Shahani, G. Sridevi, et al. 1997. Nonlipopolysaccharide components of *Lactobacillus acidophilus* stimulates the production of interleukin-1 alpha and tumor necrosis factor-alpha by murine macrophages. *Nutrition in Cancer* 28 (2):130–134.

Ren, S., and E. J. Lien. 1997. Natural products and derivatives as cancer chemopreventive agents. In *Progress in Drug Research*, vol. 48, edited by E. Jucker. Basel, Switz.: Birkhauser Verlag.

Riccardi, A., P. Pugliese, M. Danova, et al. 2001. A phase II study of sequentil 5-fluorouracil, epirubicin and cyclophosphamide (FEC), and paclitaxel in advanced breast cancer (Protocol PV BC 97/01). *British Journal of Cancer* 85 (2):141–146.

Riggs, D. R., I. DeHaven, and D. L. Lamm. 1997. Allium sativum (garlic) treatment for murine traditional cell carcinomas. *Cancer* 79:1987–1994.

Rose, D. P. 1997. Dietary fat, fatty acids, and breast cancer. *Breast Cancer* 4 (1):7–16.

Rostom, A. Y., J. Powe, A. Kandil, et al. 1999. Positron emission tomography in breast cancer: A clinico-pathological correlation of results. *British Journal of Radiology* 72 (863):1064–1068.

Sai, R. M., B. Anju, T. Pauline, et al. 2000. Effect of kombucha tea on chromate (VI)-induced oxidative stress in albino rats. *Journal of Ethnopharmacology* 71 (1–2):235–240.

Sancho-Garnier, H. 1998. Epidemiology of breast cancer. *Bulletin of the Academy of National Medicine* 182 (8):1621–1632.

Schatzkin, A., Y. Jones, R. N. Hoover, et al. 1987. Alcohol consumption and breast cancer in the epidemiologic follow-up study of the first national health and nutrition examination survey. *New England Journal of Medicine* 316:1169–1173.

Schwartz, L. M., S. Woloshin, H. C. Sox, et al. 2000. U.S. women's attitudes to false positive mammography results and detection of ductal carcinoma *in situ*: cross-sectional survey. *British Medical Journal* 320 (7250):1635–1640.

Sen, P., N. M. Bailey, F. B. Hagemeister, et al. 1990. Induction of chromosome breaks and sister chromatid exchanges in patients with Hodgkin's disease by two combination chemotherapy regimens of different leukemogenic potential. *Cancer Research* 50 (3):558–562.

Serraino, M., and L. Thompson. 1992. The effect of flaxseed supplementation on the initiation and promotional stages of mammary tumorigenesis. *Nutrition in Cancer* 17:153–159.

Silverstein, M. J. 2000. Ductal carcinoma *in situ* of the breast. *Annual Review of Medicine* 51:17–32.

Simopoulos, A. P. 1987. Obesity and carcinogenesis: Historical perspective. *American Journal of Clinical Nutrition* 45:271–276.

Singer, S. R., and S. Grismaijer. 1995. *Dressed to kill: The link between breast cancer and bras.* Garden City Park, N.Y.: Avery Publishing Group.

Sivam, G. P., J. W. Lampe, and B. Ulness. 1997. Helicobacter pylori—*in vitro* susceptibility to garlic *(Allium satibum)* extract. *Nutrition in Cancer* 27 (2):118–121.

Slattery, M. L., J. Benson, T. D. Berry, et al. 1997. Dietary sugar and colon cancer. *Cancer Epidemiology Biomarkers in Prevention* 6 (9):677–685.

Slattery, M. L., J. Benson, and K. Curtin. 2000. Carotenoids and colon cancer. *American Journal of Clinical Nutrition.* 71:575–582.

Slattery, M. L., S. L. Edwards, K. M. Boucher, et al. 1999. Lifestyle and colon cancer: An assessment of factors associated with risk. *American Journal of Epidemiology* 150 (8):869–877.

Slattery, M. L., J. D. Potter, A. Coates, et al. 1997. Plant foods and colon cancer: An assessment of specific foods and their related nutrients. *Cancer Causes Control* 8 (4):575–590.

Spratt, J. S., B. M. Gaines, W. S. Aaron, et al. 1996. What are the benefits and costs of screening mammograms on Kentucky women aged 40–49? *Journal of Surgical Oncology* 63 (2):71–76.

Spratt, J. S., R. A. Greenberg, L. S. Heuser, et al. 1986. Geometry, growth rates, and duration of cancer and carcinoma-*in-situ* of the breast before detection by screening. *Cancer Research* 46:970–974.

Spratt, J. S., and D. von Fournier. 1993. Mammographic assessment of human breast cancer growth and duration. *Cancer* 71:2020–2026.

Stein, M. B., and E. Barett-Connor. 2000. Sexual assault and physical health: Findings from a population-based study of older adults. *Psychosomatic Medicine* 62 (6):838–843.

Stellman, J. M., and Stellman, S. D. 1992. Health effects of phenoxy herbicides and Agent Orange. In *Environmental and Occupational Medicine,* 2nd ed., edited by W. Rom. Boston: Little, Brown.

Stoll, B. A. 1997. Macronutrient supplements may reduce breast cancer risk: How, when, and which? *European Journal of Clinical Nutrition* 5 (19):573–577.

————. 2000. Biological mechanisms in breast cancer invasiveness: Relevance to preventive interventions. *European Journal of Cancer Prevention* 9 (2):73–79.

Surh, Y. J., K. S. Chun, H. H. Cha, et al. 2001. Molecular mechanisms underlying chemopreventive activities of anti-inflammatory phytochemicals: down-regulation of COX-2 and iNOS through suppression of NF-kappa B activation. *Mutation Research* 480–481:243–268.

Talbott, E. O., A. O. Youk, K. P. McHugh, et al. 2000. Mortality among the residents of the Three Mile Island accident area: 1979–1992. *Environmental Health Perspectives* 108 (6):545–552.

Tamoxifen unsuitable for primary prevention of breast cancer: Uncertain efficacy, clear risks. 2000. *Prescrire International* 9 (46):56–58. No author.

Taussig, S. J., and S. Batkin. 1998. Bromelain, the enzyme complex of pineapple (*Ananas comosus*), and its clinical applicaition: An update. *Journal of Ethnopharmacology* 22 (2):191–203.

Thompson, L. U., S. E. Rickard, L. J. Orcheson, et al. (1996). Flaxseed and its lignan and oil components reduce mammary tumor growth at a late stage of carcinogenesis. *Carcinogenesis* 17 (6):1372–1376.

Thompson, L. U., M. M. Seidl, S. E. Rickard, et al. 1996. Antitumorigenic effect of mammalian lignan precursors from flaxseed. *Nutrition in Cancer* 26 (2):159–165.

Thun, M. 1992. Risk factors for fatal colon cancer in a large prospective study. *Journal of the National Cancer Institute* 84 (19):1491–1500.

Tou, J. C., and L. U. Thompson. 1999. Exposure to flaxseed or its lignan component during different developmental stages influences rat mammary gland structures. *Carcinogenesis* 20 (9):1831–1835.

Trentham-Dietz, A., P. A. Newcomb, K. M. Egan, et al. 2000. Weight change and risk of postmenopausal breast cancer. *Cancer Causes Control* 11 (6):533–542.

Trichopoulou, A., K. Katsouyanni, S. Stuver, et al. 1995. Consumption of olive oil and specific food groups in relation to breast cancer risk in Greece. *Journal of the National Cancer Institute* 87 (2):110–116.

U.S. Department of Health and Human Services. 1994. *Progress report for: Cancer.* No city.

Vachon, C. M., I. H. Kushi, J. R. Cerhan, et al. 2000. Association of diet mammographic breast density in the Minnesota breast cancer family cohort. *Cancer and Epidemiological Biomarkers and Prevention* 9 (2):151–160.

Van Netten, J. P., S. A. Cann, and D. W. Glover. 1999. Mammographic compression: A force to be reckoned with. *British Journal of Cancer* 81 (8):1426–1427.

Van Netten, J. P., T. Mogentale, M. J. Smith, et al. 1994. Physical trauma and breast cancer. *Lancet* 343 (8903):978–979.

Veierod, M. B., P. Laake, and D. S. Thelle. 1997. Dietary fat intake and risk of prostate cancer: A prospective study of 25,708 Norwegian men. *International Journal of Cancer* 73 (5):634–638.

Von Fournier, D., U. Abel, J. A. Spratt, et al. 1994. Growth rate of breast cancer: Implication for early detection and therapeutic effects. *Geburtshilfe Frauenheilkd* 54 (5):286–290.

Whysner, J., and M. Mohan. 2000. Perineal application of talc and cornstarch powders: Evaluation of ovarian cancer risk. *American Journal of Obstetrics and Gynecology* 182 (3):720–724.

Witte, J. S., M. P. Longnecker, C. L. Bird, et al. 1996. Relation of vegetable, fruit, and grain consumption to colorectal adenomatous polyps. *American Journal of Epidemiology* 144 (11):1015–1025.

Wright, C. J., and C. B. Mueller. 1995. Screening mammography and public health policy: The need for perspective. *The Lancet* 346:29–32.

Wu, A. H., M. C. Yu, and T. M. Mack. 1997. Smoking, alcohol use, dietary factors, and risk of small intestinal adencarcinoma. *International Journal of Cancer* 70 (5):512–517.

Wu, A. H., R. G. Ziegler, P. L. Horn-Ross, et al. 1996. Tofu and risk of breast cancer in Asian Americans. *Cancer Epidemiological Biomarkers and Prevention* 5 (11):901–906.

Yo, A. 1997. Diet and stomach cancer in Korea. *International Journal of Cancer* (Supplement 10):7–9.

Yoshida, S. H., S. S. Teuber, J. B. German, et al. 1994. Immunotoxicity of silicone: Implications of oxidant balance towards adjuvant activity. *Food and Chemical Toxicology* 32 (11):1089–1090.

Zang, S. M., E. L. Giovannucci, D. J. Hunter, et al. 2001. Vitamin supplement use and the risk of non-Hodgkin's lymphoma among women and men. *American Journal of Epidemiology* 153 (11):1056–1063.

Zava, D. T., M. Blen, and G. Duwe. 1997. Estrogenic activity of natural and synthetic estrogens in human breast cancer cells in culture. *Environmental Health Perspectives* 105 (Supplement 3): 637–645.

Zheng, T., T. R. Holford, S. T. Mayne, P. H. Owens, et al. 1999. Beta-benzene hexachloride in breast adipose tissue and risk of breast carcinoma. *Cancer* 85 (10): 2212–2218.

Zheng, T., T. R. Holford, S. T. Mayne, J. Tessari, et al. 2000. Risk of female breast cancer associated with serum polychlorinated biphenyls and 1,1-dichloro-2,2'-bis (p-chlorophenyl) ethylene. *Cancer Epidemiological Markers and Prevention* 2:167–174.

Zheng, W., L. H. Kushi, J. D. Potter, et al. 1995. Dietary intake of energy and animal foods and endometrial cancer incidence: The Iowa women's health study. *American Journal of Epidemiology* 142 (4):388–394.

Carpal Tunnel Syndrome

Branco, K., and M. A. Naeser. 1999. Carpal tunnel syndrome: Clinical outcome after low-level laser acupuncture, microamps transcutaneous electrical nerve stimulation, and other alternative therapies—an open protocol study. *Journal of Alternative and Complementary Medicine* 5 (1):5–26.

Castleman, M. 2000. Carpal tunnel syndrome. In *Blended medicine*. Rodale, distributed by St. Martin's Press, pp. 179–183.

Feuerstein, M., L. M. Burrell, V. I. Miller, et al. 1999. Clinical management of carpal tunnel syndrome: A 12-year review of outcomes. *American Journal of Industrial Medicine* 35 (3):232–245.

Hay, L. 1984. *Heal your body: The mental causes for physical illness and the metaphysical way to overcome them.* Carlsbad, Calif.: Hay House.

Worwood, V. A. 1991. *The complete book of essential oils & aromatherapy.* San Rafael, Calif.: New World Library.

Young, J. 1992. *Self-Massage.* London: HarperCollins, Thorson.

Chronic Fatigue Syndrome

Ax, S., V. N. Gregg, and D. Jones. 1997. Chronic fatigue syndrome: Sufferers' evaluation of medical support. *Journal of Social Medicine* 90 (5):250–254.

Deale, A., T. Chalder, and S. Wessely. 1998. Illness beliefs and treatment outcome in chronic fatigue syndrome. *Journal of Psychosomatic Research* 45 (1 spec no.):77–83.

Fulcher, K. Y., and P. D. White. 1997. Randomised controlled trial of graded exercise in patients with the chronic fatigue syndrome. *British Medical Journal* 314 (7095): 1647–1652.

Hay, L. 1984. *Heal your body: The mental causes for physical illness and the metaphysical way to overcome them.* Carlsbad, Calif.: Hay House.

Keenoy, M. Y., G. Moorkens, J. Verommen, et al. 2000. Magnesium status and parameters of the oxidant-antioxidant balance in patients with chronic fatigue: effects of supplementation with magnesium. *Journal of the American College of Nutrition* 19 (3):374–382.

Landis, R. 1997. *Herbal defense.* New York: Warner Books.

Manuel, K. B., G. Moorkens, J. Vertommen, et al. 2000. Magnesium status and parameters of the oxidant-antioxidant balance in patients with chronic fatigue: Effects of supplementation with magnesium. *Journal of the American College of Nutrition* 19 (3):374–382.

Prins, J. B., G. Bleijenberg, E. Bazelmans, et al. 2001. Cognitive behaviour therapy for chronic fatigue syndrome: A multicentre randomised controlled trial. *Lancet* 357 (9250):841–847.

See, D. M., N. Broumand, L. Sahl, et al. 1997. *In vitro* effects of echinacea and ginseng on natural killer and antibody-dependent cell cytotoxicity in healthy subjects and chronic fatigue syndrome or acquired immunodeficiency syndrome patients. *Immunopharmacology* 35 (3):229–235.

Simpson, M. 1997. A body with chronic fatigue syndrome as a battleground for the fight to separate from the mother. *Journal of Analytic Psychology* 42 (2):201–216.

Werbach, M. R. 2000. Nutritional strategies for treating chronic fatigue syndrome. *Alternative Medical Review* 5 (2):93–108

Whiting, P., A. M. Banall, A. J. Sowden, et al. 2001. Interventions for the treatment and management of chronic fatigue syndrome: A systematic review. *Journal of the American Medical Association* 286 (11):1360–1368

Depression

Beauchemin, K. M., and P. Hays. 1997. Phototherapy is a useful adjunct in the treatment of depressed in-patients. *Acta Psychiatry Scandinavia* 95 (5):424–427.

Beck, C. T. 1998. A checklist to identify women at risk for developing postpartum depression. *Journal of Obstetric, Gynecologic, and Neonatal Nursing* 27 (1):39–46.

Bell, K. M., L. Pion, W. E. Bunney, Jr., et al. 1988. S-adenosylmethionine treatment of depression: A controlled clinical trial. *American Journal of Psychiatry* 145:1110–1114.

Bolin, S. 1986. The role of pets in comforting the pet-owning widow. Delta Society International Conference, August 23, Boston.

Breslau, N., E. L. Peterson, L. R. Schultz, et al. 1998. Major depression and stages of smoking. *Archives of General Psychiatry* 55 (2):161–166.

Brodsky, B. S., M. Oquendo, S. P. Ellis, et al. 2001. The relationship of childhood abuse to impulsivity and suicidal behavior in adults with major depression. *American Journal of Psychiatry* 158:1871–1877.

Brozovic, B., and K. Wold. 2000. Managing depression in nursing home elderly. *The Clinical Advisor* (November/December):42–51.

Depressed smokers ride immune downer. 1999. *Science News* 155:358.

Depression among teens. 2001. *American Journal of Nursing* 101(1):21. No author.

Depression Guideline Panel. 1993. *Depression in primary care,* vol. 2, *Treatment of major depression.* Clinical Practice Guideline. Rockville, Md.: U.S. Department of Health and Human Services, Public Health Service, Agency for Health Care Policy and Research.

De Souza, M.C., A. F. Walker, P. A. Robinson, et al. 2000. A synergistic effect of a daily supplement for 1 month of 200 mg magnesium plus 50 mg vitamin B_6 for the relief of anxiety-related premenstrual symptoms: A randomized, double-blind, crossover study. *Journal of Women's Health and Gender-Based Medicine* 9 (2):131–139.

Exercise may be as effective as sertraline in the treatment of major depression. 2001. *American Journal of Nursing* 101 (2):19.

Fava, G. A., C. Rafanelli, A. Grandi, et al. 1998. *Archives of General Psychiatry* 55:816–820.

Feeling better with fish oil. 1999. *Science News* 155:362.

Gelfand, D. M., D. M. Teti, S. A. Seiner, et al. 1996. Helping mothers fight depression: Evaluation of a home-based intervention program for depressed mothers and their infants. *Journal of Clinical and Child Psychology* 25:406–422.

Grant, M., and V. Morrison. 2001. Primary care of major depression: Psychopharmacology strategies. *American Journal for Nurse Practitioners* (July/August):39–48.

Hay, L. 2000. *Heal Your Body.* Carlsbad, Calif.: Hay House.

Hays, J. C., D. C. Steffens, E. P. Flint, et al. 2001. Does social support buffer decline in elderly patients with unipolar depression? *American Journal of Psychiatry* 158:1850–1855.

Herzog, A. R., M. M. Franks, H. R. Markus, et al. 1998. Activities and well-being in older age: Effects of self-concept and educational attainment. *Psychology and Aging* 13 (2):179–185.

Hibbein, J. R. 1997. Essential fatty acids predict biomarkers of aggression and depression. *PUFA Newsletter* 1 (3):2.

Kupfer, D. J. 1995. Complicated grief and bereavement—related depression as distinct disorders. *American Journal of Psychiatry* 152 (1):22–30.

Lai, Y. M. 1999. Effects of music listening on depressed women in Taiwan. *Issues in Mental Health* 3:229–246.

Mazurek, B. M., and Z. Moldenbauer. 1999. Current approaches to depression in children and adolescents. *Advance for Nurse Practitioners* (February):24–29, 97.

McCoy, D. L., and S. K. Holmberg. 2001. Antidepressant medications during breastfeeding: Safety and efficacy for mother and infant. *American Journal for Nurse Practitioners* (February):9–15.

McKinney, C. H., M. H. Antoni, M. Kumar, et al. 1997. Effects of guided imagery and music (GIM) therapy on mood and cortisol in healthy adults. *Health Psychology* 16 (4): 390–400.

Miller, L. G. 1998. Herbal medicinals: Selected clinical considerations focusing on known or potential drug-herb interactions. *Archives of General Medicine* 158:2200–2211.

Mindell, E., and V. Hopkins. 1998. *Prescription alternatives* New Canaan, Conn.: Keats.

National Institute of Mental Health. 1994. *Plain talk about depression.* Rockville, Md.: U.S. Department of Health and Human Services, National Institutes of Health, Office of Scientific Information.

Oakley, I. D. 1994. Striving for "sugar 'n' spice" may produce depression in some women. *Nursing Dimensions* (Fall):5

Penninx, B. W., B. T. van Tilburg, A. J. P. Deeg, et al. 1998. Predicting depression in the chronically ill. *Health Psychology* 17: 551–558.

Penninx, B. W., J. H., J. M. Gurainik, L. Ferrucci, et al. 2000. Vitamin B_{12} deficiency and depression in physically disabled older women: Epidemiologic evidence from the Women's Health and Aging Study. *American Journal of Psychiatry* 157:715–721.

Pettigrew, J. W., J. Levine, and R. J. McClure. 2000. Acetyl-L-carnitine physical-chemical, metabolic, and therapeutic properties: Relevance for its mode of action in Alzheimer's disease and geriatric depression. *Molecular Psychiatry* 5 (6):616–632.

Philpot, V. D., and J. W. Bamburg. 1996. Restructuring negative thoughts can improve self-esteem and reduce depression. *Psychological Reports* 79:83.

Prigerson, H. G., S. V. Kasl, C. F. Reynolds III, et al. 2001. Mindfulness-based stress reduction and health-related quality of life in a heterogeneous patient population. *General Hospital Psychiatry* 23 (4):183–192.

Rief, W., S. Trenkamp, C. Auer, et al. 2000. Cognitive behavior therapy in panic disorder and comorbid major depression. *Psychotherapy and Psychosomatics* 69 (2):70–80.

Rodriguez, J. J., J. R. Rodriguez, and M. J. Gonzalez. 1998. Indicators of anxiety and depression in subjects with different kinds of diet: Vegetarians and omnivores. *Bulletin of the Medical Association of Puerto Rico* 90 (4–6):58–68.

Rosch, P. J. 1999. Depression and other diseases. *Health & Stress* 4:6

Sanchez, V. C., P. M. Lewinsohn, and D. W. Larson. 1980. Assertion training: Effectiveness in the treatment of depression. *Journal of Clinical Psychology* 36 (2):526–529.

Schubert, H., and P. Halama. 1993. Depressive episode primarily unresponse to therapy in elderly patients: Efficacy of Ginkgo biloba (Egb 761) in combination with antidepressants. *Geriatric Forsch* 3:45–53.

Singh, N. A., K. M. Clements, and M. A. Fiatarone. 1997. A randomized controlled trial of progressive resistance training in depressed elders. *Journal of Gerontology in Biological Science and Medical Science* 52 (1):M2–M35.

Sommers-Flanagan, J., and R. Sommers-Flanagan. 1996. Efficacy of antidepressant medication with depressed youth: What psychologists should know. *Professional Psychology: Research and Practice* 27:145–153.

Velting, V. 1999. Parents "clueless" about teen suicide, study shows. *Ball State University News*, press release.

Yang, X., X. Liu, H. Luo, et al. 1994. Clinical observation on needling extrachannel points in treating mental depression. *Journal of Traditional Chinese Medicine* 14 (1):14–18

Diabetes

Anderson, R. A., N. Chen, N. Bryden, et al. 1997. Elevated intakes of supplemental chromium improve glucose and insulin variables of individuals with type 2 diabetes *Diabetes* 46:1786–1791

Anderson, R. A., A. M. Roussel, N. Zouari, et al. 2001. Potential antioxidant effects of zinc and chromium supplementation in people with type 2 diabetes mellitus. *Journal of the American College of Nutrition* 20 (3):212–218.

Augusti, K. T. 1996. Therapeutic values of onion and garlic. *Indian Journal of Experimental Biology* 34 (7):634–640.

Chang, T. J., H. H. Lei, J. I. Yeh, et al. 2000. Vitamin D receptor gene polymorphisms influence susceptibility to type 1 diabetes mellitus in Taiwanese population. *Clinical Endrocrinology* 52 (5):575–580.

Childhood type 2 diabetes running rampant. 2000. *Clinician Reviews* 10 (1):156–159.

Cows' milk, diabetes connection bolstered. 1999. *Science News* 155:404–405.

Diabetes Control and Complications Trial Research Group. 1993. The effect of intensive treatment of diabetes on the development and progression of long-term complications in insulin-dependent diabetes mellitus. *New England Journal of Medicine* 329:977–986.

Facchini, F., A. M. Coulston, and G. M. Reaven. 1996. Relationship between dietary vitamin intake and resistance to insulin-mediated glucose disposal in healthy volunteers. *American Journal of Clnical Nutrition* 63 (6):946–949.

Folsom, A. R., L. H. Kushi, and C. P. Hong. 2000. Physical activity and incident diabetes mellitus in postmenopausal women. *American Journal of Public Health* 90:134–138.

Fuller, C. J., M. Chandalia, A. Garg, et al. 1996. RRR-alpha-tocopheryl acetate supplementation at pharmacologic dose decreases low-density lipoproprotein oxidative susceptibility but not protein glycation in patients with diabetes mellitus. *American Journal of Clinical Nutrition* 63 (5):753–759.

Ho, E., N. Quan, Y. H. Tsai, et al. 2001. Dietary zinc supplementation inhibits NFkappaB activation and protects against chemically induced diabetes in CD1 mice. *Experimental Biological Medicine* 226 (2):103–111.

Hu, F. B., J. E. Manson, J. Meir, et al. 2001. Diet, lifestyle, and the risk of type 2 diabetes in women. *New England Journal of Medicine* 345 (1):790–794.

Mangan, M. M. 1999. Diabetic neuropathy, clinical evaluation, and pain management. *Clinician Reviews* 9 (9):61–78.

Manson, J. E., D. M. Nathan, A. S. Krolewski, et al. 1992. A prospective study of exercise and incidence of diabetes among U.S. male physicians. *Journal of the American Medical Association* 268 (1):63–67.

Monetini, L., M. G. Cavallo, L. Stefanini, et al. 2001. Bovine beta-casein antibodies in breast- and bottle-fed infants: Their relevance in type 1 diabetes. *Diabetes Metabolism Research Review* 17 (1):51–54.

Murray, J. T. 1994. Are botanical medicines useful in diabetes? *American Journal of Natural Medicine* 1 (3):5–7.

Pettit, J. L. 2001. Alternative medicine: Chromium. *Clinician Reviews* 11 (10):66–68.

Rodriguez-Moran, M., and F. Guerrero-Romero. 2001. Low serum magnesium levels and foot ulcers in subjects with type 2 diabetes. *Archives of Medical Research* 32 (4):300–303.

Salmeron, J., J. E. Manson, and M. J. Stampfer. 1997. Dietary fiber, glycemic load, and risk of non-insulin-dependent diabetes mellitus in women. *Journal of the American Medical Association* 277 (6):472–477.

Sharma, R. D., T. C. Raghuram, and N. S. Rao. 1990. Effect of fenugreek seeds on blood glucose and serum lipids in type 1 diabetes. *European Journal of Clinical Nutrition*, 44:301–306.

Sheela, C. G., and K. T. Augusti. 1992. Antidiabetic effects of S-ayyl cysteine suphoxide isolated garlic. *Indian Journal of Experimental Biology* 30:523–526.

Shvets, N. V., L. D. Kramerenko, S. V. Vydyborets, et al. 1994. Disordered trace element content of the erthrocytes in diabetes mellitus. *Lik Sprava* (January):52–55.

Suresh, B. P., and K. Srinivasan. 1998. Amelioration of renal lesions associated with diabetes by dietary curcumin in streptozotocin diabetic rats. *Molecular Cell Biochemistry* 181 (1–2):87–96.

Ting, H. H., F. K. Timini, and K. S. Boles. 1996. Vitamin C improves endothelium-dependent vasodilation in patients with non-insulin-dependent diabetes mellitus. *Journal of Clinical Investigation* 97 (1):22–28.

Velussi, M., A. M. Cernigoi, A. D. De Monte, et al. 1997. Long-term (12 months) treatment with an antioxidant (silymarin): Its effect on hyperinsulinemia, exogenous insulin, and malondialdehyde levels in cirrhotic diabetic patients. *Journal of Heptology* 16:871–879.

Vincent, J. B. 2000. Quest for the molecular mechanism of chromium action and its relationship to diabetes. *Nutrition Reviews* 58 (3 pt. 1):67–72.

Virtanen, S. M., E. Laara, E. Hypponen, et al. 2000. Cow's milk consumption, HLA-DQB1 genotype, and type 1 diabetes: A nested case-control study of siblings of children with diabetes. Childhood Diabetes in Finland Study Group. *Diabetes* 49 (6):912–917.

Vuksan, V., M. P. Stavro, J. L. Sievenpiper, et al. 2000. American ginseng improves glycemia in individuals with normal glucose tolerance. *Journal of the American College of Nutrition* 1 (19):738–744.

Digestive Problems

Ahmed, D. S., and A. M. Karch. 2000. Hidden factors in occult blood testing. *American Journal of Nursing* 100 (12):25.

Aldoori, W. H., E. L. Giovannucci, E. B. Rimm, et al. 1995. *Gut* 36 (2):276–282.

Ali, A., B. B. Toner, N. Stuckless, et al. 2000. Emotional abuse, self-blame, and self-silencing in women with irritable bowel syndrome. *Psychosomatic Medicine* 62 (1):76–82.

Bliss, D. Z., H. J. Jung, K. Savik, et al. 2001. Supplementation with dietary fiber improves fecal incontinence. *Nursing Research* 50 (4): 203–213.

Borrelli, F., and A. A. Izzo. 2000. The plant kingdom as a source of antiulcer remedies. *Phytotherapy Research* 14 (8):581–591.

Broide, E., S. Pintov, S. Portnoy, et al. 2001. Effectiveness of acupuncture for treatment of childhood constipation. *Digestive Diseases and Science* 46 (6):1270–1275.

Chewing away heartburn. 1996. *Psychology & Health Update* 6 (2):4.

Coutino-Rodriguez, R., P. Hernandez-Cruz, and H. Giles-Rios. 2001. Lectins in fruits having gastrointestinal activity: Their participation in the hemagglutinating property of *Escherichia coli* O157:H7. *Archives of Medical Research* 32 (4):251–257.

Cruz, T., J. Galvez, E. Crespo, et al. 2001. Effects of silymarin on the acute stage of the trinitrobenzenesulphonic acid model of rat colitis. *Planta Medica* 67 (1):94–96.

Dyspepsia patients respond to herbal formulation. 1999. *Clinician Reviews* 9 (9):123–124.

Emmanuel, A. V., and M. A. Kamm. 2001. Response to a behavioural treatment, biofeedback in constipated patients is associated with improved gut transit and autonomic innervation. *Gut* 49 (2):214–219.

Field, S. 2001. Approaches to diverticular disease. *The Clinical Advisor* (September):25–31.

Friedman, H. S. 1991. *The self-healing personality.* New York: Henry Holt.

Galovski, T. E., and E. B. Blanchard. 1998. The treatment of irritable bowel syndrome with hypnotherapy. *Applied Psychophysiology and Biofeedback* 23 (4):219–232.

Girodon, F., M. Lombard, P. Galan, et al. 1997. Effect of micronutrient supplemention on infection in institutionalized elderly subjects: A controlled trial. *Annals of Nutrition and Metabolism* 41 (2):98–107.

Keefer, L., and E. B. Blanchard. 2001. The effects of relaxation reponse meditation on the symptoms of irritable bowel syndrome: Results of a controlled treatment study. *Behavior Research and Therapy* 39 (7):801–811.

Key, T. J., G. K. Davey, and P. N. Appleby. 1999. Health benefits of a vegetarian diet. *Proceedings of the Nutrition Society* 58 (2):271–275.

Lin, O. S., M. S. Soon, S. S. Wu, et al. 2000. Dietary habits and right-sided colonic diverticulosis. *Diseases of the Colon and Rectum* 43 (10):1412–1418.

Liu, J. H., G. H. Chen, H. A. Yeh, et al. 1997. Enteric-coated peppermint-oil capsules in the treatment of irritable bowel syndrome: A prospective, randomized trial. *Journal of Gastroenterology* 32:765–768.

Mahalanabis, D., and M. K. Bhan. 2001. Micronutrients as adjunct therapy of acute illness in children: Impact on the episode outcome and policy implications of current findings. *British Journal of Nutrition* 85 (Supplement 2):S151–S158.

McDonald-Hail, J., L. A. Bradley, M. A. Bailey, et al. 1994. Relaxation training reduces symptom reports and acid exposure in patients with gastroesophageal reflux disease. *Gastroenterology* 107 (1):61–69.

Merchant, R. E., and C. A. Andre. 2001. A review of recent clinical trials of the nutritional supplement *Chlorella pyrenoidosa* in the treatment of fibromyalgia, hypertension, and ulcerative colitis. *Alternative Therapies in Health and Medicine* 7 (3):79–81.

Mindell, E., and V. Hopkins. 1998. Drugs for the digestive tract and their natural alternatives. *Prescription Alternatives.* New Canaan, Conn.: Keats Publishing.

Murphy, J. 2001. *Nurse practitioners' prescribing reference* 8 (3):135–153.

Nair, P., and J. F. Mayberry. 1994. Vegetarianism, dietary fibre and gastro-intestinal disease. *Digestive Diseases* 12 (3):177–185.

Owen, R. W., A. Giacosa, W. E. Hull, et al. 2000. The antioxidant/anticancer potential of phenolic compounds isolated from olive oil. *European Journal of Cancer* 36 (10):1235–1247.

Rahman, M. M., S. H. Vermund, M. A. Wahed, et al. 2001. Simultaneous zinc and vitamin A supplementation in Bangladeshi children: Randomised double blind controlled trial. *British Journal of Medicine* 323 (7308):314–318.

Rogers, S. 1994. *Wellness against all odds.* Syracuse, N.Y.: Prestige Publishing.

Simopoulos, A. P. 1999. Essential fatty acids in health and chronic disease. *American Journal of Clinical Nutrition* 70 (3 Supplement):560S–569S.

Sivam, G. P. 2001. Protection against *Helicobacter pylori* and other bacterial infections by garlic. *Journal of Nutrition* 131 (3s):1106S–1108S.

Sturniolo, G. C., V. De Leo, A. Ferronato, et al. 2001. Zinc supplementation tightens "leaky gut" in Crohn's disease. *Inflammatory Bowel Disease* 7 (2):94–98.

Van Dulmen, A. M., et al. 1996. Cognitive-behavioral group therapy for irritable bowel syndrome effects and long-term follow-up. *Psychosomatic Medicine* 58:508–514.

Williams, D. G. 1990. What and where is this (illeocecal) valve? *Alternatives* 1 (3): 1–4.

Fibromyalgia

Bassleer, C., P. Gysent, and Bassleer R., et al. 1987. Proteoglycans synthesized by human chondrocytes cultivated in clusters. *American Journal of Medicine* 83 (5A):25–28.

Bell, K. M., L. Plon, W. E. Bunney Jr., et al. S-adenosylmethionine treatment of depression: A controlled clinical trial. *American Journal of Psychiatry* 145:1110–1114.

Brandt, K. D. 1987. Effects of nonsteroidal anti-inflammatory drugs on chondrocyte metabolism *in vitro* and *in vivo*. *American Journal of Medicine* 83 (5A):29–34.

Capodaglio, P., and G. Vicenzi. 2000. Efficacy of a chair with magnets in the prevention of musculoskeletal disorders caused by prolonged sitting. *Journal of Italian Medical Laboratory of Ergonomics* 22 (4):332–225.

Caruso, I., and V. Petrogrande. 1987. Italian double-blind multicenter study of comparing S-adensylmethionine, naproxen, and placebo in the treatment of degenerative joint disease. *American Journal of Medicine* 83 (5A):66–71.

Dingle, J. T. 1991. Cartilage maintenance in osteoarthritis interaction of cytokines, NSAID, and prostaglandins in articular cartilage damage and repair. *Journal of Rheumatology Supplement* 28:30–37.

Domijan, Z., B. Vrhovac, T. Dumgi, et al. 1989. A double-blind trial of ademetionine vs. Naproxen in activated gonarthrosis. *International Journal of Clinical Pharmacology and Toxicology* 27:329–333.

Goldenberg, D. I., D. T. Felson, and H. Dineman. 1986. A randomized, controlled trial of amitriptyline and naproxen in the treatment of patients with fibromyalgia. *Arthritis and Rheumatism* 29:1371–1377.

Goldenberg, D., M. Mayskly, C. Mossey, et al. 1996. A randomized, double-blind crossover trial of fluoxetine and amitriptyline in the treatment of fibromyalgia. *Arthritis and Rheumatism* 39:1851–1859.

Harmon, C. E. 1996. Fibromyalgia: Treatments worth trying. *Internal Medicine* 17:64–75.

Hassett, A. I., J. D. Cone, S. J. Patella, et al. 2000. The role of catastrophizing in the pain and depression of women with fibromyalgia syndrome. *Arthritis and Rheumatism* 43 (11):2493–2500.

Kagan, B. L., D. L. Sultzer, N. Rosenlicht, et al. 1990. Oral S-adenosylmethionin in depression: A randomized, double-blind, placebo-controlled trial. *American Journal of Psychiatry* 147 (5):591–595.

Kaplan, K. H., D. L. Goldenberg, and M. Galvin-Nadeau. 1992. The impact of a meditation-based stress reduction program on fibromyalgia. *General Hospital Psychiatry* 15 (5):284–289.

Manicourt, D. H., A. Druetz-Van Egeren, L. Haazen, et al. 1994. Effects of tenoxicam and aspirin on the metabolism of proteoglycans and hyaluronan in normal and osteoarthritic human and articular cartilage. *British Journal of Pharmacology* 113: 1113–1120.

Muller-Fassbender, H. 1987. Double-blind clinical trial of S-adensylmethionine versus ibuprofen in the treatment of osteoarthritis. *American Journal of Medicine* 83 (5A): 81–83.

Murray, M. T. 1996. *Encyclopedia of nutritional supplements*. Roseville, Calif.: Primar Publishing.

Rosch, P. 1998. The amazing power of magnets. *Newsletter of the American Institute of Stress* 2:7–8.

Saputo, L. 1998. Drug-free relief from fibromyalgia. *Greatlife* (April):28–31.

Sephton, S. E., G. Lynch, I. Weissbecker, et al. 2001. Effects of a meditation program on symptoms of illness and neuroendocrine responses in women with fibromyalgia. Presented at the fifty-ninth Annual Scientific Meeting of the American Psychosomatic Society, Monterey, Calif., March 6–10th.

Smith, J. D., C. M. Terpening, S. Schmidt, et al. 2000. Relief of fibromyalgia symptoms following dietary excitotoxins. *The American Journal for Nurse Practitioners* (July/August): 51–59.

Thompson, R. C. Jr., and T. R. Oegema Jr. 1979. Metabolic activity of articular cartilage in osteoarthritis. An *in vitro* study. *American Journal of Bone and Joint Surgery* 61:407–416.

Vahora, S. A., and P. Malek-Ahmadi. 1988. S-adenosylmethione in the treatment of depression. *Neuroscience and Biobehavioral Review* 12 (2):139–141.

Van Houdenhove, B., E. Neerinckx, R. Lysens, et al. 2001. Victimization in chronic fatigue syndrome and fibromyalgia in tertiary care: A controlled study on prevalence and characteristics. *Psychosomatics* 42 (1):21–28.

Vetter, G. 1987. Double-blind comparative clinical trial with S-adenosylmethionine and Indomethacin in the treatment of osteoarthritis. *American Journal of Medicine* 83 (5A):78–80.

Wolfe, F., J. Anderson, D. Harkness, et al. 1997. A prospective, longitudinal, multicenter study of service utilization and costs in fibromyalgia. *Arthritis and Rheumatism* 40:1560–1570.

Wolfe, F., M. A. Cathey, and D. J. Hawley. 1994. A double-blind placebo-controlled trial of fluoxetine in fibromyalgia. *Scandinavian Journal of Rheumatology* 23:255–259.

Yunus, M. B., A. T. Masi, and J. C. Aldag. 1989. Short-term effects of ibuprofen in primary fibromyalgia syndrome: A double-blind, placebo-controlled trial. *Journal of Rheumatology* 16:527–532.

Heart and Blood Vessel Disorders

Bensky, D., and A. Gamble. 1993. *Chinese herbal medicine, materia medica*. Seattle, Wash.: Eastland Press.

Castillo-Richmond, A., R. H. Schneider, C. N. Alexander, et al. 2001. Effects of stress reduction on carotid atherosclerosis in hypertensive African Americans. *Stroke* 31 (3):568–573.

Dal Porto, R., F. Faletra, E. Picano, et al. 2001. Safety, feasibility, and diagnostic accuracy of accelerated high-dose dipyridamole stress echocardiography. *American Journal of Cardiology* 87 (5):520–524.

Elhendy, A., C. Shub, R. B. McCully, et al. 2001. Exercise echocardiography for the prognostic stratification of patients with low pretest probability of coronary artery disease. *American Journal of Medicine* 111 (1):73–74.

Engel, G. I. 1971. Sudden and rapid death during psychological stress: Folklore and folk wisdom. *Annals of Internal Medicine* 74:771–782.

Everson, S. A., D. E. Goldberg, G. A. Kaplan, et al. 1996. Hopelessness and risk of mortality and incidence of myocardial infarction and cancer. *Psychosomatic Medicine* 58:113–121.

Farella, C. 2001. Is popular heart scan sound or scam? *Nursing Spectrum* 11 (20FL):8–9.

Frangolias, D., and E. Rhodes. 1995. Maximal and ventilatory threshold responses to treadmill and water immersion running. *Medicine and Science in Sports and Exercise* 27 (7):1007–1013.

Frankish, H. 2001. Air pollutants can trigger heart attacks. *Lancet* 357 (9272):1952.

Goldberg, J. G. 1991. *Deceits of the mind and their effects on the body*. New Brunswick, N.J.: Transaction.

Gullette, E. C. D., J. A. Blumenthal, M. Babyak, et al. 1997. Effects of mental stress on myocardial ischemia during daily life. *Journal of the American Medical Association* 277 (20):1521–1526.

Hashimoto, A., E. L. Palmar, J. A. Scott, et al. 1999. Complications of exercise and pharmacologic stress tests: Differences in younger and elderly patients. *Journal of Nuclear Cardiology* 6 (6):612–619.

Hendler, S. S. 1990. *The doctor's vitamin and mineral encyclopedia*. New York: Simon & Schuster.

Iwane, M., M. Aita, S. Tomimoto, et al. 2000. Walking 10,000 steps/day or more reduces blood pressure and sympathetic nerve activity in mild essential hypertension. *Hypertension Research* 23 (6):573–580.

Kane, G. C., and J. J. Lipsey. 2000. Drug-grapefruit juice interactions. *Mayo Clinic Proceedings* 75:933–942.

Kim, J., A. Oberman, G. F. Fletcher, et al. 2001. Effect of exercise intensity and frequency on lipid levels in men with coronary heart disease: Training level comparison trial. *American Journal of Cardiology* 87:942–946.

Kra, S. J. 1996. *What every woman must know about heart disease*. New York: Warner Books.

Lakka, T. A., J. A. Laukkanen, R. Rauramaa, et al. 2001. Cardiorespiratory fitness and the progression of carotid atherosclerosis in middle-aged men. *Annals of Internal Medicine* 134 (1):12–20.

Larrue, V., R. R. von Kummer, A. Muller, et al. 2001. Risk factors for severe hemorrhagic transformation in ischemic stroke patients treated with recombinant tissue plasminogen activator: A secondary analysis of the European-Australasian Acute Stroke Study (ECASS II). *Stroke* 32 (20):438–441.

Masaki, K. H. et al. 2000. Association of vitamin E and C supplement use with cognitive function and dementia in elderly men. *Neurology* 54:1265–1272.

Mathias, W., A. Arruda, F. C. Santos, et al. 1999. Safety of dobutamine-atropine stress echocardiography: A prospective experience of 4,033 consecutive studies. *Journal of the American Society of Echocardiography* 12 (10):785–791.

Moore, T. J., P. R. Conlin, J. Ard, et al. 2001. DASH (Dietary Approaches to Stop Hypertension) diet is effective treatment for stage 1 isolated systolic hypertension. *Hypertension* 38 (2):155–158.

Myers, J., L. Voodi, T. Umann, et al. 2000. A survey of exercise testing: Methods utilization, interpretation, and safety in the VFAHCS. *Journal of Cardiopulmonary Rehabilitation* 20 (4):251–258.

National Heart, Lung, and Blood Institute. 2000. Hypertension. Accessed at www.nhlbi. nih.gov. NHLBI stops trial of estrogen plus progestin due to increased breast cancer risk, lack of overall benefit. Press release, July 9, 2002, the National Heart, Lung and Blood Institute of the National Institutes of Health.

Nygard, O., H. Refsum, P. M. Ueland, et al. 1997. Coffee consumption and plasma total homocysteine: The Hordaland Homocysteine Study. *American Journal of Clinical Nutrition* 65 (1):136–141.

Ornish, D. 1990. *Dr. Dean Ornish's program for reversing heart disease, the only system scientifically proven to reverse heart disease without drugs or surgery*. New York: Random House.

Paganini-Hill, A., and M. Perez Barreto. 2001. Stroke risk in older men and women: Aspirin, estrogen, exercise, vitamins, and other factors. *Journal of Gender Specific Medicine* 4 (2):18–28.

Rao, V., G. T. Christakis, R. D. Weisel, et al. 1995. Risk factors for stroke following coronary bypass surgery. *Journal of Cardiac Surgery* 10 (4 Supplement):468–474.

Rodriguez, A., V. Bernardi, J. Navia, et al. 2001. Argentine randomized study: Coronary angioplasty with stenting versus coronary bypass surgery in patients with multiple-vesssel disease (ERACI II): 30-day and one-year follow-up results. ERACI II investigators. *Journal of the American College of Cardiology* 37 (1):51–58.

Ross, M. F. 1995. UF researchers study link between emotions and heart disease. Presented at the spring 1995 annual meeting of the American College of Cardiology, New Orleans.

Saloheimo, P., S. Juvela, and M. Hillbom. 2001. Use of aspirin, epistaxis, and untreated hypertension as risk factors for primary intracerebral hemorrhage in middle-aged and elderly people. *Stroke* 32 (2):399–404.

Serruys, P. W., et al. Bypass surgery vs. stenting. *New England Journal of Medicine* 344 (15):1117–1124.

Shannahoff-Khalsa, D. S., and B. Kennedy. 1993. The effects of unilateral forced breathing on the heart. *International Journal of Neuroscience* 73 (1–2):47–60.

Sinatra, S. T. 1996. *Heartbreak and heart disease.* New Canaan, Conn.: Keats Publishing.

Srivastava, K. 1984. Aqueous extracts of onion, garlic, and ginger inhibit platelet aggregation and alter arachidoic acid metabolism. *Biomedical Biochemistry Acta* 43 (8–9):335–336.

Stampfer, M. J., R. M. Krauss, J. Ma, et al. 1997. A prospective study of triglyceride level, low-density lipoprotein particle diameter, and risk of myocardial infarction. *Journal of the American Medical Association* 276 (11):882–888.

Wardell, D. W., and J. Engebretson. 2001. Biological correlates of Reiki Touch healing. *Journal of Advanced Nursing* 33 (4):439–445.

Weiss, S. J. 1992. Psychophysiologic and behavioral effects of tactile stimulation on infants with congenital heart disease. *Research in Nursing and Health* 15 (2):93–101.

Wenneberg, S. R., R. H. Schneider, K. G. Walton, et al. 1997. A controlled study of the effects of the Transcendental Meditation program on cardiovascular reactivity and ambulatory blood pressure. *International Journal of Neuroscience* 89 (1–2):15–28.

Whelton, P. K., J. He, J. A. Culter, et al. 1997. Effects of oral potassium on blood pressure: Meta-analysis of randomized controlled clinical trials. *Journal of the American Medical Association* 277 (20):1624–1632.

Kidney Disease

Borghi, L., T. Meschi, T. Schianchi, et al. 1999. Urine volume: Stone risk factor and preventive measures. *Nephron* 81 (Supplement 1):31–37.

Chang, S. T. 1986. *The complete system of self-healing internal exercises.* San Francisco: Tao Publishing.

Curhan, G. C., W. C. Willett, E. B. Rimm, et al. 1996. Prospective study of beverage use and the risk of kidney stones. *American Journal of Epidemiology* 143 (3):240–247.

Curhan, G. C., W. C. Willett, F. E. Speizer, et al. 1997. Comparison of dietary calcium with supplemental calcium and other nutrients as factors affecting the risk for kidney stones in women. *Annals of Internals Medicine* 126 (7):497–504.

DeSwart, P. M. J. R., E. B. Sokole, and J. M. Wilmink. 1998. The interrelationship of calcium and magnesium absorption in idiopathic hypercalciuria and renal calcium stone disease. *Journal of Urology* 159:669–672.

Donadio, J. V., R. T. Holman, S. B. Johnson, et al. 1994. Essential fatty acid deficiency profiles in idiopathic immunoglobin A nephropathy. *American Journal of Kidney Disease* 23 (5):648–654.

Friedman, H. S. 1991. *The self-healing personality.* New York: Henry Holt.

Hay, L. 2000. *Heal your body.* Carlsbad, Calif.: Hay House.

Hiatt, R. A., B. Ettinger, B. Caan, et al. 1996. Randomized controlled trial of a low animal protein, high fiber diet in the prevention of recurrent calcium oxalate kidney stones. *American Journal of Epidemiology* 144 (1):25–33.

Hobbs, L. M., T. E. Rayner, and P. R. Howe. Dietary fish oil prevents the development of renal damage in salt-loaded stroke-prone spontaneously hypertensive rats. *Clinical & Experimental Pharmacology & Physiology* 23 (6–7):508–513.

Jariwalla, R. J. 2001. Rice-bran products: phytonutrients with potential applications in preventive and clinical medicine. *Drugs in Experimental and Clinical Research* 27 (1):17–26.

Mindell, E., and V. Hopkins. 1998. *Prescription alternatives.* New Canaan, Conn.: Keats Publishing.

Naidu, M. U., A. A. Shifow, K. V. Kumar, et al. (2000). Ginkgo biloba extract ameliorates gentamicin-induced nephrotoxicity in rats. *Phytomedicine* 7 (3):191–197.

Okada, H., K. Moriwaki, Y. Kianno, et al. 2000. Vitamin B_6 supplementation can improve peripheral polyneuropathy in patients with chronic renal failure on high-flux haemodialysis and human recombinant erthyropoietin. *Nephrology, Dialysis, and Transplants* 15 (9):1410–1413.

Parivar, F., R. K. Low, and M. L. Stoller. 1996. The influence of diet on urinary stone disease. *Journal of Urology* 155 (2):432–440.

Patra, R. C., D. Swarup, and S. K. Dwivedi. 2001. Antioxidant effects of alpha tocopherol, ascorbic acid and L-methionine on lead-induced oxidative stress to the liver, kidney, and brain in rats. *Toxicology* 162 (2):81–88.

Pedraza-Chaverri, J., P. D. Maldonado, O. N. Medina-Campos, et al. 2000. Garlic ameliorates gentamicin nephrotoxicity: Relation to antioxidant enzymes. *Free Radical Biological Medicine* 29 (7):602–611.

Pedraza-Chaverri, J., O. N. Medina-Campos, M. A. Granados-Silvestre, et al. 2000. Garlic ameliorates hyperlipidemia in chronic aminonucleoside nephrosis. *Molecular and Cell Biochemistry* 211 (1–2):69–77.

Pierratos, A., N. Dharamsi, L. K. Carr, et al. 2000. Higher urinary potassium is associated with decreased stone growth after shock wave lithotripsy. *Journal of Urology* 164:1486–1489.

Siener, R., and A. Hesse. 1995. Influence of a mixed and a vegetarian diet on urinary magnesium excretion and concentration. *British Journal of Nutrition* 73 (5):783–790.

Simopoulos, A. P. 1999. Essential fatty acids in health and chronic disease. *American Journal of Clinical Nutrition* 70 (Supplement 3):560S–569S.

Stampfer, M. J. 1993. A prospective study of dietary calcium and other nutrients and the risk of symptomatic kidney stones. *New England Journal of Medicine* 328 (12): 833–838.

Trinchieri, A., R. Nespoli, F. Ostini, et al. 1998. A study of dietary calcium and other nutrients in idiopathic renal calcium stone formers with low bone mineral content. *Journal of Urology* 159:654–657.

Velasquez, M. T., and S. J. Bhathena. 2001. Dietary phytoestrogens: A possible role in renal disease protection. *American Journal of Kidney Disease* 37 (5):1056–1068.

Williams, D. G. 1998. How to protect yourself from one of the next big epidemics. *Alternatives for the Health Conscious Individual* 7 (10):73–75.

Yin, D., X. Dai, and X. Rao. 1998. Yishen huanshuai recipe retards progression of chronic renal failure. *Zhongguo Zhong Xi Yi Jie He Za Zhi* 18 (7):402–404.

Liver and Gallbladder Diseases

Arase, Y., K. Ikeda, N. Murashima, et al. 1997. The long-term efficacy of glycyrrhizin in chronic hepatitis C patients. *Cancer* 79 (8):1494–1500.

Badulici, S., Z. Chirulescu, P. Chirila, et al. Treatment with zincum metallicum CH5 in patients with liver cirrhosis. *Romanian Journal of Internal Medicine* 32 (3):215–219.

Bell, G. D., and J. Doran. 1979. Gallstone dissolution in man using an essential oil preparation. *British Medical Journal* 278:24.

Berkow, R., and A. J. Fletcher. 1992. *The Merck manual of diagnosis and therapy*. Rahway, N.J.: Merck Research Laboratories.

Berkson, D. 1977. *The food book: Healing the body through reflexology*. New York: Harper & Row.

Chang, S. T. 1991. *The complete system of self-healing internal exercises*. San Francisco: Tao.

Choosing foods for emotional health. 1980. *East West Journal* (September):43.

Escarce, J. J. 1995. Gallbladder surgery: Overuse of laparoscopy. *Journal of the American Medical Association* 273:1581, 1621.

Holst, B. 2001. Managing viral hepatitis. *Clinician Reviews* 11 (1):51–66.

Hubbard, P. 1998. Hepatitis C. *American Journal for Nurse Practitioners* 2 (11):17–31.

Leitzmann, M. F., E. L. Giovannucci, M. J. Stampfer, et al. The relation of physical activity to risk for symptomatic gallstone disease in men. *Annals of Internal Medicine* 128 (6):417–425.

Luper, S. 1998. A review of plants used in the treatment of liver disease. Part 1. *Alternative Medical Review* 3 (6):410–421.

Mehta, R. 1994. Phytopharmacology of licorice food forms. *Designer foods III, proceedings*. Washington, D.C.: Georgetown University Conference Center, May 25.

Misciagna, G., C. Leoci, V. Guerra, et al. 1996. Epidemiology of cholelithiasis in southern Italy. Part II: Risk factors. *European Journal of Gastroenterology & Hepatology* 8 (6):585–593.

Nair, P., and J. F. Mayberry. 1994. Vegetarianism, dietary fibre, and gastro-intestinal disease. *Digestive Diseases* 12 (3): 177–185.

Pettit, J. L. 2000. Alternative medicine: SAMe. *Clinician Reviews* 10 (5):124–128.

Simon, J. A., and E. S. Hudes. 2000. Serum ascorbic acid and gallbladder disease prevalence, U.S. adults: The Third National Health and Nutrition Examination Survey (NHANES III). *Archives of Internal Medicine* 160 (7):931–936.

Singh, A., and A. R. Rao. 1993. Evaluation of the modulatory influence of black pepper on the hepatic detoxification system. *Cancer Letters* 72:5–9.

Syngal, S., E. H. Coakley, W. C. Willett, et al. 1999. Long-term weight patterns and risk for cholecystectomy in women. *Annals of Internal Medicine* 130 (6):471–477.

Whitcomb, D. C., and G. Block. 1994. Association of acetaminophen-induced liver toxicity with fasting and ethanol use. *Journal of the American Medical Association* 272 (23):1845–1850.

Worden, B. 1981. Treating hepatitis. *Vegetarian Times/Well Being* 46:52–53.

Yamashiki, M., A. Nishimura, H. Suzuki, et al. 1997. Effects of the Japanese herbal medicine "Sho-saiko-to" (TH-9) on in vitro interleukin-10 production by peripheral blood mononuclear cells of patients with chronic hepatitis C. *Hepatology* 25 (6):1390–1397.

Multiple Sclerosis

Branas, P., R. Jordan, A. Fry-Smith, et al. 2000. Treatments for fatigue in multiple sclerosis: A rapid and systematic review. *Health Technology Assessment* 4 (27):1–61.

Clark, C. C. 1999. Multiple sclerosis. *In Encyclopedia of complementary health practice.* New York: Springer.

Fawcett, J., J. Sideny, K. Riley-Lawless, et al. 1966. An exploratory study of the relationship between alternative therapies, functional status, and symptom severity among people with multiple sclerosis. *Journal of Holistic Nursing* 14 (2):115–120.

Frozenza, C. 1997. Multiple sclerosis. *American Journal of Nursing* 97 (11):48.

Goodkin, D. E., R. M. Ransohoff, and R. A. Rudick. 1992. Experimental therapies for multiple sclerosis. *Cleveland Clinic Journal of Medicine* 59:63–74.

Gross, R. E., and A. M. Lozano. 2000. Advances in neurostimulation for movement disorders. *Neurological Research* 22 (3):247–258.

Hay, L. 2000. *Heal your body: The mental causes for physical illness and the metaphysical way to overcome them.* Carlsbad, Calif.: Hay House.

Hickling, L. 2001. Multiple sclerosis: Treatment tips. Accessed September 6 at http://www.drkoop.com/dvncon/article.asp?

Huntley, A., and E. Ernst. 2000. Complementary and alternative therapies for treating multiple sclerosis symptoms: A systematic review. *Complementary Therapies in Medicine* 8 (2): 97–105.

Husted, C., L. Pham, A. Hekking, et al. 1999. Improving quality of life for people with chronic conditions: The example of t'ai chi and multiple sclerosis. *Alternative Therapy in Health and Medicine* 5 (5):70–74.

Leussink, V. I., S. Jung, U. Merschdorf, et al. 2001. High-dose methylprednisolone therapy in multiple sclerosis induces apoptosis in peripheral blood leukocytes. *Archives of Neurology* 58 (1):91–97.

Lozano, B., C. Valle, and A. Galindo. 2001. Applied neurophysiology in the deep brain stimulation treatment of multiple sclerosis tremor. *Review of Neurology* 32 (6):559–567.

McCarty, M. F. 2001. Upregulation of lymphocyte apoptosis as a strategy for preventing and treating autoimmune disorders: A role for whole-food vegan diets, fish oil, and dopamine agonists. *Medical Hypotheses* 57 (2):258–275.

Murphy, J. L. 2001. *Nurse practitioners' prescribing reference*. New York: Prescribing Reference.

Nordvik, I., K. M. Myhr, H. Nyland, et al. 2000. Effect of dietary advice and n-3 supplementation in newly diagnosed MS patients. *Acta Neurology Scandinavia* 102 (3):143–149.

Petajan, J. H., E. Gappmaier, A. T. White, et al. 1996. Impact of aerobic training on fitness and quality of life in multiple sclerosis. *Annals of Neurology* 39 (4):432–441.

Peterson, C. 2001. Exercise in 94 degrees F water for a patient with multiple sclerosis. *Physical Therapy* 81 (4):1049–1058.

Somerset, M., R. Campbell, D. J. Sharp, et al. 2001. What do people with MS want and expect from healthcare services? *Health Expectations* 4 (1):29–37.

Sutcher, H. 1997. Hypnosis as adjunctive therapy for multiple sclerosis: A progress report. *American Journal of Clinical Hypnosis* 39 (4):283–290.

Westarp, M. E. 2000. Medical rehabilitation of chronic progressive disseminated encephalomyelitis (MS). *Journal of Neurovirology* 6:S176–S178.

Wiens, M. E., M. A. Reimer, and H. L. Guy. 1999. Music therapy as a treatment method for improving respiratory muscle strength in patients with advanced multiple sclerosis: A pilot study. *Rehabilitation Nursing* 24 (2):74–80.

Wiesel, P. H., C. Norton, A. J. Roy, et al. 2000. Gut focused behavioural treatment (biofeedback) for constipation and fecal incontinence in multiple sclerosis. *Journal of Neurosurgical Psychiatry* 69 (2):240–243.

Osteoporosis

Alekel, D. D. I., A. S. Germain, C. T. Peterson, et al. 2000. Isoflavone-rich soy protein isolate attenuates bone loss in the lumbar spine of perimenopausal women. *American Journal of Clinical Nutrition* 72 (3):844–852.

Allolio, B. 1996. Osteoporosis and nutrition. *Z Arztl Fortbild* 90 (1):19–24.

Anderson, J. J. 1999. Plant-based diets and bone health: Nutritional implications. *American Journal of Clinical Nutrition* 70 (Supplement 3):539S–542S.

Baeksgaard, L., K. P. Anderson, and L. Hyldstrup. 1998. Calcium and vitamin D supplementation increases spinal BMD in healthy, postmenopausal women. *Osteoporosis International* 8 (3):255–260.

Cappuccio, F. P., E. Meilahn, J. M. Zmuda, et al. 1999. High blood pressure and bone-mineral loss in elderly white women: A prospective study. *Lancet* 354 (9183):971–975.

Crane, S. T. *The complete system of self-healing, internal exercises*. San Francisco: Tao.

Cummings, S. R., M. C. Nevitt, W. S. Browner, et al. 1995. Risk factors for hip fracture in white women. *New England Journal of Medicine* 332 (12):767–773.

Dohn, N. E. 1996. Lifting weight shown to reverse effects of osteoporosis in heart transplant patients. Gainesville: University of Florida.

Hay, L. L. *Heal your body*. Carlsbad, Calif.: Hay House.

Hunter, D., P. Major, N. Arden, et al. 2000. A randomized controlled trial of vitamin D supplementation on preventing postmenopausal bone loss and modifying bone metabolism using identical twin pairs. *Journal of Bone Mineral Research* 15 (11):2276–2283.

Kujala, U. M., J. Kapno, P. Kannus, et al. 2000. Physical activity and osteoporotic hip fracture risk in men. *Archives of Internal Medicine* 160:705–708.

Kruger, M., and D. Horrobin. 1997. Calcium metabolism, osteoporosis, and esential fatty acids: A review. *Progress in Lipid Research* 36 (2):131–151.

Kruger, M. C., H. Coetzer, R. deWinter, et al. 1998. *Aging* 10 (5):385–394.

Lewis, R. D., and C. M. Modlesky. 1998. Nutrition, physical activity, and bone health in women. *International Journal of Sport Nutrition* 8 (3):250–284.

Maton, P. N., and M. E. Burton. 1999. Antacids revisited: A review of their clinical pharmacology and recommended therapeutic use. *Drugs* 57 (6):855–870.

Murphy, J. L. 2001. Fosamax, bisphosphonate, Alendronate. In *Nurse practitioners' prescribing reference.* New York: Prescribing Reference.

Murray, M. T. 1995. Menopause: Is estrogen necessary? *American Journal of Natural Medicine* (November):15.

NHLBI stops trial of estrogen plus progestin due to increased breast cancer risk, lack of overall benefits. Press release, July 9, 2002, the National Heart, Lung and Blood Institute of the National Institutes of Health.

Pinnell, S. R. 1985. Regulation of collagen biosynthesis by ascorbic acid: A review. *Yale Journal of Biological Medicine* 58:553–559.

Puntila, E., H. Kroger, T. Lakka, et al. 1997. Physical activity in adolescence and bone density in peri- and postmenopausal women: A population-based study. *Bone* 21 (4):363–367.

Review of fluoride: Benefits and risks. 1991. Report of the ad hoc subcommittee on fluoride of the committee to coordinate environmental health and related programs. Washington, D.C.: Department of Health and Human Services, Public Health Service.

Reynolds, T. M., P. D. Marshall, and A. M. Brain. 1992. Hip fracture patients may be vitamin B_6 deficient. *Acta Orthop Scandinavia* 83:635–638.

Scheiber, M. D., J. H. Liu, M. T. Subbiah, et al. Dietary inclusion of whole soy foods results in significant reductions in clinical risk factors for osteoporosis and cardiovascular disease in normal postmenopausal women. *Menopause* 8 (5):384–392.

Scopacasa, F., A. G. Need, M. Horowitz, et al. 2000. Inhibition of bone resorption by divided-dose calcium supplementation in early postmenopausal women. *Calcification Tissue International* 67 (6):440–442.

Stacewicz-Sapuntzakis, M., P. E. Bowen, E. A. Hussain, et al. 2001. Chemical composition and potential health effects of prunes: A functional food. *Critical Review of Food Science Nutrition* 41 (4): 251–286.

Tinker, D., and R. B. Rucker. 1985. Role of selected nutrients in synthesis, accumulation, and chemical modification of connective tissue proteins. *Physiological Review* 65:607–657.

Turner, L. 2000. Effect of gardening on bone strength. Presented at the annual meeting of the American Alliance for Health, Physical Education, Recreation, and Dance, Orlando, Florida, March 25.

Uusi-Rasi, K., H. Sievanen, I. Vuori, et al. 1999. Long-term recreational gymnastics, estrogen use, and selected risk factors for osteoporotic fractures. *Journal of Bone Mineral Research* 14 (7):1231–1238.

Wyshak, G., and R. E. Frisch. 1994. Carbonated beverages, dietary calcium, the dietary calcium/phosphorous ratio, and bone fractures in girls and boys. *Journal of Adolescent Health* 15 (3):210–215.

Overweight/Obesity

Benton, D., and R. T. Donohoe. 1999. The effects of nutrients on mood. *Public Health Nutrition* 2 (3A):403–409.

Bernardot, D., R. C. Deutz, D. E. Martin, et al. 2000. Relationship between energy deficits and body composition in elite female gymnasts and runners. *Medicine and Science in Sports and Exercise* 32 (3):659–668.

Bolumar, F., J. Olsen, M. Rebagliato, et al. 1997. Caffeine intake and delayed conception: A European multicenter study on infertility and subfecundity. *American Journal of Epidemiology* 145 (4):324–334.

Bruinsma, K., and D. C. Taren. 1999. Chocolate: Food or drug? *Journal of the American Dietetic Association* 99 (10):1249–1256.

Chait, A., M. R. Malinow, D. C. Morris, et al. 1999. Increased dietary micronutrients decrease serum homocysteine concentrations in patients at high risk of cardiovascular disease. *American Journal of Clinical Nutrition* 70:881–887.

Christensen, L. 1991. The role of caffeine and sugar in depression. *Nutrition Reports* 9 (3):17–24.

———. 1993. Effects of eating behavior on mood: A review of the literature. *International Journal of Eating Disorders* 14:171–183.

Christensen, L., and R. Burrows. 1990. Dietary treatment of depression. *Behavior Therapy* 21:183–194.

El-Khairy, L., P. M. Ueland, O. Nygard, et al. 1999. Lifestyle and cardiovascular disease risk factors as determinants of total cysteine in plasma. The Hordaland Homocysteine Study. *American Journal of Clinical Nutrition* 70 (6):1016–1024.

Fraser, G. E. 1999. Diet as primordial prevention in Seventh-Day Adventists. *Preventive Medicine* 29 (6, pt. 2):S18–S22.

———. 1999. Association between diet and cancer, ischemic heart disease, and all-cause mortality in non-Hispanic white Caucasian Seventh-Day Adventists. *American Journal of Clinical Nutrition* 70 (Supplement 3):532S–538S.

Halliwell, B. 1993. The role of oxygen radicals in human disease, with particular reference to the vascular system. *Haemostatis* 23 (Supplement 1):118–126.

Hart, K. E., and P. Chiovari. 1998. Inhibition of eating behavior: Negative cognitive effects of dieting. *Journal of Clinical Psychology* 54 (4):427–430.

Hay, L. 2000. *Heal your body*. Carlsbad, Calif.: Hay House.

Homocysteine study. *American Journal of Clinical Nutrition* 70 (96):1016–1024.

Key, T. J., G. E. Fraser, M. Thorogood, et al. 1998. Mortality in vegetarians and non-vegetarians: An analysis of 8,300 deaths among 76,000 men and women in prospective studies. *Public Health Nutrition* 1 (1):33–41.

———. 1999. Mortality in vegetarians and nonvegetarians: Derived from a collaborative analysis of five prospective studies. *American Journal of Clinical Nutrition* 70 (Supplement 3):516S–524S.

Kinzl, J. F., C. Traweger, B. Trefalt, et al. 1999. Binge eating disorder in females: A population-based investigation. *Journal of Eating Disorders* 25 (3):287–292.

Kynast-Gales, S. A., and L. K. Massey. 1994. Effect of caffeine on circadian excretion of urinary calcium and magnesium. *Journal of the American College of Nutrition* 13 (5):467–472.

Lee, I. M., and R. S. Paffenbarger. 1992. Change in body weight and longevity. *Journal of the American Medical Association* 268 (15):2045–2049.

Mantzoros, C. S., A. S. Prasad, F. W. Beck, et al. 1998. Zinc may regulate serum leptin concentrations in humans. *Journal of the American College of Nutrition* 17:270–275.

Miller, W. C., M. G. Niederpruem, J. P. Wallace, et al. 1994. Dietary fat, sugar, and fiber predict body fat content. *Journal of the American Dietary Association* 94 (6):612–615.

Milner, J. A. 1986. Dietary antioxidants and cancer. *ASDC Journal of Dentistry and the Child* 53 (2):140–143.

Oliver, G., and J. Wardel. 1999. Perceived effects of stress on food choice. *Physiological Behavior* 66 (3):511–513.

Olney, J. W., N. B. Farber, E. Spitznagel, et al. 1996. Increasing brain tumor rates: Is there a link to aspartame? *Journal of Neuropathology and Experimental Neurology* 55 (11):1115–1123.

Pasman, W. J., W. H. Saris, and M. S. Westerterp-Plantenga. 1999. Predictors of weight maintenance. *Obesity Research* 7(1):43–50.

Polivy, J., and C. P. Herman. 1999. The effects of resolving to diet on restrained and unrestrained eaters: The "false hope syndrome." *International Journal of Eating Disorders* 26 (4):434–437.

Rolls, B. J., and D. L. Miller. 1997. Is the low-fat message giving people a license to eat more? *Journal of the American College of Nutrition* 16 (6):535–543.

Rosch, P. 1999. Oxidized trans-fats and margarines. *Health and Stress* 8:4–5.

Rosch, R. J., and C. C. Clark. 2001. *De-Stress, Weigh Less.* New York: St. Martin's Press.

Samaras, K., P. J. Kelyu, M. N. Chiano, et al. Gene versus environment: The relationship between dietary fat and total and central abdominal fat. *Diabetes Care* 21 (12):2069–2076.

Stice, E., P. Cameron, and C. Hayward. 1999. Naturalistic weight-reduction efforts prospectively predict growth in relative weight and onset of obesity among female adolescents. *Journal of Consulting and Clinical Psychology* 67:967–974.

Syngal, W., E. H. Coakley, W. C. Willett, et al. 1999. Long-term weight patterns and risk for cholecystectomy in women. *Annals of Internal Medicine* 130 (6):471–477.

Thornburn, A. W., and J. Proietto. 1998. Neuropeptides, the hypothalamus, and obesity: Insights into the central control of body weight. *Pathology* 30 (3):229–236.

Trocho, C., R. Pardo, I. Rafecas, et al. 1998. Formaldehyde derived from dietary aspartame binds to tissue components in vivo. *Life Science* 63 (5):337–339.

Van den Eeden, S. K., T. D. Koepsell, W. T. Longstreth, et al. 1994. Aspartame ingestion and headaches: A randomized crossover trial. *Neurology* 44 (10):1787–1793.

Walton, R., R. Hudak, and R. J. Green-Waite. 1993. Adverse reactions to aspartame double-blind challenge in patients from a vulnerable population. *Biological Psychiatry* 34 (1–2):13–17.

Pain

AGS Panel on Chronic Pain in Older Persons. 1998. The management of chronic pain in older persons: New guidelines from the American Geriatrics Society. *Clinician Reviews* 8 (9):69–106.

Aloisi, P., A. Marrelli, C. Porto, et al. 1997. Visual evoked potentials and serum magnesium levels in juvenile migraine patients. *Headache* 37 (6):383–385.

Are headaches a warning sign? 1998. *Clinician Reviews* 8 (10):38.

Bearman, D., and S. Shafarman. 1999. The Feldenkrais Method in the treatment of chronic pain: A study of efficacy and cost effectiveness. *American Journal of Pain Management* 9:22–27.

Blumenthal, M., ed. 1998. *The complete German Commission E monographs, therapeutic guide to herbal medicine.* Austin, Tex.: The American Botanical Council and Boston Integrative Medicine Communications.

Cooner, E., and S. Amorosi. 1997. *The study of pain in older Americans.* New York: Louis Harris & Associates.

Deen, H. G. Jr. 1996. Diagnosis and management of lumbar disk disease. *Mayo Clinic Proceedings* 71 (3):283–287.

Ferrell, B. A., K. R. Josephson, A. M. Pollan, et al. 1997. A randomized trial of walking versus physical methods for chronic pain management. *Aging* 9 (1–2):99–105.

Field, T. 1998. Massage therapy and burn debridement. *Journal of Burn Care Rehabilitation* 10:241–244.

Gallai, L. D., S. M. Baker, and R. K. McLellan. 1986. Magnesium deficiency in the pathogenesis of mitral valve prolapse. *Magnesium* 5:165–174.

Gaston-Johansson, F., F. Johansson, and J. Johansson. 1996. Pain in the elderly: Prevalence attitudes and assessment. *Nursing Home Management* 4(11):325–331.

Hay, L. 2000. *Heal your body.* Carlsbad, Calif: Hay House.

Holden, E. W., M. M. Deichmann, and J. D. Levy. 1999. Empirically supported treatments in pediatric psychology: Recurrent pediatric headache. *Journal of Pediatric Psychology* 24 (2):91–109.

Hooker, G. A. 1996. Chronic pain can be managed. *Emotional Wellness Matters* (May/June):1–3.

Klein, B. J., R. T. Radecki, M. P. Foris, et al. 2000. Bridging the gap between science and practice in managing low back pain: A comprehensive spine care system in a health maintenance organization setting. *Spine* 25 (6):738–740.

Kropp, P., W. D. Gerber, A. Keinath-Specht, et al. 1997. Behavioral treatment in migraine: Cognitive-behavioral therapy and blood-volume-pulse biofeedback: A crossover study with a two-year follow-up. *Functional Neurology* 12 (1):17–24.

Matthew, N. T. 1993. Transformed migraine. *Cephalgia* 13 (Supplement 12):78–83.

Matthew, N. T., R. Kurman, and F. Perez. 1990. Drug-induced refractory headache: Clinical features and management. *Headache* 30:634–638.

Merskey, H., and N. Bogduk, eds. 1994. *Classification of chronic pain,* 2nd ed. Seattle, Wash.: IASP Press.

Mills, S. Y., R. K. Jacoby, M. Chacksfield, et al. 1996. Effect of a proprietary herbal medicine on the relief of chronic arthritic pain: A double-blind study. *British Journal of Rheumatology* 35 (9):874–878.

Murphy, J. J., S. Heptinstall, and J. R. Mitchell. 1988. Randomised double-blind placebo-controlled trial of feverfew in migraine prevention. *Lancet* 2 (8604):189–192.

Murray, M. T. 1994. Do headache medicines cause chronic headaches? *American Journal of Natural Medicine* 1 (2):5–7.

National Institutes of Health, Technology Assessment Panel. 1996. Integration of behavioral and relaxation approaches into the treatment of chronic pain and insomnia. *Journal of the American Medical Association* 276 (4):313–318.

New standards for assessment and treatment of pain instituted by JCAHO. 2001. *American Journal for Nurse Practitioners* (January):43.

Nilsson, N., H. W. Christensen, and J. Hartvigsen. 1997. The effect of spinal manipulation in the treatment of cervicogenic headache. *Journal of Manipulative Physiological Therapy* 20 (5):326–330.

Olson, K., and J. Hanson. 1997. Using Reiki to manage pain: A preliminary report. *Cancer Prevention and Control* 1 (2):108–113.

Paiva, T., A. Farinha, A. Martins, et al. 1997. Chronic headaches and sleep disorders. *Archives of Internal Medicine* 157 1701–1705.

Peikert, A., C. Wilimzig, and R. Kohne-Volland. 1996. Prophylaxis of migraine with oral magnesium: Results from a prospective, multicenter, placebo-controlled, and double-blind randomized study. *Cephalalgia* 16 (4):257–263.

Perin, M. L. 2000. Problems with propoxyphene. *American Journal of Nursing* 100 (6):22.

Pittler, M. H., and E. Ernst. 2000. Gingko biloba for intermittent claudication. *American Journal of Medicine* 108:276–281.

Ramadan, N. M., H. Halvorson, A. Vande-Linde, et al. 1989. Magnesium deficiency in migraine patients. *Headache* 34:160–165.

Rappoport, A. M. 1985. Analgesic-rebound headache: Theoretical and practical implications. *Caphalgia* 5 (Supplement 3):448–449.

Rosch, P. 1999. Stress, headache, and other head pain. *Health and Stress* 3:1–8.

Ross, M. F. 2000. UF pilot study shows massage, relaxation reduce sickle cell anemia pain. Gainesville: University of Florida.

Sanders, M. R., R. W. Shepherd, G. Cleghorn, et al. 1994. The treatment of recurrent abdominal pain in children: A controlled comparison of cognitive-behavioral family intervention and standard pediatric care. *Journal of Clinical Psychology* 62 (2):306–314.

Swanson, D. R. 1988. Migraine and magnesium: Eleven neglected connections. *Perspectives in Biological Medicine* 31 (4):526–557.

White, C. L., S. M. LeFort, R. Amsel, et al. 1997. Predictors of the development of chronic pain. *Research in Nursing and Health* 29 (4):309–318.

Wipf, J. E., and R. A. Deyo. 1995. Low back pain. *Medical Clinics of North America* 79 (2):231–246.

Parkinson's Disease

Chung, W., R. Poppen, and D. A. Lundervold. 1995. Behavioral relaxation training for tremor disorders in older adults. *Biofeedback and Self-Regulation* 20 (2):1123–1135.

de Rijk, M. C., M. M. Breteler, J. H. den Breeijen, et al. 1997. Dietary antioxidants and Parkinson's disease: The Rotterdam Study. *Archives of Neurology* 54 (6):762–765.

Forsleff, L., A. G. Schauss, I. D. Bier, et al. 1999. Evidence of functional zinc deficiency in Parkinson's disease. *Journal of Alternative and Complementary Medicine* 5 (1):57–64.

Iwasaki, K., Q. Wang, H. Seki, et al. 2000. The effects of the traditional Chinese medicine "Banxia Houpo Tang (Hange-Kobku T)": on the swallowing reflex in Parkinson's disease. *Phytomedicine* 7 (4):259–263.

Levites, Y., O. Weinreb, G. Maor, et al. 2001. Green tea polyphenol-epigallo-catechin-3-gallate prevents N-methyl-4-phenyl-1,2,3,6-tetrahydrophridine-induced dopaminergic neurodegeneration. *Journal of Neurochemistry* 78 (5):1073–1082.

Mazzio, E., J. Huber, S. Darling, et al. 2001. Effect of antioxidants on L-glutamate and Nmethyl-4-phenylpyridinium ion induced-neurotoxicity in PC12 cells. *Neurotoxicology* 22 (2):283–286.

McCarty, M. F. 2001. Does a vegan diet reduce risk for Parkinson's disease? *Medical Hypotheses* 57 (3):318–323.

Pacchetti, C., F. Mancini, R. Aglieri, et al. 2000. Active music therapy in Parkinson's disease: An integrative method for motor and emotional rehabilitation. *Psychosomatic Medicine* 62 (3):386–393.

Parkinson's Disease Study Group. 1995. An alternative medicine treatment for Parkinson's disease: Results of a multicenter clinical trial. *Journal of Alternative and Complementary Medicine* 1 (3):249–255.

Redman, D. A. 2000. *Ruscus aculeatus* (butcher's broom) as a potential treatment for orthostatic hypotension, with a case report. *Journal of Alternative Complementary Medicine* 6 (6):539–549.

Reis, J. G. 1995. A Parkinson's primer. *Nursing Spectrum* (June 26):12–14.

Scheider, W. L., L. A. Hershey, J. E. Vena, et al. 1997. Dietary antioxidants and other dietary factors in the etiology of Parkinson's disease. *Movement Disorders* 12 (2):190–196.

Schenkman, M., T. M. Cutson, M. Kuchibhatia, et al. 1998. *Journal of the American Geriatric Society* 46 (1d):1207–1216.

Smolowitz, J. and C. Waters. 2001. Clinical management of the adult with Parkinson's disease. *American Journal for Nurse Practitioners* (July–August):9–34.

Stallibrass, C. 1997. An evaluation of the Alexander Technique for the management of disability in Parkinson's disease—a preliminary study. *Clinical Rehabilitation* 11 (1):8–12.

Tissingh, G., J. Booij, A. Winogrodzka, et al. 1997. IBZM- and CIT-SPECT of the dopaminergic system in Parkinsonism. *Journal of Neurological Transmission* 50:31–37.

Tuchsen, F., and A. A. Jensen. 2000. Agricultural work and the risk of Parkinson's disease in Denmark 1981–1993. *Scandinavian Journal of Work and Environmental Health* 26 (4):359–362,

Wells, M. R., S. Giantinoto, D. D'Agate, et al. 1999. Standard osteopathic manipulative treatment acutely improves gait performance in patients with Parkinson's disease. *Journal of the American Osteopathic Association* 99 (2):92–98.

Zhuang, X., and L. Wang. 2000. Acupuncture treatment of Parkinson's disease—a report of 29 cases. *Journal of Traditional Chinese Medicine* 20 (4):265–267.

Sleep Disorders

American Sleep Disorders Association. 1994. Practice parameters for the use of laser-assisted uvulopalatoplasty. *Sleep* 17:744–748.

Aubert-Tulkens, G., M. Hamoir, J. van den Eeckhaut, et al. 1989. Failure of tonsil and nose surgery in adults with long-standing severe sleep apnea syndrome. *Archives of Internal Medicine* 149:2118–2121.

Azar, B. 1996. Intrusive thoughts proven to undermine our health. *American Psychological Association Monitor* 27:10.

Brown, D. B. 1999. Managing sleep disorders. *Clinician Reviews* 9 (10):51–70.

Chase, J. E., and B. E. Gidal. 1997. Melatonin: Therapeutic use in sleep disorders. *Annals of Pharmacotherapy* 31:1218–1226.

Chen, M. L., L. C. Lin, S. C. Wu, et al. 1999. The effectiveness of acupressure in improving the quality of sleep of institutionalized residents. *Journal of Gerontology and Biological Science and Medical Science* 54 (8):M389–M394.

Cornell University. 1998. The effect of light exposure on release of melatonin. *Science* 279 (5349):333–334, 396–399.

Fletcher, E. C., and D. A. Munafo. 1990. Role of nocturnal oxygen therapy in obstructive sleep apnea: When should it be used? *Chest* 98:1497–1504.

Gerhard, U., N. Linnenbrink, C. Georghiadou, et al. 1996. Vigilance-decreasing effects of two plant-derived sedatives. *Schweiz Rundsch Med Prax* 85 (15):473–481.

Graedon, J. 1994. Graedon's guide to getting a good night's sleep. In *The People's Pharmacy*. N.p. King Features, Graedon Enterprises.

Hay, L. 2000. *Heal your body.* Carlsbad, Calif.: Jay House.

Hughes, R. J., R. L. Sack, and J. Levy. 1998. The role of melatonin and circadian phase in age-related sleep-maintenance insomnia: Assessment in a clinical trial of melatonin replacement. *Sleep* 21:52–68.

Kennan, S. P., H. Burt, C. F. Ryan, et al. 1994. Long-term survival of patients with obstructuctive sleep apnea treated by uvulopalato-pharyngoplasty or nasal CPAP. *Chest* 105:155–159.

Lee, K. A., M. E. Baffke, and K. Baratte-Beebe. 2001. The effect of folate and iron on restless legs syndrome. *Journal of Women's Health and Gender-Based Medicine* 10 (4):335–341.

Mendelson, W., M. A. Cohn, W. C. Dement, et al. *Don't Take Sleep Problems Lying Down.* N.p. Upjohn. N.d.

National Center on Sleep Disorders Research. 1995. *Sleep apnea: Is your patient at risk?* Bethesda, Md.: U.S. Department of Health and Human Services.

———. 1998. *Insomnia.* Bethesda, Md.: National Institutes of Health, Public Health Service, National Heart, Lung, and Blood Institute.

Phillips, B. A., F. A. Schmitt, D. T. R. Berry, et al. 1990. Treatment of obstructive sleep apnea: A preliminary report comparing nasal CPAP to nasal oxygen in patients with mild OSA. *Chest* 98:325–330.

Sack, R. L., A. J. Lewy, and R. J. Hughes. 1998. Use of melatonin for sleep and circadian rhythm disorders. *Annals of Medicine* 30:115–120.

Schmitz, M., and M. Jackal. 1998. N.t. *Wien Med Wochenschar* 148 (13):291–298.

Stradling, J., D. Robers, A. Wilson, et al. 1998. Controlled trial of hypnotherapy for weight loss in patients with obstructive sleep apnea. *International Journal of Obesity and Related Metabolic Disorders* 22 (3):278–281.

Stradling, J. R., G. Thomas, A. R. H. Warley, et al. 1990. Effect of adenotonsillectomy on nocturnal hypoxaemia, sleep disturbance, and symptoms in snoring children. *Lancet* 335:249–253.

Tousignant, P., M. G. Cosio, R. D. Levy, et al. 1994. Quality adjusted life years added by treatment of obstructive sleep apnea. *Sleep* 17:52–60.

Weaver, E. M. 2001. Obstructive sleep apnea syndrome: What to suspect, how to help. *Consultant* (March):397–405.

Williams, D. G. 1995. Safe "shuteye"—natural remedies for insomnia. *Alternatives* 6 (4):25.

Index

About the AHNA

The American Holistic Nurses' Association (AHNA) is a professional nursing organization dedicated to the promotion of holism and healing. The AHNA believes that holistic nurses engage in therapeutic partnerships with clients, their families, and their communities to serve as facilitators in the healing process. The holistic caring process supported by AHNA is one exemplified by nurses:

- Recognizing each person as a whole comprised of body, mind, and spirit
- Assessing clients holistically, using appropriate traditional and holistic methods
- Creating a plan of care in collaboration with clients and their significant others consistent with cultural background, health beliefs, sexual orientation, values, and preferences that focuses on health promotion, recovery or restoration, or peaceful dying so that the person obtains the highest level of independence
- Providing care and guidance to individuals through nursing interventions and therapies consistent with research findings and other sound evidence
- Acquiring and maintaining current knowledge and competencies in holistic nursing practice, including the integration of selected complementary therapies within that practice
- Preserving the wholeness and dignity of self and others
- Engaging in self-care

The AHNA is involved in various activities to promote holistic nursing, which include sponsorship of an annual conference, publication of the *Journal of Holistic Nursing*, scholarships, research grants, and an endorsement process for educational programs related to holistic nursing practice. More information on the AHNA can be obtained by visiting their Web site at www.AHNA.org or by contacting their headquarters at P.O. Box 2130, Flagstaff, AZ 86003.

About the Author

Carolyn Chambers Clark, A.R.N.P., Ed.D., H.N.C., F.A.A.N., D.A.B.F.N., F.A.A.I.M., is on the Health Services Doctoral Faculty at Walden University and has been on the graduate and undergraduate nursing faculty at several other universities. Dr. Clark is the founder of The Wellness Institute, and edited *The Wellness Newsletter* for fifteen years. She is founding editor of *Alternative Health Practitioner: The Journal of Complementary and Natural Care* (now called *Complementary Health Practice Review*). Her book *Wellness Practitioner: Concepts, Research, and Strategies* won an *American Journal of Nursing* Book-of-the-Year Award. She has published widely on complementary, holistic, and self-care topics for both academic and consumer audiences. She is the editor in chief of *The Encyclopedia of Complementary Health Practice* and the author of *Integrating Complementary Health Procedures into Practice*, both *AJN* Book-of-the-Year Award winners. Dr. Clark is certified as a holistic nurse by the American Holistic Nurses' Certification Corporation and serves on the advisory board for the American Association of Integrative Medicine. She has been a Fellow of the American Academy of Nursing since 1980 and has maintained a wellness/holistic practice with clients since 1976.

Contact Dr. Clark

Dr. Clark is interested in hearing your questions, comments, and suggestions for a second edition or a related book. She also offers workshops, consultation, and retreats based on the principles and practices presented in this book. (These programs are appropriate for couples, individuals, health professionals, and others interested in self-care and complementary procedures.) If you have questions or suggestions about the book, or wish to receive information about her programs, please write to her at cccwellness@earthlink.net or visit http://home.earthlink.